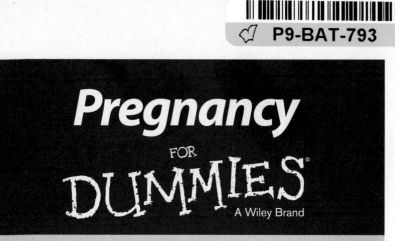

Pregnancy

FOR DUMMIES®
A Wiley Brand

4th Edition

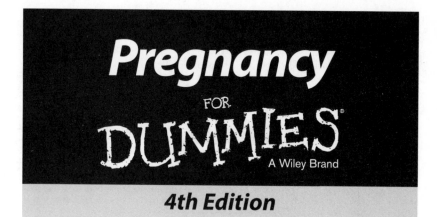

Pregnancy

FOR DUMMIES®

A Wiley Brand

4th Edition

by Joanne Stone, MD, and
Keith Eddleman, MD

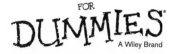

FOR DUMMIES®

A Wiley Brand

Pregnancy For Dummies,® 4th Edition

Published by: **John Wiley & Sons, Inc.,** 111 River Street, Hoboken, NJ 07030-5774, www.wiley.com

Contents at a Glance

Table of Contents

Chapter 7: The Third Trimester 151

Part III: The Big Event: Labor, Delivery, and Recovery...................................... 189

Chapter 8: Honey, I Think I'm in Labor!..............191

Chapter 9: Special Delivery: Bringing Your Baby into the World 223

Chapter 10: Hello, World! Meet Your Newborn. 245

Chapter 11: Taking Care of Yourself after Delivery . . . 263

Introduction

●●

*I*t's ironic that this book is called *Pregnancy For Dummies,* because the whole idea behind it is that couples today *aren't* dummies (in the traditional sense) and are quite capable of understanding complex medical information when it's presented clearly. Our goal, in fact, has been to write a scientifically correct, comprehensive guide to what is one of the most memorable experiences in anyone's life — pregnancy. The *For Dummies* books are known for being accurate and informative, yet easy to read. That's why we found this format to be the perfect one in which to present the medical facts of pregnancy and still acknowledge, and even encourage, the humor and light-heartedness that are part of the miraculous process of having babies.

About This Book

We know from our experience caring for thousands of women at Mount Sinai Medical Center in New York City that prospective parents are truly interested in and curious about everything related to pregnancy, from when the baby's heart is formed to whether eating sushi or dyeing your hair is okay. In this book, we incorporate our responses to many commonly asked questions. Our approach to some of the more controversial ones is to provide answers based on *real,* medically based data. We make sure to provide not just the party-line answer, or the safe answer, but the response that is based on the medical literature. Sometimes, no solid data exists to indicate whether something is safe or unsafe, and when this is the case, we tell you.

Too often, our patients come to us incredibly worried about something they've read in another book that is either outdated, lacks any real scientific basis, or is exaggerated way out of proportion. Sometimes, other pregnancy books present info in such a way as to be alarmist, or they're not properly in perspective. The trouble is that pregnant women are, by nature, already anxious about whether anything they do or eat may hurt the baby. The guiding principle of our approach has been to put all the facts into perspective and not to create needless anxiety or fear. Pregnancy should be a joy, not a worry. A big part of our philosophy in writing this book is to reassure pregnant women whenever medically possible, rather than to add to the unnecessary worries they already have.

Our experience has shown us that prospective parents also want to know about the real medical aspects of pregnancy. When are fingers developed? What blood tests should be done, and why? What options are available for detecting various problems? In addressing these topics, we have attempted to write a book that is essentially a medical text on obstetrics for the layperson.

We are practicing obstetricians who are also board certified in the subspecialty of maternal-fetal medicine (high-risk pregnancies), and we also teach residents, medical students, and other doctors about pregnancy and prenatal care. So we came into this project with a certain amount of expertise. Also, we consulted many of our colleagues in areas of medicine outside obstetrics — in pediatrics, internal medicine, and anesthesia, for example. For many topics, we conducted comprehensive searches of the medical literature to make sure the information we provide is based on the most recent studies available. Working with Mary Duenwald on the text has been enormously helpful in making sure that the medical information we provide is comprehensible to someone who isn't in the medical field. In addition, as a mother of twins, Mary has been able to provide her own unique insight into various aspects of pregnancy.

In most pregnancy books, the father of the baby is, sadly, overlooked. We think that's a shame. Dads are, of course, welcome to read any part of the book that interests them (or that the Moms-to-be direct them to), but we also include insightful commentary that is intended specifically for dads.

We designed *Pregnancy For Dummies,* 4th Edition, to be used gradually, as you enter into each stage of pregnancy. Many women are curious about what lies ahead and may want to read the whole book right off the bat. But the information is organized in such a way that you can take things week by week, if you want. You can also consult it as needed if you run into some particular question or problem.

We trust that you will use this book as a companion to regular medical care. Perhaps some of the information in it will lead you to ask your practitioner questions that you may not otherwise have thought to ask. Because there isn't always just one answer or even a right answer to every question, you may find that your practitioner holds a different point of view than we do in some areas. This difference of opinion is only natural, and, in fact, we even occasionally disagree with each other. The bottom line is that this book provides a lot of factual information, but it is not "gospel." Remember, also, that many topics we discuss apply to pregnancy in general, but your particular situation may have unique aspects to it that warrant different or extra consideration.

What's New in This Edition

Writing this book was very much like giving birth to a baby. It took a lot of planning, discovering, labor, and love and resulted in tremendous pride and joy for the two of us. Medicine, and specifically the field of obstetrics, is changing constantly. In order to keep up with the latest trends and medical news, we have updated and revised the information for this fourth edition.

What's also new in this edition is the way we organized the book. The first part is an overview about preparing for pregnancy, lifestyle issues during pregnancy, and the overall "game plan." Next we divided up information by trimesters because that's the traditional way of thinking about pregnancy. But in this edition, we have also given you a week-by-week account of what's going on and what you should do. We focused an entire section of the big event — labor and delivery — and then all the important newborn issues, such as breastfeeding and things you should know before you take that cute little bundle home. In Part IV, we focus on special concerns, so that if need be, you will be prepared in case of certain pregnancy complications. Finally the last section is load with fun facts. Also, with the advancements in obstetrical ultrasound, we have provided new ultrasound images so that you can know what to anticipate when you go for your OB ultrasound!!

As in the first three editions, we rely on scientific data rather than opinion or hearsay. Recent medical research has answered some earlier questions, helping us to give better care to pregnant women. For example, we've added new information about revised dietary recommendations from the U.S. Department of Agriculture. Societal and cultural trends that affect us all also affect pregnant women. Topics like Botox and thimerisol weren't important issues when we wrote the first edition, but we discuss them in this edition because they come up more frequently today. Most importantly, we have listened to our patients' comments and suggestions for a fourth edition, and incorporated many of those ideas into this book.

Foolish Assumptions

As we wrote this book, we made some assumptions about you and what your needs may be:

- ✔ You may be a woman who is considering pregnancy, planning to have a baby, or already pregnant.
- ✔ You may be the partner of the mother-to-be.
- ✔ You may know and love someone who is or plans to be pregnant.
- ✔ You want to find out more about pregnancy but have no interest in becoming an expert on the topic.

If you fit any of these criteria, then *Pregnancy For Dummies,* 4th Edition, gives you the information you're looking for!

Icons Used in This Book

Like other *For Dummies* books, this one has little icons in the margins to guide you through the information and zero in on what you need to find out. The following paragraphs describe the icons and what they mean.

 This icon signals that we're going to delve a little deeper than usual into a medical explanation. We don't mean to suggest the information is too difficult to understand — just a little more detailed.

We flag certain pieces of information with this icon to let you know something is particularly worth keeping in mind.

 This icon marks bits of advice we give you about handling some of the minor discomforts and other challenges you encounter during pregnancy.

Throughout this book, we try to avoid being too alarmist, but there are some situations and actions that a pregnant woman clearly should avoid. When this is the case, we show you the Warning icon.

 Many things you may feel or notice while you're pregnant beg the question, "Is this important enough for my practitioner to know about?" When the answer is yes, you see this icon.

We know from experience that pregnancy can bring out the instinct to worry. Feeling a little anxious from time to time is normal, but some women go overboard working themselves up over things that really aren't a problem. We use this icon — more than any other one — to point out the countless things that you really need not fret about.

Beyond the Book

In addition to the material in the print or e-book you're reading right now, this product also comes with some access-anywhere goodies on the web. Check out the free Cheat Sheet at www. dummies.com/cheatsheet/pregnancy for a handy schedule of prenatal visits and tests, a list of common medical abbreviations, a look at how your baby grows during pregnancy, a checklist of items to have for your hospital stay, and a reference of important phone numbers and addresses to have on hand.

Also included are some bonus articles that can be accessed at www.dummies.com/extras/pregnancy. These little "extras" cover topics from genetic testing and the benefits of skin-to-skin contact to placenta previa and the whys of when ultrasounds are scheduled.

Where to Go from Here

If you're the particularly thorough type, go ahead and read this book from cover to cover. If you just want to find specific information and then close the book, take a look at the table of contents or at the index. Dog-ear the pages that are especially interesting or relevant to you. Write little notes in the margins. Have fun and, most of all, enjoy your pregnancy!

Part I
Getting Started with Pregnancy

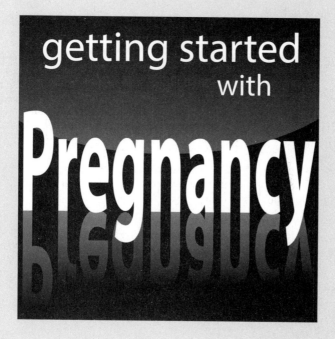

In this part . . .

✔ You're pregnant! Or, at least, you think so! Find out how to recognize the signs of pregnancy and what to do about getting your pregnancy confirmed.

✔ Check out how your pregnancy will progress week by week.

✔ Discover how your daily life will change now that you're pregnant. Gain insight on how to plan for everything from taking medications to visiting the hairdresser.

✔ Understand how eating right and exercising is just as important for mom as it is for baby.

Chapter 1

Seeing Double Lines: I Think I'm Pregnant!

So you think you may be pregnant! Or maybe you're hoping to become pregnant soon. Either way, you want to know what to look for in the early weeks of pregnancy so that you can know for sure as soon as possible. In this chapter, we take a look at some of the most common signals that your body sends you in the first weeks of pregnancy, and offer advice for confirming your pregnancy and getting it off to a great start.

Recognizing the Signs of Pregnancy

So assume it has happened: A budding embryo has nestled itself into your womb's soft lining. How and when do you find out that you're pregnant? Quite often, the first sign is a missed period. But your body sends many other signals — sometimes even sooner than that first missed period — that typically become more noticeable with each passing week.

✔ **Honey, I'm late!** You may suspect that you're pregnant if your period hasn't arrived as expected. By the time you notice you're late, a pregnancy test will probably yield a positive result (see the next section, "Determining Whether You're Pregnant," for more on pregnancy tests). Sometimes, though, you may experience one or two days of light bleeding, which is known as *implantation bleeding,* because the embryo is attaching itself to your uterus's lining.

✔ **You notice new food cravings and aversions.** What you've heard about a pregnant woman's appetite is true. You may become ravenous for pickles, pasta, and other particular foods, yet turn up your nose at foods you normally love to eat. No one knows for sure why these changes in appetite occur, but experts suspect that these changes are, at least partly, nature's way of ensuring that you get the proper nutrients. You may find that you crave bread, potatoes, and other starchy foods, and perhaps eating those foods in the early days is actually helping you store energy for later in pregnancy, when the baby does most of its growing. As with any other time in life, though, be careful not to overeat. You may also be very thirsty early in pregnancy, and the extra water you drink is useful for increasing your body's supply of blood and other fluids.

✔ **Your breasts become tender and bigger.** Don't be surprised by how large your breasts grow early in pregnancy. In fact, large and tender breasts are often the first symptom of pregnancy that you feel because very early in pregnancy, levels of estrogen and progesterone rise, causing immediate changes in your breasts.

Joanne's story

One day a couple of years after my first daughter was born, I found myself heading to the grocery store to buy pickles and ketchup, intent on mixing them together to make a lovely, tasty, green-and-red meal. I was craving it so much that it didn't even occur to me what an odd dish it is. In fact, it wasn't until I had cleaned up the dishes that I realized that pickles and ketchup had been my only craving during the early months of my first pregnancy. I had no other reason to think I was pregnant again; I hadn't even missed a period. But the next morning I tested myself, and sure enough, it was time for round two.

Determining Whether You're Pregnant

Well, are you or aren't you? These days, you don't need to wait to get to your practitioner's office to find out whether you're pregnant. You can opt instead for self-testing. Home tests are urine tests that give simply a positive (often two lines — hence the title of this chapter) or negative result (only one line). (By the way, these tests are very accurate for most people.) Your practitioner, on the other hand, may perform either a urine test similar to the one you took at home or a blood test to find out whether you're pregnant.

Getting an answer at home

Suppose you notice some bloating or food cravings, or you miss your period by a day or two. You want to know whether you're pregnant, but you aren't ready to go to a doctor yet. The easiest, fastest way to find out is to go to the drugstore and pick up a home pregnancy test. These tests are basically simplified chemistry sets, designed to check for the presence of *human chorionic gonadotropin* (hCG, the hormone produced by the developing placenta) in your urine. Although these kits aren't as precise as laboratory tests that look for hCG in blood, in many cases they can provide positive results very quickly — by the day you miss your period, or about two weeks after conception.

The results of home pregnancy tests aren't a sure thing. If your test comes out negative but you still think you're pregnant, retest in another week or make an appointment with your doctor. A urine test is positive at a level of about 20-50 IU/L while a blood test is positive at a level of 5-10 IU/L, depending on the test. So a blood test will be positive a little earlier than a urine test. An ultrasensitive blood test can even detect an hCG level of about 1-2 IU/L. hCG is found in the maternal blood at 6-12 days after ovulation (20-26 days from last menstrual period of ovulation occurs on day 14).

Going to your practitioner for answers

Even if you had a positive home pregnancy test, most practitioners want to confirm this test in their office before beginning your prenatal care. Your practitioner may decide to simply repeat a urine pregnancy test or to use a blood pregnancy test instead.

A blood pregnancy test checks for hCG in your blood. This test can be either qualitative (a simple positive or negative result) or quantitative (an actual measurement of the amount of hCG in your blood). The test your practitioner chooses depends on your history and your current symptoms and on her own individual preference. Blood tests can be positive even when urine tests are negative.

Calculating your due date

Only 1 in 20 women actually delivers on her due date — most women deliver anywhere from three weeks early to two weeks late. Nonetheless, it's important to pinpoint the due date as precisely as possible to ensure that the tests you need along the way are performed at the right time. Knowing how far along you are also makes it easier for your doctor to see that the baby is growing properly.

The average pregnancy lasts 280 days — 40 weeks — counting from the first day of the last menstrual period. Your due date — what doctors once referred to as the EDC, for estimated date of confinement (in the old days, women were actually "confined" to the hospital around the time of their delivery) — is calculated from the date on which your last menstrual period (LMP) started.

If your cycles are 28 days long, you can use a shortcut to determine your due date. Simply subtract three months from your LMP and add seven days. If your last period started on June 3, for example, your due date would be March (subtract three months) 10 (add seven days). If your periods don't follow 28-day cycles, don't worry. You can establish your due date in other ways. If you've been tracking ovulation and can pinpoint the date of conception, add 266 days to that date (the average time between the first day of your LMP and ovulation is about 14 days, or 2 weeks).

If you're unsure of the date of conception or the date your last period started, an ultrasound exam during the first three months can give you a good idea of your due date. A first-trimester ultrasound predicts your due date more accurately than a second- or third-trimester one.

You can also use a pregnancy wheel to calculate how far along you are. To use this handy tool, line up the arrow with the date of your last menstrual period and then look for today's date. Just below the date you see the number of weeks and days that have gone by. (If you know the date of conception, rather than your last period, there is a line on the wheel corresponding to this, too.) There are now online wheels (`http://www.premierus.com/wheel/`) as well as apps that you can download to calculate your due date.

Selecting the Right Practitioner for You

Finding the right practitioner to care for you (and your baby) is a decision you shouldn't take lightly. Your healthcare is always important, but your new and sometimes overwhelming condition means you want a practitioner who's in sync with your approach to pregnancy. This person should be someone you trust and feel safe with. You may already have a practitioner if you've had a previous child. If not, there's no need to feel overwhelmed. This section helps you make that important decision.

Considering your options

Many kinds of professionals can help you through pregnancy and delivery. Be sure to choose a practitioner with whom you feel comfortable. Review this list of the basic five:

- ✔ **Obstetrician/gynecologist:** After completing medical school, this physician receives another four years of special training in pregnancy, delivery, and women's health. She should be *board certified* (or be in the process of becoming board certified) by the American Board of Obstetrics and Gynecology (or an equivalent program if you're from a country other than the United States).

- ✔ **Maternal-fetal medicine specialist:** Also known as a *perinatologist* or *high-risk obstetrician,* this type of doctor has completed a two- to three-year fellowship in the care of high-risk pregnancies, in addition to the standard obstetrics residency, to become board certified in maternal-fetal medicine. Some maternal-fetal medicine specialists act only as consultants, and some also deliver babies. You might seek the care or even a consultation with a high-risk specialist if you have had a history of problem pregnancies (prior preterm delivery, history of preeclampsia, or multiple miscarriages), if you have underlying medical problems (like diabetes or chronic hypertension), or if your fetus has been diagnosed with a disorder.

✔ **Family practice physician:** This doctor provides general medical care for families — men, women, and children. She is board certified in family practice medicine. This kind of doctor is likely to refer you to an obstetrician or maternal-fetal medicine specialist if complications arise during your pregnancy.

✔ **Nurse-midwife:** A nurse-midwife is a registered nurse who has completed additional training to obtain a master's degree in nursing and is also licensed to perform deliveries. A certified nurse-midwife typically practices in a setting where there is a physician available and refers patients when complications occur.

✔ **Nurse practitioner:** A nurse practitioner is a registered nurse who has completed additional training to obtain a master's degree in nursing and is trained to provide routine prenatal care, but typically does not perform deliveries. She usually practices in conjunction with a physician; whether you see the nurse practitioner or the physician for your prenatal visits depends on the individual practice and where you are in your pregnancy.

Determining whether you're at high risk

The question of whether you and your pregnancy are at high risk has no black-and-white answer, especially at the beginning. But it helps to be aware of the kinds of situations (which you may either have or develop) that can put a pregnancy at high risk:

✔ Diabetes

✔ High blood pressure

✔ Lupus

✔ Blood disorders

✔ Heart, kidney, or liver disorders

✔ Twins, triplets, or other multiple fetuses

✔ A premature delivery in a prior pregnancy

✔ A previous child with birth defects

✔ A history of miscarriage

✔ An abnormally shaped uterus

✔ Epilepsy

✔ Some infections

✔ Bleeding

✔ Advanced maternal age (over age 35)

Remember that midwives and most family practice physicians are not equipped to handle high-risk pregnancies. If you have or develop any of these conditions, consult an obstetrician or a maternal-fetal medicine specialist.

Asking questions before you choose

Before you make a decision, you want to be complete and thorough in your search. Make sure you know what you want out of the experience. When you're deciding on a practitioner, ask yourself the following key questions:

✔ **Am I comfortable with and do I have confidence in this person?** You should trust and feel at ease not only with your practitioner but also with the whole constellation of people who work in the practice. Would you feel free to ask questions or express your anxieties to them? Another point to keep in mind is how your general personality fits in with the practice's philosophy. For example, some women prefer a low-key, low-tech approach to prenatal care, while others want to have every possible diagnostic test under the sun. Does this practitioner deliver in a setting where you feel most comfortable having your baby? Your past medical and obstetrical history can also influence the approach you take to your pregnancy and the provider you choose.

✔ **How many practitioners are involved in the practice?** You may end up choosing between a practitioner who works with one or more partners and one who is in solo practice. Many group practices rotate you through appointments with each of the doctors, getting to know them all so that you feel comfortable having any one of them deliver your baby. Some practices utilize nurse practitioners to help render prenatal care (see previous section). Practically speaking, you're likely to bond more with one or two people in the practice than with others, which is natural, given that most women and most practitioners have many varied personalities. A provider who practices alone should tell you who handles deliveries when she is ill, off duty, or out of town.

Ask your practitioner about her policy for after-hours problems or emergencies — including questions you may need to ask by telephone during evening or weekend hours.

✓ **Where do I want to deliver?** If your pregnancy is uncomplicated, any good hospital or birthing center will work just fine. Some women may even choose a home birth. If you're at risk for some complications, however, you should consider a hospital delivery and ask whether the hospital you'll be delivering in has a labor and delivery suite and a nursery equipped to handle any problems that may arise if, for example, the baby is born early. You may also want to ask the following questions:

- Is an anesthesiologist on-site 24 hours a day, or can your doctor call in an anesthesiologist quickly in case of an emergency?

- Can the hospital provide you with *epidural* anesthesia (a form of pain control during labor)? If epidural anesthesia isn't readily available, or you're not interested in this form of pain relief, find out what other options are available for pain management.

- Are you allowed to *room in* — that is, keep the baby in your room as much as possible — after delivery? Also, are accommodations available for your partner to stay with you during your postpartum hospitalization?

✓ **Can this practitioner refer me to a nearby specialist if needed?** Consider whether you may need the services of a maternal-fetal medicine specialist or a *neonatologist,* a physician who specializes in the care of infants who are born early or who have other medical problems. Ideally, your practitioner can refer you to someone quickly if anything comes up.

✓ **Will my insurance plan cover this practitioner?** Now that managed care has become an important part of the health insurance industry, check to see whether your plan covers your practitioner of choice. Some places allow you to select an "out-of-network" physician if you pay part of the cost yourself.

Weeks versus months

Most of us think of pregnancy as lasting nine months. But face it — 40 weeks is a little longer than nine times four weeks. It's closer to ten lunar months (in Japan, they actually speak of pregnancy as lasting ten months) and a bit longer than nine 30-to-31-day calendar months. That's why your doctor is more likely to talk in terms of weeks.

Because you start counting from the date of your last menstrual period, the count actually begins a couple of weeks before you conceive. So when your doctor says you're 12 weeks pregnant, the fetus is really only 10 weeks old!

Keeping Your Medicines and Vaccinations in Check

After you find out you're pregnant, you may wonder about the risks involved with certain medications and vaccinations. Maintaining good health throughout your pregnancy is a critical step in delivering a healthy baby. Review the following sections to see what risks and benefits are associated with certain medicines and vaccinations.

Reviewing your medications

Many medicines — both over-the-counter and prescription — are safe to take during pregnancy. If you're taking medications essential for your health, discuss them with your physician prior to stopping them or changing your dose or regimen. But a few medications can cause problems for the baby's development. So let your doctor know about *all* the medications you take. If one of them is problematic, you can probably switch to something safer. Keep in mind that adjusting dosages and checking for side effects may take time.

Exposure to the following drugs and chemicals is considered to be safe during pregnancy:

- ✔ Pain medications (for example, acetaminophen)
- ✔ Anti-viral medications (for example, acyclovir)

✔ Antiemetics/anti-nausea medications (for example, phenothiazines, trimethobenzamide, and Diclegis, a combination of doxylamine and vitamin B6, which has recently been approved by the Food and Drug Administration for morning sickness and is in the safest drug classification for pregnancy [category A])

✔ Antihistamines (for example, doxylamine)

✔ Low-dose aspirin — often used to decrease risk for preeclampsia in patients at risk

✔ Minor tranquilizers and some antidepressants (for example, meprobamate, chlordiazepoxide, and fluoxetine)

✔ Antibiotics (for example, penicillin, cephalexin, trimethoprim-sulfamethoxazole, and erythromycin)

✔ Anti-viral agent used in patients with HIV: Zidovudine

The following are some of the common medications that women should ask about before they get pregnant:

✔ **Birth control pills:** Women sometimes get pregnant while they're on the Pill (because they missed or were late taking a couple of pills during the month) and then worry that their babies will have birth defects. But oral contraceptives haven't been shown to have any ill effects on a baby. Two to three percent of *all* babies are born with birth defects, and babies born to women on oral contraceptives are at no higher risk.

✔ **Ibuprofen (Motrin, Advil):** Occasional use of these and other *nonsteroidal anti-inflammatory agents* during pregnancy (for pain or inflammation) is okay and hasn't been associated with problems in infants. However, avoid chronic or persistent use of these medications during pregnancy (especially during the last trimester) because they have the potential to affect platelet function and blood vessels in the baby's circulatory system, and because your baby's kidneys process them just like your own kidneys do.

✔ **Vitamin A:** This vitamin and some of its derivatives can cause miscarriage or serious birth defects if too much is present in your bloodstream when you get pregnant. The situation is complicated by the fact that vitamin A can remain in your body for several months after you consume it. Discontinuing any drugs that contain vitamin A derivatives — the most common is the anti-acne drug Accutane — at least one month before trying to conceive is important. Scientists don't know whether topical creams containing vitamin A derivatives — anti-aging creams like Retin A and Renova, for example — are as problematic as drugs that you swallow, so consult your physician.

Some women take vitamin A supplements because they're vegetarians and don't get enough from their diet, or because they suffer from vitamin A deficiency. The maximum safe dose during pregnancy is 5,000 international units (IU) daily. (You need to take twice that amount to reach the danger zone.) Multiple vitamins, including prenatal vitamins, typically contain 5,000 IU of vitamin A or less. Check the label on your vitamin bottle to be sure.

If you're worried that your prenatal vitamin plus your diet will put you into that "danger zone" of 10,000 IU per day, rest assured that it would be extremely difficult to get that much vitamin A in your diet.

✔ **Blood thinners:** Women who are prone to developing blood clots or who have artificial heart valves need to take blood-thinning agents every day. One type of blood thinner, *Coumadin,* or its derivatives can trigger miscarriage, impair the baby's growth, or cause the baby to develop bleeding problems or structural abnormalities if taken during pregnancy. Women who take this medicine and are thinking of getting pregnant should switch to a different blood thinner. Ask your practitioner for more information.

✔ **Drugs for high blood pressure:** Many of these medications are considered safe to take during pregnancy. However, because a few can be problematic, you should discuss any medications to treat high blood pressure with your doctor (see Chapter 15).

✔ **Antiseizure drugs:** Some of the medicines used to prevent epileptic seizures are safer than others for use during pregnancy. If you're taking any of these drugs, discuss them with your doctor. Don't simply stop taking any antiseizure medicine, because seizures may be worse for you — and the baby — than the medications themselves (see Chapter 15).

✔ **Tetracycline:** If you take this antibiotic during the last several months of pregnancy, it may, much later on, cause your baby's teeth to be yellow.

✔ **Antidepressants:** Many antidepressants (like Prozac and Zoloft) have been studied extensively and are considered safe during pregnancy. Recent studies on selective serotonin reuptake inhibitors (SSRIs) showed a small increase in certain birth defects, particularly with paroxetine, while other studies showed no increased risk. Most doctors believe that the absolute risk is very small. Although most data doesn't show an increase in prematurity or low birth weight, some data suggests a possible small increased chance of miscarriage in the first trimester. Some reports also show a very small risk (0.6 to 1.2 percent) of a newborn condition called persistent pulmonary hypertension with exposure in the latter half of pregnancy. Some of the newer antidepressants like Cymbalta, Celexa, Lexapro, and Effexor appear to be safe in pregnancy, but because they are new, data is limited. If you need to start an antidepressant during pregnancy, many doctors feel that sertraline (Zoloft) is the best first-line drug. But if you're already taking an antidepressant, ask your doctor whether you'll be able to keep taking the medication while you're pregnant or need to switch to something safer.

Aside from birth defects, there's also been concern that SSRIs were associated with an increased risk for autism. More recent studies, however, did not find a significant increase in the risk of this disorder in women taking SSRIs during pregnancy.

✔ **Bupropion:** Bupropion is an antidepressant, but it's also prescribed to help people stop smoking (for example, Wellbutrin or Zyban). Very little info exists on its use during pregnancy, but the available data doesn't suggest any significant problems with fetal development. Although you shouldn't use it as a first line for depression, its use for smoking cessation may be beneficial.

✔ **Fluconazole:** Fluconazole is an oral medication used to treat yeast or other fungal infections. A recent study showed that oral fluconazole used during the first trimester was not associated with an increased risk of birth defects overall, but that it may be associated with an increased risk of a specific heart defect known as Tetralogy of Fallot.

✔ **Decongestants:** A mounting body of recent evidence suggests that decongestants like phenylephrine and phenylpropanolamine, when used during the first trimester, may be associated with an increased risk of birth defects. If possible, you should avoid taking these medications until you have completed your first trimester, but if you inadvertently took some before you found out that you were pregnant, the likelihood of a birth defect resulting from it is still very low.

✔ **Lithium:** Lithium is a medication that is used occasionally to treat bipolar disorder. It is thought that this medication places women who take it during pregnancy at an increased risk for having a child with a specific cardiac abnormality known as Ebstein's anomaly. If possible, an alternative medication should be chosen for the first trimester, but if lithium is inadvertently taken during the first trimester, the risk is still quite low. Women taking lithium during early pregnancy should have a fetal echocardiogram around 20 weeks. This is a special type of ultrasound done to diagnose cardiac abnormalities, including Ebstein's anomaly.

Recognizing the importance of vaccinations and immunity

People are immune to all kinds of infections, for one of two reasons:

✔ **They've suffered through the disease.** Most people are immune to chicken pox, for example, because they had it when they were kids, causing their immune systems to make antibodies to the chicken pox virus.

✔ **They've been vaccinated.** That is, they've been given a shot of something that causes the body to develop antibodies.

Many vaccines are safe, and in fact recommended, while you're pregnant. (See Table 1-1 for information on several vaccines.) Here is some further information on some common vaccinations:

✔ **Rubella:** Your practitioner tests to see whether you're immune to *rubella* (also known as *German measles*) by drawing a sample of blood and checking to see whether it contains antibodies to the rubella virus. (*Antibodies* are immune system agents that protect you against infections.) If you are not immune to rubella, your practitioner is likely to recommend that you be vaccinated against rubella at least three months *before* becoming pregnant. Getting pregnant before the three months are over is highly unlikely to be a problem. No cases have been reported of babies born with problems due to the mother having received the rubella vaccine in early pregnancy. If you are already pregnant when you learn that you are not immune to rubella, your practitioner will recommend that you get the vaccine after you deliver your baby, just before you go home from the hospital.

✔ **Flu:** The influenza vaccine is safe and recommended during pregnancy. Pregnant women who get the flu are at increased risk of complications as a result of it. The vaccine poses no harm to your developing baby.

✔ **Tetanus, diphtheria, and pertussis:** It is recommended that women get an adult tetanus, diphtheria, and per-tussis (Tdap) vaccine during each pregnancy, ideally between weeks 27 and 36 of pregnancy.

✔ **Measles, mumps, and poliomyelitis:** Most people are immune to measles, mumps, and poliomyelitis, and your practitioner is unlikely to check your immunity to all these illnesses. Besides, these illnesses aren't usually associated with significant adverse effects for the baby.

✔ **Chicken pox:** Chicken pox carries a small risk that the baby can contract the infection from her mother. If you've never had chicken pox, tell your practitioner so you can discuss possible vaccination before you get pregnant, or if you are already pregnant, after delivery before you go home.

✔ **Human papilloma virus:** Vaccines are available for the human papilloma virus (HPV), which is associated with some kinds of abnormal pap smears, genital warts, and cervical cancer. Studies suggest it's similar to other vac-cinations that are safe in pregnancy; however, it is still recommended that you not receive this vaccination during pregnancy. If you inadvertently got vaccinated before real-izing that you were pregnant, the risk to your developing baby is very low, but you should not get subsequent doses until after delivery.

Testing for HIV

If you're at risk for HIV infection, get tested before contemplating pregnancy. Some states now require that doctors discuss and offer HIV testing to *all* pregnant women. If you have contracted HIV, taking certain medications throughout pregnancy will decrease the chances that your baby will also contract HIV.

Table 1-1   Safe and Unsafe Vaccines before or during Pregnancy

Disease	Risk of Vaccine to Baby during Pregnancy	Immunization Recommendations	Comments
Cholera	None confirmed	Same as in non-pregnant women	
Hepatitis A (inactivated)	None confirmed	Okay if high risk for infection or for prevention due to recent exposure	
Hepatitis B	None confirmed	Okay if high risk for infection	Used with immuno-globulins for acute exposure; newborns need vaccine
Human papil-loma virus	None con-firmed, but little data	If found to be pregnant after ini-tiating series, give remaining doses postpartum	
Influenza (inactivated)	None confirmed	Recommended	
Measles	None confirmed	No	Vaccinate postpartum
Mumps	None confirmed	No	Vaccinate postpartum

(continued)

Table 1-1 *(continued)*

Disease	Risk of Vaccine to Baby during Pregnancy	Immunization Recommendations	Comments
Plague	None confirmed	Selected vaccination if exposed	
Pneumococcus	None confirmed	Okay if high risk	
Poliomyelitis	None confirmed	Only if exposed	Get if traveling to endemic area
Rubella	None confirmed	No	Vaccinate postpartum
Rabies	Unknown	Indication same as for nonpregnant women	Consider each case separately
Smallpox	Possible miscarriage	No, unless emergency situation arises or fetal infection	
Tetanus, diphtheria, and pertussus (Tdap)	None confirmed	Recommended for each pregnancy between 27 and 36 weeks	
Typhoid	None confirmed	Only for close, continued exposure or travel to endemic area	
Varicella (chicken pox)	None confirmed	Immunoglobulins recommended in exposed nonimmune women; should be given to newborn if around time of delivery	If nonimmune, vaccinate postpartum (second dose four to eight weeks later)
Yellow fever	Unknown	No, unless exposure is unavoidable	

Debunking old wives' tales

Pregnancy has a certain mystique. Millions of women have been through it, yet predicting in detail what any one woman's experience will be like is difficult. Perhaps that's why so many myths have formed (and survived) over the centuries, most of which are designed to foresee the unknowable future. Here are 12 tales that, alas, are really nothing but nonsense:

✔ **Old Heartburn Myth: If a pregnant woman frequently experiences heartburn, her baby will have a full head of hair.** Simply not true. Some babies have hair; some don't. Most lose it all within a few weeks, anyway.

✔ **Mysterious Umbilical Cord Movement Myth: If a pregnant woman lifts her hands above her head, she will choke the baby.** Give us a break. People used to think (and, alas, some still believe) that the mother's movement could cause the baby to become tangled in the umbilical cord, but that's just not true.

✔ **Curse Myth: Anyone who denies a pregnant woman the food that she craves will get a sty in his eye.** Nope. This myth doesn't mean that someone who stands between a pregnant woman and her craving is in the clear, though: He will most certainly be subjected to threats, name-calling, or icy glares, but no sties.

✔ **Heart Rate Myth: If the fetal heart rate is fast, the baby is a girl, and if the heart rate is slow, the baby is a boy.** Medical researchers actually looked into this myth. They did find a very slight difference between the average heart rate of boys and that of girls, but it wasn't significant enough to make heart rate an accurate predictor of sex.

✔ **Ugly Stick Myth: If a pregnant woman sees something ugly or horrible, she will have an ugly baby.** How could this possibly be true? There's no such thing as an ugly baby!

✔ **Java Myth: If a baby is born with café au lait spots (light-brown birthmarks), the mother drank too much coffee or had unfulfilled cravings during her pregnancy.** Nope. Drinking 150-200 mg caffeinated beverages/day is considered safe (about 1 ½ cups coffee/day – but we are not talking about Starbucks Trenta though). Higher consumption of caffeine has been linked to miscarriage and low-birth weight.

✔ **Myth of International Cuisine: Eating spicy food brings on labor.** It doesn't, but it may be an effective marketing tool: We know of an Italian restaurant that advertises its Chicken Fra Diavolo as a surefire labor-inducer. The dish may be delicious, but it simply

(continued)

(continued)

can't bring on labor. Nope. Niet. Nunca. Nein. Non.

✔ **Great Sex Myth: Having passionate sex brings on labor.** What got you into this mess will also get you out? That's just wishful thinking, but go ahead and try it (if you feel like it when you're nine months pregnant). It's likely to be worth the effort.

✔ **Round Face Myth: If a pregnant woman gains weight in her face, the baby is a girl, and if a woman gains weight in her butt, the baby is a boy.** Neither statement is true, obviously. The baby's sex has no influence whatsoever on the way the mother stores fat.

Another related myth is that if the mother's nose begins to grow and widen, the baby is a girl. The so-called reasoning here is that a daughter always steals her mother's beauty. Strange concept — and quite untrue.

✔ **Moon Maid Myth: More women go into labor during a full moon.** Although many labor and delivery personnel insist that the labor floor is busier during a full moon (police say their precinct

houses are livelier then, too), the scientific data just doesn't support the idea.

✔ **Belly Shape Myth: If a pregnant woman's belly is round, the baby is a girl, and if the woman's belly is more bulletlike, it's a boy.** Forget about it. Belly shape differs from woman to woman, but the child's sex has nothing to do with it.

✔ **Ultrasound Tells All Myth: Ultrasound can always tell the baby's sex.** Nope, not always. Often, by about 18 to 20 weeks' gestation, seeing a fetus's genitalia on ultrasound is possible. But being able to determine the baby's sex depends on whether the baby is in position to give you a good view. Sometimes the sonographer can't see between the uncooperative baby's legs and therefore can't determine the sex. Sometimes, too, the sonographer may be wrong, especially if the ultrasound is done very early in the pregnancy. So even though you can find out the baby's sex through ultrasound in most cases, it's not 100 percent guaranteed.

Chapter 2

Your Pregnancy at a Glance: Overview of Pregnancy Week-by-Week

In This Chapter

▶ Knowing what to expect as your pregnancy progresses

▶ Scheduling doctor appointments and routine tests

▶ Getting ready for your baby's birth

*A*s we indicate throughout this book, pregnancy is usually referred to as a 40-week enterprise, which is a tad misleading. The pregnancy starts at conception, which — with a normal 28-day cycle — is two weeks after the first day of your last menstrual period (LMP). So, if you start at conception, pregnancy is only 38 weeks, but obstetricians use 40 weeks because most women don't know when they conceive but do remember when their LMP was.

Many of the things we mention in a particular week may still be important at other times throughout the pregnancy. So, just because we mention ultrasound at 20 weeks doesn't mean it can't be done at any time throughout the pregnancy. Feel free to find where you are in your pregnancy and check off each important item after you do it.

Some things we include in this chapter are optional and may not be necessary for everyone. We include them for the sake of completeness and so that you'll have some information to frame a discussion with your provider about whether they're right for you. Also, the week/weeks we assign to prenatal tests or pregnancy events are an approximation. Don't be overly alarmed if, in your pregnancy, they are off by a week or so.

Weeks 0–4

If you suspect that you're pregnant, you're probably excited and want to know definitively whether you are pregnant. The first four weeks are important because the pregnancy is getting established as the implantation process is underway.

During these initial weeks, do the following:

✔ Record your last menstrual period (LMP). Doing so helps your provider better estimate your due date (40 weeks from your LMP). Be sure to tell him if your cycles are irregular.

✔ Begin taking a daily prenatal vitamin if you haven't already. Check to see that the vitamin has at least 400 micrograms of folic acid to make sure your baby is as healthy as possible.

✔ Check for ovulation. Some women know when they ovulate by a sensation known as *mittelschmerz* (German for "middle pain" due to the mild pain that may be felt when the egg is released from the ovary, typically 14 days after the LMP). Others know they've ovulated due to a change in the cervical mucus or a positive reading from an ovulation prediction kit (see Chapter 1).

Fertilization usually occurs within the fallopian tube. The embryo starts as one cell. During the first week, that cell divides many times as it moves down the fallopian tube toward the uterine cavity.

✔ **Take your first pregnancy test.** Pregnancy tests check for a hormone called human chorionic gonadotropin (hCG), which is produced by the embryo as it implants into the wall of the uterus — usually five to seven days after conception. By the time you miss a period, around ten days after conception, your pregnancy test will most likely be positive.

Don't be too concerned if you have a little spotting around the time when you would expect your period. This is most likely due to the embryo implanting in the womb (implantation bleeding).

At the end of the fourth week, your baby measures 0.2 inches (4 mm) in length.

Weeks 5–8

By this time, the pregnancy is well established and you're feeling the typical signs and symptoms of pregnancy, such as nausea and fatigue. It's an important time to make any necessary lifestyle changes, if you haven't already done so (like stopping smoking or speaking with your doctor abut adjusting medications).

During this time, begin making these necessary medical appointments:

✔ **Call your doctor to make an appointment for your first prenatal visit.** Most doctors want to see their patients before 8 to 10 weeks.

✔ **Talk to your healthcare provider about scheduling an ultrasound or obtaining a heartbeat by Doppler to confirm a healthy pregnancy.** An ultrasound during this period is very accurate at establishing your due date (it is sometimes called a "dating scan") and can also tell you whether you're having one, two, or even more babies! Your due date is most accurate when it is established by an ultrasound between 8 and 12 weeks.

This is when most of the organ systems are beginning to form. The first organ to start working is the heart. It's amazing to realize it starts beating at just 5 weeks, although you can't see it beating on ultrasound until 6 weeks. The baby's arms and legs are beginning to develop at this stage. The head is the biggest part of the embryo because the brain is the fastest-growing organ at this time. (Check out Chapter 5 for more on what happens during the first trimester.) The placenta is rapidly growing and is now the way nutrients and oxygen get to your developing baby.

✔ **If you are taking any medications, call or see your doctor earlier than the 8 to 10 weeks mentioned.** You want to make sure that these meds aren't a problem for your developing baby. You should also discuss any over-the-counter or herbal medications you're taking to make sure they aren't a problem.

At the end of the eighth week, your baby measures 1.2 inches (30 mm) in length. Your uterus is about the size of a medium orange.

Weeks 9–12

Although you won't be feeling it this early, this is the time when your baby starts to move around. If you're having an ultrasound at this time, you may actually see these movements on the screen. Before 10 weeks, male and female embryos look the same. After 10 weeks, their external genitalia start to develop differently, although your practitioner may not be able to see this difference on ultrasound until after 14 to 15 weeks. By the end of the tenth week, all the organ systems have formed. The brain is unique in that it continues to develop throughout pregnancy and even into childhood.

You want to consider the following counseling and testing at this time:

- ✔ **Schedule an appointment for genetic counseling if you have a family history of genetic problems.** Your doctor may also recommend it depending on varying circumstances.

- ✔ **Make sure you schedule your first trimester screen for Down syndrome.** Remember, the best time to do this is at 11 to 12 weeks (see Chapter 5). This is a combination of measuring a fluid-filled region behind the fetal neck called a "nuchal translucency," which is combined with your age and blood tests (hCG and PAPPP-A) and gives a specific risk for Down syndrome, as well as Trisomy 13 and 18 (and extra chromosome 13 and 18). Talk to your provider to see if he thinks you are a candidate for a different type of screening for Down syndrome by one of the newer tests that extracts fetal genetic material from your blood (see Chapter 5). This blood sample can be drawn as early as 9 weeks.

- ✔ **If you're considering having a chorionic villus sampling (CVS), weeks 10 to12 are the best time to do this.** See Chapter 5 for more information on this test.

At the end of week 12, your baby is 2.13 inches (5.4 mm) long and weighs less than half an ounce (around 14 g). Your uterus is the size of a large orange.

Weeks 13–16

Congratulations! You and your baby made it through the first trimester. You're starting to feel more like yourself — you have more energy and less nausea. After week 14, the majority of the amniotic fluid surrounding your baby is made up of the baby's urine. By week 15, an experienced sonographer can tell by ultrasound whether you're having a boy or a girl. By week 16, your baby starts to grow fine, soft hair (called *lanugo*) and fingernails.

The following considerations apply during this time period:

- ✔ **Between weeks 15 and 18, have your blood drawn to check the alpha-fetoprotein (AFP) level.** This blood test helps to identify fetal abnormalities such as spina bifida. This is also the time to have the second part of your Down syndrome screening (quad screen).

- ✔ **Schedule your amniocentesis between weeks 16 and 18 if you're planning on having one.** See Chapter 6 for the reasons to consider an amniocentesis.

- ✔ **Consider shopping at a maternity store.** Many women start to show at this time. If you aren't showing, don't worry because some body types hide pregnancy better than others.

At the end of week 16, your baby is 4.6 inches (11.6 cm) long and weighs about 3½ ounces (100 g). Your uterus is the size of a large grapefruit.

Weeks 17–20

During weeks 17 to 20, your baby begins to put on some fat and looks more like a real baby. The baby's skeleton, which starts out mostly as cartilage, is now transforming into bone. Often you may notice a little fluttering sensation in your abdomen. This could be gas, but more likely it's early fetal movement. By 20 weeks, the top of the uterus (called the *fundus*) is at the level of your belly button. Twenty weeks is the halfway mark, so you should congratulate yourself. The second half usually flies by faster than the first.

You want to keep the following in mind:

- ✔ **Schedule your anatomy ultrasound.** This is the ultrasound where the doctor is able to check the baby's anatomy and make sure he is growing properly and is surrounded by normal amniotic fluid.

- ✔ **Pay attention to the baby's movements.** This period is when many women start to feel the baby move, which is called quickening. First-time moms, though, don't always feel quickening this early, so don't be alarmed if you haven't.

Your baby now weighs about 10 ounces (300 g) and is about 10 inches (26 cm) long.

Weeks 21–24

During this time, there aren't any actual tasks that you have to schedule with your provider, other than your routine prenatal visits (which should be about every four weeks during this period). Your baby's lungs are going through a very important phase of development. The lining of the lungs is beginning to thin out enough to allow for oxygen exchange. You may be experiencing discomfort on either side of your lower abdomen (in the groin area) known as *round ligament pain*. The round ligaments are actual ligaments that attach from the top of the uterus to the labia. At this time, many women feel an uncomfortable pulling sensation, which tends to worsen upon standing and improve upon sitting or lying down. The good news is that after 24 weeks, round ligament pain usually goes away.

At this time your baby is regularly swallowing large amounts of amniotic fluid, and excreting urine back into the amniotic cavity. The baby's fingernails are almost fully formed, and he has started to grow eyelashes and eyebrows. The lanugo is turning from a pale color to a darker hue.

By 24 weeks, your baby is considered *viable*. This means survival on the outside is possible, although the baby would need a great deal of medical attention. The top of your uterus is usually at or above the level of your belly button.

At the end of this period, your baby weighs about 1 pound, 5 ounces (600 g) and measures about 12 inches (30 cm) long.

Weeks 25–28

Your baby's bones are continuing to harden, and his fingernails, toes, eyebrows, and eyelashes are fully present. Meanwhile, your baby's skin is still fairly see-through, although it is changing from transparent to a more opaque look. You should still be seeing your provider about every four weeks during this period of pregnancy.

The following considerations are typically addressed during this time:

- ✔ **Get your glucose screen.** This is the blood test to screen for gestational diabetes. You're instructed to drink a 50-gram glucose drink (it tastes like flat soda), and your blood is drawn one hour later. If the glucose level is above a certain value, a definitive test called a GTT (glucose tolerance test) is needed. You're instructed to fast the night before this test so that your fasting glucose level can be determined with the initial blood draw. You then drink a 100-gram glucose drink and have your blood drawn every hour for the next three hours. Two abnormal values are needed for a diagnosis of gestational diabetes. During the glucose screening process, your doctor may draw some additional blood to check for conditions like anemia.

- ✔ **If your blood type is Rh negative (see Chapter 14), you need to get a shot of Rh immune globulin.** This shot (sometimes called by the brand name Rhogam or Rhophylac) can prevent any effects of incompatibility between you and your baby.

The top of your uterus is a couple of inches above your belly button. By 28 weeks your baby weighs about 1 pound, 4 ounces (1 kg). He is about 13.8 inches (35 cm) long.

Weeks 29–32

Your baby's eyes can now open. His permanent teeth have developed, and the lungs and digestive tract are nearly mature. In order to keep a closer eye on you and your baby, your practitioner will start to schedule your prenatal visits every two weeks during this time.

The following steps are recommended during this time:

- ✔ **If you haven't started childbirth classes, begin them now.** Many alternatives are available, so check with your doctor or the hospital where you will deliver. Chapter 7 discusses several options. If you'll have help taking care of your newborn, remember that it's a good idea for all caregivers (including you and your partner) to take an infant CPR class to be as prepared as possible for your newborn.

- ✔ **Pay closer attention to your baby's movements.** Although fetuses still spend most of their time sleeping, they start to develop clear sleep and wake cycles. A good general rule is that feeling about six movements in an hour is a sign of fetal well-being. You don't have to feel these movements every hour, but if you're ever concerned that you're not feeling your normal fetal movement, lie down and count the movements. If you can feel six movements in an hour, you can rest assured that this is normal.

   The nature of the fetal movements may also change. Instead of the big punches and kicks you were feeling earlier, the movements during this time may be gentler, rolling type of movements.

- ✔ **Undergo a follow-up ultrasound if your practitioner orders one.** This ultrasound can confirm that the baby is growing normally and has a good amount of amniotic fluid. Most practitioners also follow growth by measuring your uterine height every time you visit.

The top of your uterus is midway between your navel and your sternum. By 32 weeks, your baby weighs about 3 pounds, 11 ounces to 4 pounds (1.7 kg) and is 16 to 17 inches (40 cm) long.

Weeks 33–36

If you're having twins, you should be well prepared for their arrival now, because on average, twins deliver at about 35 to 36 weeks. During this time, you may be feeling lots of rhythmic fetal movements, which are really the baby hiccupping, a normal occurrence. These hiccups can continue even after the baby is born.

The following considerations come into play now:

- ✔ **Get a culture taken for GBS (group B strep).** Your doctor tests for these common bacteria that can be found in the vagina or rectum. If your GBS culture is positive, your doctor will place you on antibiotics during labor to prevent the baby from contracting the infection. There isn't any point in treating it earlier, because it can just come back again.

- ✔ **Continue to pay attention to the baby's movements.** Even though you're used to feeling kicks and punches, it's normal for the intensity of these movements to decrease during these last weeks of pregnancy. It's the *number* that is important, though, rather than the intensity. See Chapter 7 for more about fetal movements in the third trimester.

The top of your uterus is a couple of inches below your sternum. At or just after 36 weeks, your doctor will see you at least once a week until you deliver. Your baby weighs about 5 pounds, 2 ounces (2.3 kg) and is almost 18 inches (45 cm) long.

Weeks 37–40

Congratulations — you are now considered *"term."* Even though you may not yet be at your due date, any delivery that occurs at or after 37 weeks is called full-term. You may notice irregular contractions that come and go in spurts. The big event can happen any time during this period, so be prepared — day or night.

Do the following to ensure that you're ready for the big day to arrive:

- ✔ **Make sure your bags are packed, and you have the phone numbers of your practitioners handy!** If you have other children at home, make sure you have all the arrangements set for their care, in case you go into labor.

- ✔ **Watch for signs.** Loss of your mucous plug, bloody show, or loose stools may happen during the days before labor to indicate that labor is coming. Unfortunately, they don't determine when labor will happen with any certainty.

The average baby at full-term weighs about 7½ pounds (close to 3.5 kg), but there is a wide degree of variation in what is considered normal. At this point in pregnancy, your baby will put on about a quarter of a pound per week until delivery. The top of your uterus should be at or just below your sternum or breastbone. Babies at 40 weeks average about 20 to 21 inches (51 to 52 cm) long.

Weeks 40–42

Don't worry — the end really is in sight. If you haven't gone into labor on your own, your doctor will likely schedule you for either induction or cesarean section by 41-42 weeks. If you are older than 35, and especially older than 40, your doctor may want to deliver you sooner. Because the risks to continuing the pregnancy really increase after 41-42 weeks, your baby should be delivered by that time. Your doctor makes sure your baby remains healthy during this time:

- ✔ **Your doctor monitors you with non-stress tests to check on fetal well-being.** This is a non-invasive way to make sure the baby is tolerating the in-utero environment. (See Chapter 7 for more information.)

- ✔ **Your doctor checks the amount of amniotic fluid present to make sure it's still adequate.** The amniotic fluid volume usually tends to decrease after 36 weeks, so it is not uncommon for it to be low at this time. Low amniotic fluid volume is a common reason for labor induction during this period.

Although the baby continues to grow after 40 weeks, the rate of growth slows a little, and he may not put on the quarter-pound per week that he did in the few weeks before 40 weeks.

Common Tests during Pregnancy

Table 2-1 lists common tests that may be recommended during your pregnancy. As stated earlier, they may not be recommended for every pregnancy, but are included for the sake of those who need them.

Table 2-1	Common Tests during Pregnancy	
TEST	*GESTATIONAL AGE (weeks)*	*PURPOSE OF TEST*
Dating ultrasound	7–12	Confirm viability of pregnancy, establish due date, rule out multiple gestations
Harmony, MaterniT21, Panorama, or Verifi	9–20	These are newly available tests for some women that use a sample of maternal blood to screen for genetic defects in the fetus.
Nuchal translucency test (ultrasound)	11–12	Part of the first trimester screen for Down syndrome
Chorionic villus sampling (CVS)	10–12	Diagnostic test that samples the placental tissue for genetic abnormalities; recommended for some women but should be offered to all women
AFP/quad screen	15–18	A blood test to screen for defects such as spina bifida and to complete the second trimester screen for Down syndrome
Amniocentesis	16–18	Another diagnostic test that samples the amniotic fluid for genetic abnormalities; recommended for some women but again should be offered to all women

(continued)

Table 2-1 *(continued)*

TEST	GESTATIONAL AGE (weeks)	PURPOSE OF TEST
Anatomy ultrasound	18–22	An ultrasound to look at the baby from head to toe to make sure he is developing normally (to rule out many birth defects)
Glucose screen	24–28	A test for gestational diabetes (see Chapter 15)
Group B strep (GBS) swab	35–37	To see if the birth canal is colonized with group B strep bacteria (if so, mom will be given antibiotics during a vaginal delivery to protect the baby)
Non-stress test (NST)	40–42	A test of the baby's heart rate patterns to determine fetal well-being, despite going past his due date. Often done earlier in pregnancy for other complications like high blood pressure and diabetes.
Biophysical profile (BPP)	40–42	An ultrasound test to determine fetal well-being. Also often done earlier in pregnancy for other complications. Includes an assessment of amniotic fluid volume.

Chapter 3

Preparing for Life during Pregnancy

*E*ven though you're pregnant and your body is already undergoing miraculous changes, your day-to-day life goes on. How will you need to change your lifestyle in order to make your pregnancy go as smoothly as possible? What things in your life don't need to change, or need to be modified only slightly? You have a lot to consider: your job, the general level of stress in your life, what medications you take, whether you smoke or drink alcohol regularly, and what to do about routine things like going to the dentist or hairdresser. If you're like most normally healthy women, you'll probably find that for the most part, your life can go on largely as usual.

In this chapter and the next, we offer a general outline for how to plan your life during pregnancy, but all the issues we mention are subjects for discussion with your practitioner. If you consider from the beginning how your daily habits and health practices interact with your pregnancy, you're likely to have an easier time getting used to your new state of being. The earlier you get started on the right diet, exercise, and overall health program, the better (see Chapter 4 for more).

Planning Prenatal Visits

Your positive pregnancy test marks a new beginning. The time has come to start thinking about what lies ahead. After you decide who your practitioner will be (check out Chapter 1), give the office a call to find out how to proceed. Some practices want you to come in for a visit with the office nurse to give a medical history and confirm your good news with either a blood or urine test, whereas others schedule a first visit with the practitioner. How soon your first visit will be scheduled depends in part on your past or current history.

If you didn't have a preconceptional visit (see Chapter 1) beforehand, and you haven't been on prenatal vitamins or other vitamins containing folic acid, let the office know. A prescription for prenatal vitamins can be called in so you can start taking them even before your first prenatal visit. All over-the-counter adult multi- and prenatal vitamins should have the correct dose of folic acid so the typical patient doesn't need a prescription for them, but ask the pharmacist if you're not sure. Also, some insurance companies may cover prescription vitamins but not over-the-counter ones, and some women just simply prefer one particular type of vitamin.

Some things are consistent from trimester to trimester — like checking your blood pressure, urine, and the baby's heartbeat — so we cover these topics in this chapter. In Chapters 5, 6, and 7, we go over the specifics of what happens during prenatal visits for each trimester. See Table 3-1 for an overview of a typical schedule for prenatal visits.

Table 3-1	Typical Prenatal Visit Schedule
Stage of Pregnancy	*Frequency of Doctor Visits*
First visit to 28 weeks	Every four weeks
28 to 36 weeks	Every two to three weeks
36 weeks to delivery	Weekly

If you develop problems during pregnancy or if your pregnancy is considered "high risk" (see the risk factors we describe in Chapter 13), your practitioner may suggest that you come in more frequently.

This schedule of prenatal visits isn't set in stone. If you're planning a vacation or need to miss a prenatal visit, tell your practitioner and reschedule your appointment. If your pregnancy is going smoothly, rescheduling usually isn't a big deal. However, because some prenatal tests have to be performed at specific times during pregnancy (see Chapters 8 and 9 for details), just make sure that missing an appointment won't affect any of these tests.

Prenatal visits vary a bit according to each woman's personal needs and each practitioner's style. Some women need particular laboratory tests or physical examinations. However, the following procedures are standard during your prenatal visits:

- ✔ **A nurse checks your weight and blood pressure.** For more information on how much weight you should be gaining and when, see Chapter 4.

- ✔ **You give a urine sample (usually an easy job for most pregnant women!).** Your practitioner checks for the presence of protein or glucose, which may be a sign of preeclampsia or diabetes (see Chapters 15 and 16). Some urine tests also enable your doctor to look for any indications of a urinary tract infection.

- ✔ **Starting sometime after 14 to 16 weeks, a nurse or doctor measures your fundal height.** The practitioner uses either a tape measure or her hands to measure your uterus. This gives her a rough idea of how the baby is growing and whether you have an adequate amount of amniotic fluid (see Figure 3-1).

The nurse or doctor is measuring the *fundal height,* the distance from the top of the pubic bone to the top of the uterus (the *fundus*). By 20 weeks, the fundus usually reaches the level of the navel. After 20 weeks, the height in centimeters roughly equals the number of weeks pregnant you are. (Being above or below by 2 centimeters is usually within acceptable norms as long as you're consistent from visit to visit.)

Note: The fundal height measurement may not be useful in women who are expecting two or more babies or in women who have large fibroids (in both cases, the uterus is much bigger than normal) or in women who are very obese (because it can be difficult to feel the top of the uterus).

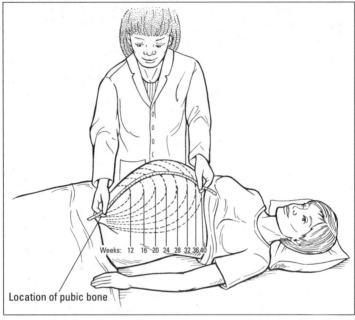

Weeks: 12 16 20 24 28 32 36 40

Location of pubic bone

Kathryn Born, MA

Figure 3-1: Your practitioner may measure your fundal height to ensure that your baby is growing properly.

✔ **A nurse or doctor listens for and counts the baby's heartbeat.** Typically, the heartbeat ranges between 120 and 160 beats per minute. Most offices use an electronic Doppler device to check the baby's heartbeat. With this method, the baby's heartbeat sounds sort of like horses galloping inside the womb. Sometimes, you can hear the heartbeat as early as 8 or 9 weeks using this method, but often it isn't clearly discernible until 10 to 12 weeks. Prior to the availability of Doppler, a special stethoscope called a *fetoscope* was used to hear the baby's heartbeat. Using this method, the doctor can hear the heartbeat around 20 weeks. A third way of checking the baby's heartbeat is by seeing it on ultrasound. The heart beating away can frequently be seen at around 6 weeks.

In some practices, a medical assistant or nurse performs tasks such as checking your blood pressure; in other practices, a doctor may perform this task. No matter who performs the technical components of the prenatal visit, you should always have the opportunity to ask a practitioner questions before leaving the office.

Preparing for Physical and Emotional Changes

When you're pregnant, your body is undergoing transformation. You can expect to experience changes, such as mood swings, leg cramps, and stress. You've probably experienced these conditions before — just not with such intensity. The following sections cover these and other problems and let you know what you may be in for. Have your family and friends read these sections, too — then tell them to consider themselves forewarned.

Coping with mood swings

Hormonal shifts affect mood, as most women, especially those who suffer from premenstrual syndrome (PMS), already know. The hormonal fluctuations that support pregnancy are perhaps the most dramatic a woman experiences in her lifetime, so it's hardly surprising that emotional ups and downs are commonplace. And the fatigue that goes along with pregnancy can easily make these ups and downs more severe. Add to this biochemical mix the normal anxieties that the average expectant mother has about whether the baby will be healthy and whether she'll be a good mother, and you have plenty of fuel to produce good old-fashioned mood swings.

You're not alone. Moodiness is a normal part of pregnancy, and you're not the first or only woman to experience it. So don't blame yourself. Your family and friends will understand.

Your moodiness may be especially pronounced during the first trimester because your body is adjusting to its new condition. You may find yourself overreacting to little things. A silly, mushy television commercial, for example, may leave you in tears. Misplacing your appointment book may send you into a panic. A grocery store clerk who accidentally smashes your loaf of bread may draw you into a teeth-clenching rage. Don't worry — you're just pregnant. Take a few deep breaths, go out for a walk, or just close your eyes and take a short break. These feelings often pass as quickly as they arise.

Living through leg cramps

Leg cramps are a common annoyance of pregnancy, and they're likely to become more frequent as the months go along. They're due to a sudden tightening of the muscles. The muscles may tighten for many different reasons, including lack of fluids, muscle strain, or staying in one position for too long. Doctors once thought that leg cramps were due to too little calcium or potassium in the diet, although that has not been shown to be true. Some studies suggest that taking an oral magnesium supplement may reduce leg cramps.

To diminish leg cramps, you may want to try one of these suggestions:

✔ Apply heat to the calves.

✔ Drink plenty of fluids.

✔ Avoid staying in one position too long.

✔ Stretch and extend your legs and feet.

✔ Take a short walk.

✔ Ask your partner to give you a foot or leg massage.

Do your stretching nightly before bed. Point your toes up toward the ceiling to really stretch your calves out. Do this about ten times. In the morning, get in the habit of doing this stretching at least a couple of times, before you even open your eyes if possible. Try to avoid extending your feet when you first wake up to avoid triggering a spasm. Also take a nice walk and ask your partner to get involved by giving you a foot or leg massage!!

Noticing vaginal discharge

During pregnancy, your vaginal discharge normally increases substantially. Some women find that they need to wear thin panty liners every day. The discharge tends to be thin, white, and virtually odorless, technically known as leucorrhea. Vaginal douches aren't a good idea because they may alter a woman's natural ability to fight off vaginal infections.

The type of vaginal discharge common in pregnancy is called *leukorrhea.* You can use this term when discussing your condition with your practitioner and really show her you've done your pregnancy research!

If your vaginal discharge takes on a brown, yellow, or green color, or if it develops a noxious odor or causes itching, let your practitioner know. (Be sure to use your judgment about how much of an emergency this is — it isn't the sort of problem that requires a 3 a.m. phone call to her office.)

Pregnancy doesn't prevent you from getting a vaginal infection, and the high levels of estrogen in your blood may predispose you to developing a yeast infection. A yeast infection usually produces a thick, white-yellow discharge, and it may, in some cases, cause itchiness or redness. Topical vaginal creams should solve the problem, and they pose no risk to the fetus. Most over-the-counter preparations come in 1-, 3-, and 7-day dosages and are completely safe for the baby. For hard-to-beat yeast infections, talk with your doctor about oral fluconazole, which may be used safely in pregnancy.

Putting up with backaches

Backaches are a common symptom that many women experience during pregnancy. They typically occur in the latter part of pregnancy, although they can occur earlier. The shift in your center of gravity can be one cause. Another can be the change in the curvature of your spine as the baby grows and the uterus enlarges. You may get some relief by getting off your feet when you can, applying mild local heat, and taking acetaminophen (Tylenol). Our patients often ask us about using a specially designed pregnancy girdle that they've seen advertised or heard about. Although some patients say this girdle helps, others don't think so.

Some women experience pain extending from their lower back to their buttocks and down one leg or the other. This pain, or less commonly, numbness, is known as *sciatica,* which is due to pressure on the sciatic nerve, a major nerve that branches from your back, through your pelvis, to your hips, and down your legs. You can relieve mild cases of sciatica with bed rest, warm baths, or heating pads. If you develop a severe case, you may need prolonged bed rest or special exercises.

Occasionally, preterm labor can present itself as low back pain. However, when it's preterm labor, the pain is more cramp-like and it comes and goes, rather than being continuous.

Handling stress

Many women wonder whether stress has any effect on pregnancy. That question is difficult to answer because stress is such an elusive concept. We all know what stress is, but each woman seems to handle it in her own way, and no one can really measure its intensity. We do know that chronic stress — unrelieved day after day — can increase the levels of stress hormones circulating in the bloodstream. Many doctors think that such elevated levels of stress hormones can promote preterm labor or blood pressure problems during pregnancy, but few studies have been able to prove this idea.

While you're pregnant, pay attention to your comfort and happiness. Everyone has her own way of relaxing — whether it's by getting a massage, going to a movie, having dinner with friends, taking a hot shower or bubble bath, or just sitting back and putting her feet up. Take the time you need to be good to yourself.

Understanding the Effects of Medications, Alcohol, and Drugs on Your Baby

Alcohol and recreational/illicit drugs can cross the placenta and get into your baby's circulatory system. Some medications can also cross the placenta. Some are completely harmless, whereas others can cause problems. The following sections outline which substances you can safely use and which you should avoid — information that's crucial to your baby's health.

Taking medications

During your pregnancy, you'll probably experience at least a headache or two and an occasional case of heartburn. The question of whether you can safely take pain relievers, antacids, and other over-the-counter medicines is bound to come up. Many women are afraid to take any medicine at all, for fear of somehow harming their babies. But most nonprescription drugs — and even many prescription drugs — are safe during pregnancy. During your first prenatal visit, go over with your practitioner what medications are okay to take during pregnancy — both over-the-counter medications and medications prescribed to you by another physician. If another physician is treating you for a medical condition, let her know that you're pregnant, in case any adjustments need to be made.

Don't stop taking a prescription medication or change the dosage on your own without talking to your doctor first.

Many medications are labeled "Don't take during pregnancy" because they haven't been adequately studied in pregnant women. However, this warning label doesn't necessarily mean that adverse effects have been reported or that you can't use these medications. Whenever you have a question about a particular medication, ask your practitioner for advice. Don't be surprised if opinions vary among practitioners, especially between non-obstetric medical people and obstetricians. Many non-obstetricians are hesitant to prescribe many medications because they're uncertain, whereas your obstetric practitioner may be more secure.

Certain medical problems, such as high blood pressure, pose more risk to the growing fetus than the medication you would take to treat it does. Even a common headache, if it's bad enough to cause you to miss a traffic signal when you're behind the wheel, can be more dangerous than a little acetaminophen (Tylenol), which actually isn't dangerous at all when taken in therapeutic doses. The fact is that we find many pregnant women suffer needlessly with common symptoms that could be treated with medications that are safe for the baby.

In Chapter 1, we list many of the drugs/chemicals that are safe for most pregnant women to take. We also discuss some of the drugs that are known to have a *teratogenic* effect, which means they have the potential to cause birth defects or problems with growth and development.

If you took any teratogenic medications before you knew you were pregnant — or before you knew that the drugs could pose a problem — don't panic. In many cases, the drugs do no harm, depending on when during pregnancy you took them and in what quantities. Some medications can cause problems in the first trimester, but are totally safe in the third trimester, and vice versa. In fact, relatively few substances are proven to be teratogenic to humans, and even those that are don't cause birth defects every time. Discuss with your practitioner the medications you've been taking and what tests are available to check on your baby's growth and development.

You can also call or go to the Web site of a number of medical information services, including those in the following list, for more data about teratogenic substances. These services get their information from medical databases (also listed), so if the information you get over the phone or on the Web site is overly technical, ask your practitioner to interpret for you:

- ✔ Micromedex, Inc., REPRODISK (REPROTEXT, REPROTOX, Shepard's Catalog of Teratogenic Agents, and TERIS), Greenwood Village, Colorado; Web site: `www.micromedex.com`

- ✔ Reproductive Toxicology Center, REPROTOX, Bethesda, Maryland; phone 301-514-3081; Web site: `http://reprotox.org`

- ✔ Teratogen Information System, TERIS and Shepard's Catalog of Teratogenic Agents, Seattle, Washington; phone 206-543-2465

Smoking and its risks

Unless you've been living on Mars for the past ten years, you no doubt are aware that smoking is a health risk for you. When you smoke, you run the risk of developing lung cancer, emphysema, and heart disease, among other illnesses. During pregnancy, however, smoking poses risks to your baby as well.

The carbon monoxide in cigarette smoke decreases the amount of oxygen that your growing baby receives, and nicotine cuts back on blood flow to the fetus. Consequently, women who smoke stand an increased chance of delivering babies with low birth weight, which may mean more medical problems for the baby. In fact, babies born to smokers are expected to weigh a half-pound less, on average, than those born to nonsmokers. The exact difference in birth weight depends on how much the mother smokes. Secondhand smoke is also a risk.

In addition to low birth weight, smoking during pregnancy is associated with a greater risk of preterm delivery, miscarriage, placenta previa (see Chapter 16), placental abruption (see Chapter 16), preterm rupture of the amniotic membranes, and even sudden infant death syndrome (SIDS) after the baby is born.

Quitting smoking can be extremely difficult. But keep in mind that even cutting back on the number of cigarettes you smoke is beneficial to your baby (and yourself).

 If you quit smoking during the first three months you're pregnant, give yourself a pat on the back and be reassured that your baby is likely to be born at a normal weight and have fewer health issues.

 Some women use nicotine patches, gum, lozenges, or inhalers to help them kick the habit. The nicotine from these products is still absorbed into the bloodstream and can still reach the fetus, but at least the carbon monoxide and other toxins in cigarette smoke are eliminated. The American College of Obstetrics and Gynecology recommends that nicotine replacements such as these may be used when non-pharmacologic treatments have failed. The total amount of nicotine absorbed from the intermittent use of the gum or inhalers may be less than the amount from the patch, which is used continuously.

The effects on fetal development with the use of bupropion (Zyban or Wellbutrin) haven't been extensively studied, but one well-designed study showed that pregnant smokers receiving bupropion were much more likely to quit than those not taking the medication.

Drinking alcohol

Clearly, pregnant women who use alcohol put their babies at risk of fetal alcohol syndrome, which encompasses a wide variety of birth defects (including growth problems, heart defects, mental retardation, or abnormalities of the face or limbs). The controversy arises because medical science hasn't defined an absolute safe level of alcohol intake during pregnancy. Scientific data shows that daily drinking and heavy binge drinking can lead to serious complications, although little information is available about occasional drinking. Two recent studies from Britain, however, demonstrated that light or moderate drinking had little effect on either neurodevelopmental outcomes or balance. In one study, up to two drinks/week was not linked with developmental problems with children. A separate study of 7,000 10-year-olds whose mothers had light (one glass/week) or moderate (three to seven glasses/week) alcohol consumption during pregnancy found that the children had no difference in balance compared to those whose mothers did not drink at all during pregnancy. The authors of the studies still say, however, that abstaining from alcohol during pregnancy is the best choice. Similarly, both the American College of Obstetricians and Gynecologists and the Food and Drug Administration (FDA) recommend avoiding any amount of alcohol during pregnancy.

If you think you may have a drinking problem, don't feel uncomfortable talking to your practitioner about it. Special questionnaires are available to help your doctor identify whether your drinking is excessive enough to pose a risk to you and the fetus. If you think you may have a problem, discussing this questionnaire with your practitioner is crucial to your baby's health — and to yours.

Expectant mothers ask . . .

Questions about alcohol consumption during pregnancy are very common, so we provide the answers to some of the most frequently asked questions:

Q: "On my Caribbean vacation, I enjoyed some piña coladas on the beach. I didn't find out I was pregnant until a few weeks later. Will my baby have birth defects?"

A: No evidence exists that a single episode of drinking has any increased risk of adverse effects on pregnancy. Now that you know you're pregnant, avoid alcohol.

Q: "Is hard liquor worse for the baby than wine or beer?"

A: They're all considered the same risk. A can of beer, a glass of wine, and a mixed drink with one ounce of hard liquor contain roughly the same amounts of alcohol.

Q: "My doctor suggested I have a glass of wine on the evening after my amniocentesis. Is this okay?"

A: While the party line is that avoiding alcohol entirely is best, occasional use is probably okay, especially under these circumstances. Alcohol is a *tocolytic,* which basically means that it relaxes the uterus. After amniocentesis, many women feel a little uterine cramping. The alcohol in a glass of wine minimizes that discomfort without hurting the baby.

Using recreational/illicit drugs

Many studies have evaluated the effects of drug use during pregnancy. But the studies can be confusing because they tend to lump all kinds of drug users together, regardless of which drugs they use and how much they use. The mother's lifestyle also influences the degree of risk to the baby, which complicates the information even more. For example, women who abuse drugs are more likely to be malnourished than other women, they are typically of lower socioeconomic status, and they suffer a higher incidence of sexually transmitted diseases. All these factors, independent of and added to drug use, can cause problems for your pregnancy and for your baby.

Looking at Lifestyle Changes

Your lifestyle inevitably changes during your pregnancy. You may wonder whether it's still okay to do some of the things you may have done on a regular basis before you were pregnant. This section provides information on activities such as whether you can safely color your hair while you're pregnant, whether you can use saunas and hot tubs, whether you can travel, and whether you can continue working.

Pampering yourself with beauty treatments

When your friends and relatives hear that you're pregnant, they'll probably tell you how beautiful you look or what a lovely maternal glow you have. And you may feel more beautiful, too, although some women feel the exact opposite. You may find that you're not happy with the physical changes that are happening to your body. Either way, if you're like most of our patients, you may wonder whether your customary beauty habits are safe to follow during pregnancy. In this section, we go over them one by one and let you know about any possible risks:

   ✔ **Botox:** The safety of Botox therapy during pregnancy and breast-feeding is controversial and the data limited. In one study involving 16 pregnant women injected mostly in the first trimester, there were no reported birth defects. One patient suffered a miscarriage, although she had a miscarriage in a prior pregnancy. A few other studies with small numbers showed no untoward effects. Our advice? Enjoy the beauty from your pregnancy glow while you're pregnant, and wait until after you deliver for the Botox. On the other hand, if there is a medical indication for Botox (severe migraines, severe cervical dystonia), it may be a reasonable option. Talk to your practitioner about it.

✔ **Injectable fillers:** Injectable skin fillers are used to smooth wrinkles and make lips fuller. Often they're made with collagen or hyaluronic acid. No good data currently exists documenting the safety of fillers during pregnancy, so at this time they are probably best avoided until safety data is available. The good news is that the fluid retention of pregnancy may lessen the wrinkles anyway!

✔ **Chemical peels:** Alpha-hydroxy acids are the main ingredients in chemical peels. The chemicals work topically, but small amounts are absorbed into your system. We haven't found any data on whether chemical peels are safe during pregnancy. They're probably okay, but first discuss it with your practitioner.

✔ **Facials:** You may notice that your complexion has changed over the past few months. Sometimes pregnancy hormones can wreak havoc on your skin. Facials may or may not help. But go ahead and have one anyway, if only to enjoy the time to sit back and relax! (See the preceding comments about chemical peels.)

✔ **Hair dyes:** Many different types of chemicals are used in hair dyes, and manufacturers typically change their formulas frequently. Limited data is available on the safety of hair dye, because these chemicals are not usually studied during pregnancy. However, remember that only a fraction of any hair treatment chemicals get absorbed into a woman's body through her skin, and this small amount is probably not enough to cause a problem for the developing baby. In addition, there is absolutely no evidence that suggests that hair dyes cause birth defects or miscarriage. Semi-permanent dyes or highlights are even less controversial. With highlights, foil surrounds the strands of hair coated with the formula so even less absorption through the skin occurs. Because of the limited hard-core scientific data available, your practitioner may tell you to stick to vegetable hair dyes during pregnancy, while your friend's practitioner may tell her that dyeing her hair is fine.

- ✔ **Standard chemical straightening treatments:** There are several standard chemical treatments available to women who wish to have silky-straight locks. Such standard treatments usually include chemicals such as lye (containing sodium hydroxide), no lye (containing calcium hydroxide and guanidine carbonate), and thio (with thioglycolic acid salts). Although the data is limited, it seems to show that these treatments are generally safe in pregnancy. One study showed no increase of preterm birth or low birth weight, but did not look at risks of birth defects. Therefore, it may be best to use after the first trimester.

- ✔ **Brazilian hair treatments:** Brazilian or Brazilian Keratin treatments are a popular method for straightening and smoothing the hair. Most of these treatments contain a chemical called formaldehyde, which can be absorbed through the skin or by breathing it in. Formaldehyde was used many years ago in hair dyes and was found to be carcinogenic (causing childhood cancers). Therefore, we suggest embracing your curls and avoiding these products, or sticking to blow-drying or flat irons for that super-straight look in pregnancy.

- ✔ **Hair waxing:** Waxing legs or the bikini line involves applying a heated wax preparation topically and then removing it along with the hair. Nothing in the wax preparations can lead to problems for the baby. So if you like, keep waxing away while you're pregnant to help you remain carefree and hair-free.

- ✔ **Laser hair removal:** The laser used for hair removal works by transmitting heat to the hair follicle and stopping hair regrowth. Often anesthetic creams are applied to the skin first to reduce pain. Although we couldn't find specific data on laser hair removal during pregnancy, we know of no reason that this therapy, which is applied locally, should cause any problem to the baby.

- ✔ **Manicures and pedicures:** Another frequently asked question is: "Can I have a manicure/pedicure or have nail tips or acrylic nails placed while I'm pregnant?" Again, the answer is yes. Common sense suggests that you go to a reputable salon where the equipment is properly cleaned and the area is well ventilated.

✔ **Massages:** Massages are fine, and you'll find that many massage therapists offer special pregnancy massages aimed at accommodating your pregnant belly. Some use special tables with the center cut out so that you can comfortably lie facedown, especially in the latter part of the pregnancy.

✔ **Permanents:** No scientific evidence suggests that the chemicals in hair permanents are harmful to the developing baby. These preparations usually do contain significant amounts of ammonia, however, so for your own safety, use them in well-ventilated areas.

✔ **Thermal reconditioning:** Thermal reconditioning, also known as the Japanese straightening technique, is a fairly new method to permanently straighten hair. The process involves applying a variety of chemicals and conditioners to the hair, and then using a flat iron to permanently straighten it. No scientific research has studied this technique in pregnancy. Some of the chemicals used are similar to those used for perming hair. The bottom line: Thermal reconditioning is likely okay during pregnancy, but we know of no definitive data. If you want to play it as safe as possible, we would avoid this treatment.

✔ **Wrinkle creams:** The two most common antiwrinkle creams used today are Retin-A and Renova. Both of these preparations contain vitamin A derivatives. Substantial data exists to suggest that oral medications containing vitamin A derivatives (for example, Accutane) can cause birth defects, but the information that's available on topical preparations such as Retin-A and Renova doesn't indicate a problem. Due to the significant effects of oral preparations, however, many practitioners discourage the use of any medications containing these compounds, oral or topical, to their patients.

Relaxing in hot tubs, whirlpools, saunas, or steam rooms

Using hot tubs, whirlpools, saunas, or steam rooms when you're pregnant can be risky because of the high temperatures involved. In laboratory animals, exposure to high levels of heat during pregnancy has been known to cause birth defects or miscarriage. Studies involving humans suggest that pregnant women whose core body temperatures rise significantly during the early weeks of pregnancy may stand an increased risk of miscarriage or having babies with neural tube defects (spina bifida, for example).

However, problems typically occur only if the mother's core temperature rises above 102 degrees Fahrenheit (or about 39 degrees Celsius) for more than ten minutes during the first seven weeks of her pregnancy.

A lot of women ask about just taking a nice relaxing warm bath. In general, soaking in a warm, soothing bath is fine during pregnancy. Just make sure that the water temperature isn't too high, for the reasons just mentioned.

Common sense suggests that after the first trimester, occasionally using hot tubs, saunas, and steam rooms for less than ten minutes is probably okay. However, remember to drink plenty of fluids to avoid dehydration. Later in the pregnancy, hot tubs and saunas are fine but we would suggest limiting to about 10 minutes.

Traveling

The main potential problem with traveling during pregnancy is that it puts distance between you and your prenatal care provider. If you're close to your due date or if your pregnancy is considered high-risk, you probably shouldn't travel far from home. Your decision to travel, though, depends on what the risk factors actually are. If you have diabetes but it's well controlled, going on a trip is probably okay. But if you're pregnant with triplets, traveling to Timbuktu probably isn't a good idea. If your pregnancy is uncomplicated, travel during the first, second, and early third trimesters is usually okay.

Traveling by car poses no special risk, aside from requiring that you sit in one place for a long time. On long trips, stop every couple of hours to get out and walk around a bit. Wear your seat belt and shoulder strap; they keep you safe, and they won't hurt the baby, even if you're in an accident. The amniotic fluid surrounding the fetus serves as a cushion against any constriction from the lap belt. Not wearing restraints clearly poses a greater risk; studies show that the leading cause of fetal death in auto accidents is death of the mother.

Wear your seat belt below your abdomen, not above it, and keep the shoulder strap in its usual position.

Most airlines allow women to fly if they're less than 36 weeks pregnant, but you may want to carry a note from your practitioner indicating that she sees no medical reason why you shouldn't fly. Flying is perfectly safe, especially if you take a couple of precautions:

- ✔ **Get up from your seat occasionally during longer flights and walk around the plane.** Prolonged periods of sitting can cause blood to pool in your legs. Walking around keeps your circulation going.

- ✔ **Carry a water bottle with you and drink water frequently.** Airplane air is always very dry. (A pilot once told us that the relative humidity in airplanes is typically lower than in the Sahara desert. Planes can't carry enough water to keep the humidity up, because the extra water would add too much cargo weight.) Because airplane air is so dry, you can easily become dehydrated during long flights.

  Drinking extra water also ensures that you get up frequently to go to the restroom, which keeps the blood from pooling in your legs.

You don't need to worry about airport metal detectors — or any other metal detectors — because they don't use ionizing radiation. (The conveyor belt that carries your luggage after you check it in does use ionizing radiation, however, so we don't recommend that you climb onto the counter and send yourself through that machine.)

If you're prone to air sickness and have found Dramamine helpful in the past, using it in normal doses while you're pregnant is okay.

If you plan to visit tropical countries, where some diseases are particularly prevalent, you may want to be vaccinated before you go. But check with your doctor to see whether any vaccines you're considering are safe to have during pregnancy. (For more information on vaccines, see Chapter 1.)

Getting dental care

Most people see their dentist for routine cleanings every 6 to 12 months, which means you'll probably need to visit your dentist at least once during your pregnancy. Pregnancy itself shouldn't affect your dental health. You don't want to avoid the dentist because neglected cavities can become infected, which is all the more reason to see your dentist when you're pregnant. Some recent studies have shown that pregnant women who suffer from *periodontal disease,* which is infection and inflammation of the gums, are at a higher risk for delivering small or premature babies. This finding is one more reason for making good oral hygiene a priority.

Pregnancy causes an increase in blood flow to the gums. In fact, about half of all pregnant women develop a condition called *pregnancy gingivitis,* which is simply a reddening of the gums caused by this increased blood flow. In this condition, gums have a tendency to bleed easily, so try to be gentle when you brush and floss your teeth.

For those of you who want whiter and brighter teeth, plenty of products are available, including whitening toothpastes and over-the-counter gels, strips, whitening systems, and trays. Although most are frequently used during pregnancy, no large studies document the safety of such treatments. Whitening toothpastes help remove surface stains without using bleach. There is no reason to think they are a problem. Over-the-counter whitening strips, gels, and whitening systems are peroxide-based and haven't been specifically studied in pregnancy. However, the safety of peroxide can be implied from other studies. In one such study, pregnant rats were fed up to 10 percent hydrogen peroxide in their diet and no problems were detected in their offspring. Similarly, when tested as a component in hair dyes, peroxide wasn't found to cause birth defects. With in-office bleaching, the technician applies the whitening product to the teeth and uses heat and/or a laser to quicken the process. Many dentists don't perform these procedures on pregnant women because they haven't been well-studied. On the bright side, seeing your dentist for cleaning not only promotes good hygiene, but also removes surface stains and leaves you with a brighter smile.

If you need routine dental work — cavities filled, teeth pulled, crowns placed — don't worry. Local anesthesia and most pain medications are safe to use during pregnancy. Some dentists also recommend antibiotics during dental procedures, most of which are also safe during pregnancy, but you should check with your prenatal care provider to make sure. Even dental X-rays pose no significant problem for the fetus, as long as a lead "apron" or shield is placed over the abdomen.

Having sex

For most couples, having sex during pregnancy is perfectly safe. In fact, some couples find that sex during pregnancy is even better than before. However, you may have some issues to consider.

In the first half of pregnancy, sex can usually continue as before because your body hasn't changed that noticeably. You may notice that your breasts are particularly sensitive to the touch, or even tender. Later, as the uterus grows, some sexual positions become more difficult. You and your partner may find that you have to be a little creative to make things work. If you find that intercourse is too uncomfortable, other forms of sexual gratification may work better for you and your partner.

Many women ask us whether having sex at the end of pregnancy is okay, even if the cervix is a little bit dilated. Having sex then is perfectly fine as long as your membranes haven't ruptured (your water hasn't broken).

Avoid intercourse if you're at a high risk for preterm labor (for example, you have been treated for preterm labor or have a cerclage in place) or if you have placenta previa (see Chapter 16) in the third trimester, or have recent bleeding. Most practitioners suggest refraining from intercourse for two reasons:

- ✔ Intercourse has the potential to introduce an infection into the uterus.

- ✔ Semen contains substances that are known to make the uterus contract.

Another important aspect to consider is how each of you feels psychologically about having sex during pregnancy. Like some women, you may find that your libido or sex drive has increased. Often, you may find that you have vivid sexual dreams and that orgasm itself is heightened. On the other hand, you may find that your interest in sex is less than it was before you got pregnant. You may feel less attractive because of the physical changes that have taken place, which is perfectly normal. Your partner may also experience changes in his desire for sex because of the excitement and normal apprehension that go along with being a father, and due to (unfounded) fears that intercourse will hurt the baby or that the baby will somehow know what Mom and Dad are up to.

Working during Pregnancy: A Different Type of Labor

Over the last half-century, the number of women who work outside the home has steadily increased. More than 75 percent of pregnant women work during the third trimester, and more than half work up to a few weeks of delivery. Many women find that working until the end of pregnancy keeps them happy and occupied and helps them not to focus on the discomforts. In addition, many women don't have a choice — they may be the main income providers for their families and their careers are top priority. Although most of the time working throughout pregnancy doesn't cause any problems for the baby, there can be some exceptions.

Stress in pregnancy, whether related to work or to home situations, isn't well-studied. Some doctors believe that very high levels of stress may increase the risk of developing pre-eclampsia or preterm labor, although no study has confirmed this risk (both of which we discuss in Chapter 14). Unusual stress may increase your risk of post-partum depression. Too much stress obviously isn't good for anyone. Do whatever you can to decrease the stress in your life and talk with your practitioner if you find you're becoming persistently blue or anxious.

Considering occupational hazards

Maybe your job requires minimal standing or walking, allows you to work regular hours, and never stresses you out. If that's the case, and if you have no previous medical problems, you can skip this section (and let us know what your job is!). But if you're like the rest of us, read on.

Occupations that are physically demanding can be problematic. Most jobs fall somewhere in between sedentary and demanding, but even then the amount of stress varies according to the individual. If your pregnancy proceeds without complications, you probably can continue to work right up until delivery. However, some complications that may arise during pregnancy may make reducing your workload or stopping work altogether advisable. For example, if you develop preterm labor, your practitioner will most likely advise you to stop working. Other conditions that may warrant a reduction in physical activity are hypertension or problems with the baby's growth.

If you work at a computer terminal, you may wonder whether you're being exposed to anything harmful. But you have no need to worry — no evidence suggests that the electromagnetic fields that computer terminals emit are a problem.

Some studies suggest that women who have jobs associated with physically demanding responsibilities, such as heavy lifting, manual labor, or significant physical exertion, may be at a slightly higher risk of preterm birth, high blood pressure, preeclampsia, or small-for-gestational-age babies. On the other hand, long working hours haven't been found to increase the chances for premature delivery. Other studies have also shown that jobs in which prolonged standing is required (more than eight hours a day) were associated with a greater chance for back and foot pain, circulatory problems, and a slightly increased risk of preterm birth. The good news: The use of support hose, although not particularly attractive, is helpful in decreasing varicose veins.

Remember that your health and your baby's health are the highest priority. Don't feel you're a wimp because you have to attend to your pregnancy. Some women believe that if they complain about certain symptoms or take time out from a busy schedule to eat or go to the restroom, they will garner

the disapproval of their superiors at work. Don't let yourself feel guilty about your special needs during this time, and don't let work cause you to ignore any unusual symptoms. If you need time off to deal with complications, take it, and don't feel bad about it. People who have never been pregnant don't completely understand the physical strains you're dealing with.

Understanding pregnancy and the law

Take the time to understand your rights as they pertain to pregnancy. In the United States, an amendment to Title VII of the Civil Rights Act of 1964, called The Pregnancy Discrimination Act, requires pregnant women to be treated in a manner equal to all employees or applicants. According to this act, employers can't refuse to hire a woman because of her pregnancy-related condition, as long as she's capable of performing the job's major functions. If an employee is temporarily unable to carry out her job due to the pregnancy, the employer must treat her the same as any other temporarily disabled employee, taking such actions as providing alternative tasks, disability leave, or leave without pay. A disability may arise due to the pregnancy itself, such as significant nausea and vomiting. A disability may also occur due to complications of pregnancy, such as bleeding, preterm labor, or high blood pressure, or may occur due to hazardous job exposures. If your healthcare provider decides that your pregnancy is disabling, you can ask that she send a letter to your employer, verifying your disability.

In the U.S., most maternity leaves are from 6-8 weeks, although you are entitled to a 12-week leave in a one-year period under the Family and Medical Leave Act, although this may not be a paid leave.

Health insurance provided by an employer should cover expenses for pregnancy-related conditions in a way that's similar to its coverage of other medical conditions, as long as obstetric services are covered. Health insurers are prohibited by law from considering pregnancy a preexisting condition, which means you cannot be denied coverage when you go from one job to another and switch health plans.

Chapter 4

Diet and Exercise for the Expectant Mother

● ●

In This Chapter

▶ Understanding healthy weight gain — yours and your baby's

▶ Optimizing your diet

▶ Taking food safety into account

▶ Staying fit during pregnancy

● ●

*T*hrough the ages, women have received all kinds of advice about what, and how much, to eat while they're expecting. Cultural traditions, religious beliefs, and scientific thinking have all had their influence. As recently as a generation ago, women were told to limit how much they ate and drank and thus keep their weight gain to a minimum. At other times, they were encouraged to eat lots of fatty foods — the notion being that the greater the weight gain, the healthier the child. These days, your practitioner's advice is likely to depend on your particular health habits and your size when your pregnancy begins. Also, if you're carrying more than one baby, you're expected to gain more than the average number of pounds.

Of course, health involves more than just eating well. Exercise is as important while you're pregnant as it was before, although what and how much you do to stay fit may change as your pregnancy progresses. This chapter provides you with the information you need in order to properly nourish yourself and your baby and to keep exercising safely.

Looking at Healthy Weight Gain

Starting pregnancy at a healthy weight and gaining weight at a moderate pace throughout pregnancy can help ensure that your baby grows and develops normally, and that you stay healthy as well. So what is healthy? This section explains in more depth the weight issues associated with pregnancy.

Determining how much is enough

The best way to figure out your ideal weight — and weight gain — is to look at a measurement that's known as *body mass index (BMI)*, a number that takes into account both height and weight.

Find your body mass index by looking up your measurements on the chart in Figure 4-1. Locate your weight on the vertical line on the left-hand side of the chart and your height on the horizontal (bottom) line. (Alternatively, use the metric measurements on the right-hand and top sides.) Find the place where those two points intersect on the chart, and then follow the diagonal line closest to that point to find your BMI.

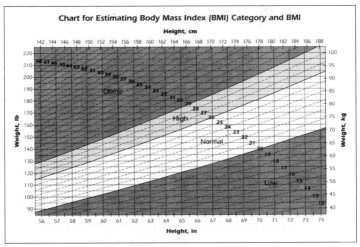

Source: Nutrition During Pregnancy and Lactation, The National Academies Press, 1992

Figure 4-1: The body mass index chart.

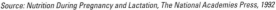

After you know your body mass index, you can figure out your ideal weight gain during pregnancy by consulting Table 4-1. (But don't forget, this number refers to women carrying only one baby!)

Table 4-1   Figuring Out Your Ideal Weight Gain

Body Mass Index	Recommended Weight Gain
Less than 19.8 (underweight)	28 to 40 pounds (12.5 to 18 kilograms)
19.9 to 26 (normal weight)	25 to 35 pounds (11.5 to 16 kilograms)
26 to 29 (overweight)	15 to 25 pounds (7 to 11.5 kilograms)
29 or more (obese)	15 pounds (6 kilograms) or less

These numbers refer to total weight gain during the entire pregnancy, so you won't know whether you've hit the target until delivery day. Scientific research hasn't determined the optimal pattern of weight gain throughout pregnancy. Gaining very little weight early on (when you may be in the throes of morning sickness) may have less effect on fetal growth than poor weight gain in the late second or third trimester. Some women gain weight inconsistently, putting on a large number of pounds early and then much less later on. Nothing is necessarily unhealthy about this pattern, either.

Avoiding weight obsession

For the most part, use the charts of optimal weight gain as a guide, but don't become fanatical about how much you weigh. Even if the amount you gain is somewhat off course, if your doctor says that the baby is growing normally, you have nothing to worry about. Women who gain more than average can still have healthy babies, and so can women who gain very little.

If your weight gain is way too high or way too low, your doctor can check the baby's growth by measuring the fundal height (see Chapter 3) or schedule you for a sonogram. If you deviate significantly from the recommended weight gain, your doctor will probably want to evaluate your diet. He may refer you to a nutritionist or dietitian who can give you specific advice about what and how much to eat.

Where does the weight go?

The good news is that the weight you gain during pregnancy doesn't all go to your thighs. Then again, it doesn't all go to the baby, either. A pregnant woman typically adds a little to her own body fat. It's a myth, however, that you can tell by a woman's pattern of weight gain — more in the hips or more in the belly — whether she's going to have a boy or a girl. (See Chapter 2 for some other myths regarding determining your baby's sex.)

Look at this realistic view of your weight gain — assuming it's 27 pounds, which is fairly average:

Baby	7 pounds (3,180 grams)
Placenta	1 pound (455 grams)
Amniotic fluid	2 pounds (910 grams)
Uterus	2 pounds (910 grams)
Breasts	1 pound (455 grams)
Fat stores	7 pounds (3,180 grams)
Body water	4 pounds (1,820 grams)
Extra blood	3 pounds (1,360 grams)

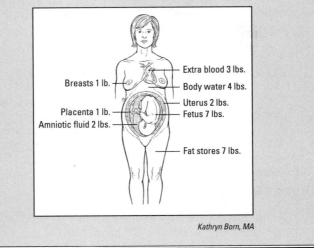

Kathryn Born, MA

 The bottom line is that you want to do all you can to improve your baby's chances of optimal growth and development, but not at the expense of driving yourself crazy.

Understanding your baby's weight gain

Although your weight gain may follow a path all its own, your baby's own bulking-up pattern is likely to progress slowly at first, and then pick up at about 32 weeks, only to slow again in the last weeks before birth. At 14 to 15 weeks, for example, the baby puts on weight at about 0.18 ounce (5 grams) per day, and at 32 to 34 weeks, 1.06 to 1.23 ounces (30 to 35 grams) per day (that's about half a pound or 0.23 kilograms each week). After 36 weeks, the fetal growth rate slows to about a quarter of a pound per week, and by 41 to 42 weeks (you're overdue at this point), minimal or no further fetal growth may occur. Check out Chapter 7 for more about how your baby grows.

In addition to your diet and weight gain, the following factors affect fetal growth:

- ✔ **Cigarette smoking:** Smoking can reduce the birth weight by about half a pound (about 200 grams).

- ✔ **Diabetes:** If the mother is diabetic, the baby can be too big or too small.

- ✔ **Genetic or family history:** In other words, basketball players usually don't have children who grow up to be professional jockeys!

- ✔ **Fetal infection:** Some infections affect growth, although others don't.

- ✔ **Illicit drug use:** Drug abuse can slow fetal growth.

- ✔ **Mother's medical history:** Some medical problems, like hypertension or lupus, can affect fetal growth.

- ✔ **Multiple pregnancy:** Twins and triplets are often smaller than single babies.

- ✔ **Placental function:** Placental blood flow that's below par can slow down the baby's growth.

Your practitioner keeps an eye on your baby's growth rate, most often by measuring fundal height and paying attention to your weight gain. If you put on too little or too much weight, if your fundal height measurements are abnormal, or if something in your history puts you at risk for growth problems, your doctor is likely to send you for an ultrasound exam to more accurately assess the situation.

Taking Stock of What You're Taking In

Sticking to a well-balanced, low-fat, high-fiber diet is important not only for your baby but also for your own health. Consuming adequate protein is also important because protein carries out many of the body's functions. The fiber in your diet helps to prevent or reduce constipation and hemorrhoids. By not consuming too much fat, you help keep your heart healthy and avoid putting on extra pounds that may be difficult to shed. Avoiding excessive weight gain also decreases your chances of developing stretch marks. To read more about stretch marks, see Chapter 7.

If your diet is balanced and not too heavy in sugar or fat, you don't need to modify the way you eat dramatically. During pregnancy, you should take in roughly 300 *extra* calories a day, on average. That means that if you're at a healthy weight and you're taking in 2,100 calories per day, while pregnant you should take in an average of 2,400 calories per day (perhaps a little less during your first trimester and a little more during your third trimester).

You should *not* increase your caloric intake by eating a hot fudge sundae every day. Filling these additional requirements with nutritious foods is key. Your practitioner will likely advise you to take some supplemental vitamins and minerals, too. Keep reading to find out which foods and supplements are best for you.

Using the USDA Choose My Plate

No single food can satisfy all your nutritional needs. The USDA Choose My Plate, shown in Figure 4-2, is a general guideline that illustrates the relative proportions of servings you should eat in each group. To get some specific recommendations tailored for your pre-pregnancy weight and activity level, go to http://www.choosemyplate.gov/pregnancy-breastfeeding/pregnancy-nutritional-needs.html and create a profile to receive a personalized "Daily Food Plan."

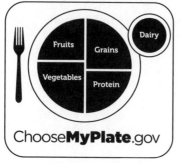

United States Department of Agriculture

Figure 4-2: Use the USDA MyPlate guide to help you eat healthily during pregnancy.

The Choose My Plate (formerly known as the food pyramid) includes the following food groups:

✔ **Grains:** While there are many different types of grains that are healthy to eat, the Choose My Plate refers to fortified dry and cooked cereals. Choose ones that are fortified with folic acid when possible. Other grains such as

✔ **Vegetables:** Vegetables are divided into five groups, based on their nutrient content. The following list orders them from highest nutrient content (dark green vegetables) to lowest (other vegetables), and includes examples within each category:

- **Dark green vegetables:** Spinach, dark green leafy lettuce, romaine lettuce, broccoli, kale, turnip greens, watercress

- **Orange vegetables:** Carrots; pumpkin; sweet potatoes; acorn, butternut, and Hubbard squash

- **Dry beans/peas:** Pinto, black, garbanzo, kidney, navy, soy, and white beans; split peas; lentils; tofu

- **Starchy vegetables:** Potatoes, corn, green peas, green lima beans

- **Other vegetables:** Cabbage, cauliflower, iceberg lettuce, green beans, celery, green and red peppers, mushrooms, onions, tomatoes, asparagus, cucumbers, eggplant

Pregnant women should try to fill half of their plate with fruits or vegetables. Any of the above vegetables or pure

vegetable juice counts toward this goal, but dark green or orange vegetables and dried beans are best because their nutrient content is higher. Eating a variety of different vegetables is also important, though.

✔ **Fruits:** A variety of fruits is an important part of your diet while you are pregnant. Fruits are not only a good source of vitamins and minerals, but they also provide fiber, which is very important during pregnancy to help reduce constipation. Fruits contain healthy amounts of vitamins A and C, as well as potassium.

You can choose fresh, frozen, canned, or dried fruits. Go easy on the fruit juices, though, because they can contain lots of extra sugar.

✔ **Dairy:** Foods that fall in this group include milk, yogurt, and cheese, and all are great sources of calcium. It's best to focus on low-fat or fat-free milk products whenever possible. An average-sized woman needs to consume about three cups of milk or milk products per day.

✔ **Protein:** Meat, poultry, fish, dry beans, and nuts fall into this category. You should focus on low-fat and lean foods in this category and vary your choices. Baking, broiling, and grilling are the healthiest ways to cook meat, poultry, and fish. During pregnancy, you should eat five to seven ounces of food from this category daily.

Considering oils and fats

Oils are fats that remain liquid at room temperature, like vegetable oil, olive oil, and corn oil. These fats are mostly unsaturated and are the healthiest type of fats to eat. Foods like nuts, avocados, fish, and olives are naturally high in unsaturated fats. Solid fats are fats that are solid at room temperature, like butter, shortening, lard, and margarine. These foods are high in saturated fats.

Trans fats are a type of saturated fats that are common in processed foods and have been associated with obesity and heart disease.

Ideally, fewer than 20 to 35 percent of your total calories should come from fats, with fewer than 10 percent coming from saturated fats. Avoid trans fats altogether.

Experiencing morning sickness during the first trimester is very common (see Chapter 5). If you're experiencing this nausea and can't eat a well-balanced diet, you may wonder whether you're getting enough nutrition for you and the baby. You actually can go for several weeks not eating an optimal diet without any ill effects on the baby. You may find that the only foods you can tolerate are foods heavy in starch or carbohydrates. If all you feel like eating are potatoes, bread, and pasta, go right ahead. Keeping something down is better than starving.

As your pregnancy progresses, your body needs a lot of extra fluid. Early on, some women who don't drink enough liquid feel weak or faint. Later in pregnancy, dehydration can lead to premature contractions. Make a point of drinking plenty of water (or milk) — about six to eight glasses a day, and a bit more if you are carrying more than one baby.

Is caffeine safe during pregnancy?

Although some women think that the only food that contains caffeine is a strong cup of coffee, in fact, you can find caffeine in many of the other things you eat and drink on a daily basis: tea, many sodas, cocoa, and chocolate. No evidence suggests that caffeine causes birth defects. However, if you consume caffeine in large amounts, it may raise the risk of miscarriage.

Most studies suggest that it takes more than 200 milligrams (mg) of caffeine a day to affect the fetus. The average cup of coffee (remember, this is an 8-ounce cup of regular coffee — not the super-mega size or an espresso or cappuccino!) has between 100 and 150 mg of caffeine. Caffeinated tea has slightly less caffeine — about 50 to 100 mg — and soft drinks have approximately 36 mg per 12-ounce serving. So drinking one 8-ounce cup of coffee (or the equivalent caffeine content in other foods or beverages) per day is usually okay during pregnancy. A lot of women ask about the caffeine content in chocolate — your sweet tooth will be happy to know that an average-sized chocolate bar or cup of hot cocoa has only about 6 mg of caffeine.

Remember, too, that consuming caffeine often increases the already frequent trips to the bathroom. If you're already bothered by frequent urination, you may want to cut your caffeine intake further. Also, you may find that, especially in the last trimester, getting a full night's rest is almost impossible because you can't find a comfortable sleeping position and, even if you do, you have to get up several times to go to the bathroom. Drinking coffee or tea at bedtime may only aggravate your inability to get some rest!

Supplementing your diet

If your diet is healthy and balanced, you get most of the vitamins and minerals you need naturally — with the exception of iron, folic acid, and calcium. To make sure you get enough of these nutrients and to guard against inadequate eating habits, your practitioner is likely to recommend prenatal vitamins. In the case of vitamins, more isn't necessarily better; take only the prescribed number of pills each day. Several different prenatal vitamins are available, and they are generally equivalent. Some are better tolerated than others, so if you find the one you're taking is not agreeable to you, try a different brand. Also, many now contain omega-3 fatty acid supplementation. Some data suggests that omega-3 supplements may decrease the risk of preterm delivery and may have a beneficial effect on the newborn brain, but this hasn't been proven with certainty.

If you miss taking a vitamin, don't worry. Nothing bad is going to happen. During the early months, if your vitamins make you nauseous, skipping them until you feel better is perfectly safe for the baby. Remember that the baby is still very small, without large nutritional requirements. If you're very early in your pregnancy (four to seven weeks), you can take just a folic acid supplement, which is sometimes easier to tolerate, until you can handle the complete prenatal vitamin pill. If later on in the pregnancy you get a stomach virus and can't tolerate vitamins for some time, that's not a problem, either. The growing baby is able to get what it needs, even at the expense of the mom (a theme that continues throughout life!).

If you find that the vitamins really make you nauseous, try eating a few crackers before you take them, or take them at bedtime.

Iron

You need more iron when you're expecting because both you and the baby are making new red blood cells every day. On average, you need 30 milligrams (mg) of extra iron every day of your pregnancy, which is what most prenatal vitamins contain. Blood counts can easily drop during pregnancy because your body gradually is making more and more blood *plasma* (fluid) and relatively fewer red blood cells (a condition that is called a *dilutional anemia*). If you do develop anemia, you may need to take an extra iron supplement.

Foods rich in iron include chicken, fish, red meat, green leafy vegetables, and enriched or whole-grain breads and cereals. You can raise the iron content of foods by cooking them in cast-iron pots and skillets.

Calcium and vitamin D

You need about 1,200 milligrams of calcium and 2,000 units of vitamin D every day while you're pregnant. (The U.S. Recommended Daily Allowance [USRDA] of calcium for *all* women is about 1,000 mg.) Most women actually get much less. If you're already starting out somewhat deficient in calcium and vitamin D, the calcium requirements of the developing baby will only make matters worse for you. A fetus can extract enough calcium from its mother, even if it means getting it at the expense of the mother's bones. So the extra calcium and vitamin D needed during pregnancy are really aimed at protecting you and your health. The vitamin D helps you store the calcium.

Prenatal vitamins contain only about 200 to 300 mg of calcium (about one-quarter of the USRDA), so you need to get calcium from other sources as well.

Getting enough calcium from your diet alone is possible if you really pay attention. You can get it from three to four servings of calcium-rich foods, such as milk, yogurt, cheese, green leafy vegetables, and canned fish with bones (if your stomach can take it). Supermarkets also stock special lactose-free foods that are high in calcium. The following list indicates portions of foods that qualify as one serving (300 mg of calcium):

✔ **1 8-ounce glass of milk**

  Choose low-fat or skim milk.

✔ **4 ounces of cooked broccoli**

✔ **4 to 5 ounces of canned salmon with bones**

✔ **1½ to 2 ounces of cheese**

  Cottage cheese has less calcium than many other cheeses.

✔ **8 ounces of yogurt**

If your diet is low in calcium, take a supplement. Tums and some other antacids contain quite a bit of calcium and, at the same time, help relieve any pregnancy heartburn you may have. (A single Tums tablet has the equivalent calcium content of an 8-ounce glass of milk.)

Determining Which Foods Are Safe

When our patients ask us about nutrition and which foods they may want to avoid, certain items come up again and again. Some of the foods we're most often asked about should be avoided, and others are unlikely to cause harm. This section identifies the potentially harmful foods and also debunks some common myths about other foods.

Eyeing potentially harmful foods

If you're healthy, you can probably confidently eat most of the foods you usually eat. Nonetheless, the following list contains some potential dangers that we feel we ought to mention:

- **Cheeses from unpasteurized or raw milk:** Cheeses made from unpasteurized or raw milk may contain certain bacteria, such as listeria, monocytogenes, salmonella, and E. coli. Listeria, in particular, has been linked to certain pregnancy complications, such as premature labor or even miscarriage. The FDA mandates that all cheeses sold in the United States be either made from pasteurized milk or aged more than 60 days (which makes the likelihood of listeria extremely low), so most cheeses you buy at your local market are safe. Just check the label to be sure. (For more on listeria, see the sidebar "Clarifying listeria," later in this chapter.)

- **Raw or very rare meat:** Steak tartare or very rare beef or pork may contain bacteria, such as listeria, or parasites, such as toxoplasma. Adequate cooking kills both bacteria and parasites. In other words, you want your food to be cooked medium-well to well done.

- **Liver:** Because it contains extremely high amounts of vitamin A (more than ten times the amount recommended for a pregnant woman), liver consumed in early pregnancy may hypothetically be linked to birth defects. Consuming more than 10,000 international units (IUs) of vitamin A daily (the recommended daily allowance for pregnant women is 2,500 IU) was linked to birth defects in one study. Scientists haven't proven this danger unequivocally, but you may want to find a substitute for that liver-and-onions craving in the first trimester. And check out

the label on your prenatal vitamins to make sure you're not getting too much vitamin A.

Debunking popular food myths

Many of the foods that have at one time or another been thought dangerous for pregnant women aren't likely to harm you or your baby. Although you don't have to avoid the following foods, they should be eaten in moderation, especially those that are manufactured (as opposed to natural) products:

- **Aspartame (Equal or NutraSweet):** Aspartame (a common component of low-calorie foods and beverages) is a type of amino acid, and the body is accustomed to amino acids because they're what all proteins are made of. No medical evidence shows that aspartame causes any problems for the growing baby.

- **Sucralose (Splenda):** Sucralose is a low-calorie sweetener, with less than 2 calories per teaspoon. It is actually a type of sugar, but it's much more potent than regular table sugar, so you only need small amounts to sweeten things up (and therefore you get fewer calories). Because it's a type of sugar, it should have no harmful effects on your developing baby.

- **Stevia leaf extract sweeteners (Truvia or Stevia):** The most recent additions to non-sugar based sweeteners are derived from the stevia leaf. While the data is somewhat limited, they appear to be completely safe to use in pregnancy.

- **Cheeses:** Not only do most people believe that processed and pasteurized cheeses are safe, but these cheeses are also a great source of both protein and calcium. See the previous section, "Eyeing potentially harmful foods," for information about unpasteurized cheeses.

- **Fish:** Fish is a great source of protein and vitamins, and is also low in fat. In fact, the high levels of protein, omega-3 fatty acids, vitamin D, and other nutrients make fish an excellent food for pregnant mothers and their developing babies. However, certain fish — shark, mackerel, swordfish, and tilefish — contain high levels of mercury. The jury's still out on whether mercury may lead to certain childhood developmental delays or problems with fine motor skills (probably not), but the FDA currently recommends you avoid fish with high levels of mercury when you're pregnant.

Clarifying listeria

Listeria, which is a bacteria that may lead to premature labor and other complications, is found primarily in unpasteurized cheeses, but also is present in other foods — some pâtés, hot dogs, and deli meats, for example, as well as prepackaged salads that have been contaminated with soil that contains listeria.

Because listeria is found in so many different foods, you can't avoid eating all foods known to contain it. The good news is that the incidence of listeria infection during pregnancy is actually very uncommon (0.012 percent).

There are some guidelines you can follow to further reduce your risk, such as eating hot food immediately after heating. Foods thought to be virtually free of listeria include chocolate, marmalade, cookies, raw carrots, raw apples, and raw tomatoes. So if you really want to avoid listeria altogether, have a marmalade, raw carrot, and cookie sandwich. Seriously, if you inadvertently eat any of the foods that may contain listeria, don't panic; your actual risk of infection is still quite low, and the problem is relatively uncommon.

The USDA guidelines say you can still enjoy up to 12 ounces (two average meals) per week of fish and shellfish lower in mercury, like salmon, haddock, tilapia, cod, sole, and shrimp, or up to 6 ounces of albacore tuna per week. (The limitations are due to the fact that even fish that is low in mercury isn't mercury-free, so mercury consumption could add up to a significant amount if fish were eaten in large quantities.) Don't let your concern for mercury make you give up fish altogether, because two recent studies looking at fish consumption in pregnant women showed that women who eat fish may actually have lower rates of preterm delivery, and their children may have higher IQs than those who do not eat fish.

- **Sushi:** Raw fish (except raw shellfish) actually carries a very small risk of a parasitic infection (about one infection in two million servings), whether you're pregnant or not (this is less than the risk of getting sick from eating chicken!). Pregnancy doesn't increase the danger, and your fetus is unlikely to suffer any harm from such an infection. Most important is to make sure that the fish comes from a reliable source and that it is stored properly.

• **Smoked meats or fish:** Many pregnant women worry about eating smoked meats and fish because they've heard that these foods are high in nitrites or nitrates. Although these foods do contain these substances, they won't hurt your baby if eaten in moderation.

Considering Special Dietary Needs

Try as you may to follow all the rules of healthy nutrition, you may encounter certain problems with digestion, such as constipation or heartburn. Or you may find that you need to tailor the rules to fit your particular eating habits — for example, if you're a vegetarian. In this section, we address some of the issues that arise for women with special nutritional needs and for all women who may experience any digestive problems.

Eating right, vegetarian-style

If you're a vegetarian, rest assured you can produce a healthy baby without eating steak. But you do have to plan your diet more carefully. Vegetables, whole grains, and legumes (peas and beans) are rich in protein, but most don't have complete proteins. (They don't contain all the essential amino acids that your body can't produce by itself.) To get all the necessary protein, you can combine various proteins; for example, whole grains with legumes or nuts, rice with kidney beans, or even peanut butter with whole-grain bread. The combination doesn't have to occur at the same meal, only on the same day, but a good rule of thumb is to try to get some protein with each meal.

If you don't eat any animal products, including milk and cheese, your diet may not provide enough of six other important nutrients: vitamin B12, calcium, riboflavin, iron, zinc, and vitamin D. Bring up the topic with your doctor. You may also want to discuss your diet with a nutritionist.

Staying healthy, vegan-style

Vegans, like vegetarians, do not consume meat, fish, or poultry, but take it even further by eliminating all animal

products from their diet. So, no milkshakes or eggs-over-easy for vegans! Because many vegans consume fewer calories and may start their pregnancy with a lower BMI, they need to pay extra attention to make sure they are getting enough calories and nutrition for themselves and their growing baby. Here are some helpful hints for those vegan preggies out there:

✔ Vitamin B12 deficiency is not unusual for vegans, so make sure you are getting enough vitamin B12, and speak with your doctor about possible supplementation.

✔ Good sources of protein can be found in soy products, beans, whole grains, lentils, and tofu.

✔ Pay attention to calcium, since calcium and vitamin D are needed for you and your baby's bones. Good sources of calcium for vegans include calcium-fortified soy milk and juice, calcium-set tofu, soybeans and soy nuts, green leafy vegetables, Chinese cabbage, kale, mustard greens, and okra. Dry cereals are a source of Vitamin D.

✔ Iron is super important during pregnancy, because your body needs to increase its blood supply for the pregnancy. You can find iron in dried beans, green leafy vegetables, and tofu.

✔ Folate is another important factor that has been shown to reduce the chance of the baby developing a condition called a neural tube defect. It's important to have enough folate on board before the pregnancy starts and especially through the first trimester. Folate can be found in enriched breads, pasta, cereals, and orange juice.

✔ DHA (docosahexaenoic acid) is great for the developing fetal brain. Many people think of DHA as occurring only in fish, but a form of DHA can also be found in flaxseed, flaxseed oil, canola oil, walnuts, and soy nuts.

Maintaining a gluten-free diet

For women with celiac disease, following a gluten-free diet is essential to maintaining good health. A gluten-free diet typically avoids foods made from gluten-containing grains such as wheat, rye, barley, and oats. Many women worry that a gluten-free diet may be problematic in pregnancy. For expectant

mothers, it's important to keep in mind that a gluten-free diet may be low in calcium, iron, fiber, zinc, B vitamins, and magnesium, and that gluten-free vitamin and mineral supplementation may be needed for adequate nutrition.

Pregnancy in general often causes constipation, and pregnant women with celiac disease may find this to be a particular issue. You can, however, find fiber in foods such as quinoa, teff, and millet. Rest assured that you can have a healthy pregnancy even if you eat gluten-free — just remember that supplementation may be key in ensuring adequate nutrition.

Combating constipation

Progesterone, a hormone that circulates freely through your body during pregnancy, can slow down your digestive system and thus cause constipation. The extra iron from your prenatal vitamin only makes matters worse. Women who are on bed rest because of pregnancy complications are at particular risk for constipation because they're so inactive.

 You can counteract constipation by drinking plenty of fluids, eating adequate fiber (in the form of fruits, vegetables, beans, bran, and other whole grains), and, if possible, getting exercise every day. Keep in mind, however, that some women experience abdominal discomfort, bloating, or gas from eating too much of foods high in fiber. You may have to use a little trial and error to see which fiber-rich foods you tolerate best. If constipation bothers you, your practitioner may recommend a stool softener.

Dealing with diabetes

If you're diabetic or if you develop diabetes during pregnancy, adjust your diet so that it includes specific quantities of proteins, fats, and carbohydrates to ensure that you maintain a normal level of blood glucose (sugar). We discuss diabetes more in Chapter 15.

Working Out for Two

The great fitness movement hasn't left pregnant women behind. You see them jogging in parks, working out in gyms,

or stretching their limbs in yoga classes. During pregnancy, exercise helps your body in many ways: It keeps your heart strong and your muscles in shape, and it relieves the basic discomforts of pregnancy — from morning sickness to constipation to achy legs and backs. The earlier in pregnancy a woman gets regular exercise, the more comfortable she is likely to feel throughout the 40 weeks. Regular exercise may even make for shorter labor.

So if you're in good health and not at risk for obstetrical or medical complications, by all means go ahead and continue with your exercise program — unless your program calls for climbing Mount Fuji, entering a professional boxing match, or some other super-strenuous activity. Go over your exercise program with your practitioner, so he knows what you're doing and so that you can ask any other questions you have.

As good as exercise is for most pregnant women, we don't advise it for everyone. If you have any of the following conditions (see Chapters 14, 15, and 16 for more details), you may be better off not working out — at least until you discuss the situation with your doctor:

✔ Bleeding

✔ Incompetent cervix

✔ Intrauterine growth restriction

✔ Low volume of amniotic fluid

✔ Placenta previa (late in pregnancy)

✔ Pregnancy-induced hypertension

✔ Premature labor or preterm rupture of the membranes

✔ Carrying triplets or more

Adapting to your body's changes

Even if you work out in moderation, remember that pregnancy causes your body to undergo real physical changes that can affect your strength, stamina, and performance. The following list details some of those changes:

✔ **Cardiovascular changes:** When you're pregnant, the amount of blood that your heart pumps through your body increases. That increase in blood volume usually

has no effect on your workout. (Some women can feel as though they hear their heartbeat in their ears because of the increased volume.) Also, if you lie flat on your back, especially after about 16 weeks of pregnancy, you may find yourself feeling dizzy or faint — or even nauseous. Known as *supine hypotension syndrome,* this dizziness sometimes happens when the enlarging uterus presses down on major blood vessels that return blood to the heart, thus decreasing the heart's output. It happens even more readily if you're carrying a multiple pregnancy and your uterus is that much heavier.

If you're doing any exercises that require you to lie on your back (or if you're accustomed to sleeping on your back), put a small pillow or foam wedge under the right side of your back or your right hip. The pillow tilts you slightly sideways and effectively lifts your uterus off the blood vessels.

✓ **Respiratory changes:** Your body is using more oxygen than usual to support the growing baby. At the same time, breathing is more work than it used to be because the enlarging uterus presses upward against the diaphragm. For some women, this difficulty makes performing aerobic exercise a little harder.

✓ **Structural changes:** As your body shape changes — bigger abdomen, larger breasts — your center of gravity shifts, which can affect your balance. You notice it especially if you dance, bicycle, ski, surf, ride horses, or do anything else (walk tightropes, maybe?) where balance is important. In addition, pregnancy hormones cause some laxness in your joints, which also can make balance more difficult and may increase your risk of injury.

✓ **Metabolic changes:** Pregnant women use carbohydrates faster than nonpregnant women do, which means that they're at a higher risk of developing *hypoglycemia* (low blood sugar). Exercise can be very useful in helping lower and control blood sugar levels, but it also increases the body's need for carbohydrates. So if you exercise, make sure you're eating an adequate amount of starch just before you work out.

✓ **Effects on the uterus:** One study of women at *term* (far enough along to deliver) showed that their contractions increased after moderate aerobic exercise. Another study indicated that exercise is associated with a lower risk of

early labor. But most studies have shown that exercise has no effect either way, and exercise does not pose a risk of preterm labor in healthy pregnant women.

✔ **Effect on birth weight:** Some studies have shown that women who work out strenuously (at high intensity) during pregnancy have lighter-weight babies. The same effect appears to occur in women who perform heavy physical work in a standing position while they're pregnant. But this decrease in birth weight seems to be due mainly to a decrease in the newborn's subcutaneous fat. In other words, more strenuous exercise has no effect on the fetus's normal growth.

Exercising without overdoing it

Your changing body is going to demand a change in exercise routine. Don't beat yourself up if you find that pregnancy makes it harder to continue the workouts you're accustomed to. Modify your program according to what you can reasonably tolerate.

Listen to your body. If weight lifting suddenly hurts your back, lighten up. You may find it easier to perform non-weight-bearing exercises like swimming or stationary bicycling. No matter what your particular exercise regimen may be, keep in mind the basic rules for working out during pregnancy:

✔ If you have a moderate exercise routine, keep it up. If you've been pretty sedentary, don't suddenly plunge into a strenuous program; ease in slowly to avoid putting too much strain on your body.

Remember that keeping up a regular schedule of moderate activity is better than engaging in infrequent spurts of intense exercise, which are more likely to cause injury.

✔ Avoid overheating, especially during the first six weeks of pregnancy.

✔ Avoid exercising flat on your back for long periods of time; doing so may reduce blood flow to your heart.

✔ Try not to overheat or become dehydrated, and if you feel fatigued, dizzy, faint, or nauseous, by all means stop. On very hot or humid days, don't exercise outdoors.

✓ Avoid anything that puts you at risk of being hurt in the abdomen, like road/mountain biking.

✓ Steer clear of high-impact, bouncy exercises that can tax your loosening joints.

✓ Throughout the nine months, low- or moderate-impact workouts make more sense than high-impact ones.

✓ Carry a bottle of water to every exercise session and stay well hydrated.

✓ Eat a well-balanced diet that includes an adequate supply of carbohydrates (see "Taking Stock of What You're Taking In," earlier in this chapter).

✓ Talk to your practitioner about what your peak exercise heart rate should be. (Many practitioners suggest 140 beats per minute as the upper limit.) Then regularly measure your heart rate at the peak of your workout to make sure it's at a safe level.

✓ Stop exercising and talk to your doctor if you experience any of these symptoms:

- • Shortness of breath that is persistent or out of proportion to the exercise you're doing

- • Vaginal bleeding

- • Rapid heartbeat (that is, more than 140 beats per minute)

- • Dizziness or feeling faint

- • Any significant pain

Comparing forms of exercise

Now isn't the time to shoot for that Ms. Fitness title, but that certainly doesn't mean you can't exercise. Because your pregnant body demands you take new precautions, choose your style of exercise carefully.

Working your heart: Aerobic exercise

Weight-bearing exercises like running, walking, aerobics, and using a stair-climbing machine or an elliptical trainer are great, as long as you don't do too much. These exercises require you to support all your weight, which is ever-increasing. Because

your joints are loosening and your center of gravity is shifting at the same time, you run a slightly higher risk of injuring yourself. Remember to do only what you know you can rather than setting off on a new exercise routine that is too demanding for your current state of fitness, not to mention your pregnancy.

Pilates is a popular mind-body conditioning program focused on strengthening the core postural muscles important in maintaining your balance and supporting your spine. For the most part, continuing Pilates classes while you are pregnant is safe, as long as you avoid lying flat on your back for long periods of time.

If you choose to take aerobics or Pilates classes, look for those designed specifically for pregnant women. If no classes are available, talk to the instructor to find modifications for exercises that are inappropriate.

You may find it easier, particularly later in pregnancy, to perform non-weight-bearing exercises. Because your weight is supported, you have less chance of injuring yourself, and your joints aren't stressed. If you're new to exercise, a low-intensity workout in the pool or on a stationary bike is ideal.

Downhill skiing, waterskiing, and horseback riding put you at risk of falling with significant impact, which could injure you or your baby. Although these activities may be fine early in pregnancy, talk to your doctor before doing them in your second or third trimester. Cross-country skiing is less risky, especially if you're experienced.

Strengthening your muscles

You won't get a great cardiac benefit from weight lifting, yoga, or body sculpting, but you can improve your muscle tone and flexibility, which comes in handy during labor and delivery.

Weight-lifting machines may be preferable to using free weights because you know you won't drop the weights onto your abdomen. But use free weights with caution, preferably with the help of a trainer or a skilled friend. A trainer can also show you the proper way to exhale and inhale during lifting. Breathing well is important because it lessens the chance that you might bear down (otherwise known as the *valsava maneuver,* a method of increasing abdominal pressure). This can reduce blood flow, raise your blood pressure, and stress your heart.

Practicing safe yoga

Yoga can be a wonderful and relaxing way to work out while you're pregnant, but only if you exercise caution. Follow these tips when doing yoga during pregnancy:

✔ If you're new to yoga, take a beginner class to ease yourself into a new exercise regime.

✔ Be careful about positions that stretch your muscles too much. Due to elevated levels of progesterone and relaxin (hormones produced during pregnancy), you can easily overstretch your muscles and ligaments.

✔ When bending forward, try to bend from the hips, not from the back. Also, try to lift your chest high to avoid putting extra pressure on your abdomen.

✔ After the mid second trimester, try to avoid performing poses that require you to lie flat on your back for extensive periods of time, because pressure from a pregnant uterus may decrease blood flow both to your heart and to the baby.

✔ As a general rule for any exercise, if you feel any pain or discomfort, stop and rest.

Avoid using very heavy weights, which can cause injury to your joints and ligaments.

Yoga, which is a great choice for pregnant women, is not only an excellent form of exercise, but may also be helpful in mastering breathing and relaxation techniques. Yoga is particularly useful in strengthening lower back and abdominal muscles and increasing stamina and physical endurance — all of which make you better equipped to handle the rigors of pregnancy.

Across the country, yoga studios are gaining in popularity, and many are offering specific classes for pregnant women. See the nearby sidebar, "Practicing safe yoga," for more about yoga.

Bikram yoga is a special type of yoga that is rapidly gaining popularity in the United States. It involves performing yoga in a room heated to 105 degrees Fahrenheit with a relative humidity of 60 to 70 percent. Although some doctors feel that this

type of yoga is safe for pregnant women during the first trimester, we believe that prolonged exposure to high temperatures during the first trimester is inadvisable, given the possible risks of causing a neural tube defect. (See Chapter 6 for more on neural tube defects, such as spina bifida.)

Part II
Pregnancy: Countdown

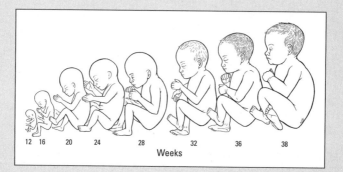

12 16   20   24   28   32   36   38

Weeks

Kathryn Born, MA

Go to www.dummies.com/extras/pregnancy for a
bonus article on genetic testing.

In this part . . .

- ✔ From inception through week 12, find out all the changes that your body is going to go through and how your baby will be developing.

- ✔ I just felt a kick! Weeks 13 through 26 are an exciting time. Prepare to have some prenatal testing done, your first ultrasound, and sharing the news with family and friends.

- ✔ Time to get ready for your new arrival. Find out about childbirth classes, preparing to go to the hospital, and bringing baby home.

Chapter 5

The First Trimester

. . . .

In This Chapter

▶ Getting a glimpse of your baby's development in the first trimester

▶ Coping with the physical symptoms of early pregnancy

▶ Addressing genetic concerns that may affect your baby

▶ Undergoing standard tests to ensure that you and your baby are healthy

▶ Knowing what constitutes cause for concern

▶ Getting dad's perspective on the pregnancy

. . . .

*T*he first trimester of your pregnancy is an exciting time, full of many changes for you and especially for your baby, which — in just 12 short weeks — grows from a single cell to a tiny being with a beating heart and functioning kidneys. With all that change going on in your baby, you can certainly expect many changes in your own body — from fatigue and nausea to newly voluptuous (va-va-va-voom!) but tender breasts. Through it all, you need to know what's normal and what's worth a call to your practitioner, whom you begin visiting regularly at this point. This chapter gives you a snapshot of what to expect.

A New Life Takes Shape

Pregnancy begins when the egg (or *oocyte*) and sperm meet, which happens in the fallopian tube. At this stage, the egg and sperm together form what we refer to as the *zygote* — a single cell. The zygote divides many times into a cluster of multiple cells called a *blastocyst,* which travels down the fallopian tube and into the *uterus* (also called the *womb*), shown in Figure 5-1. When it reaches the uterus, both you and your baby begin to experience major changes.

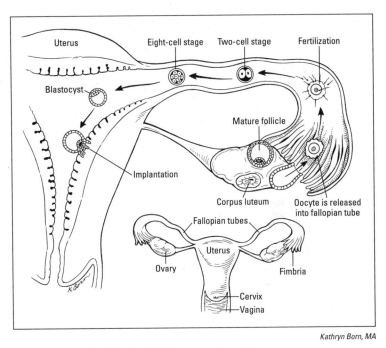

Kathryn Born, MA

Figure 5-1: The female reproductive system in action.

Following the numbers: How the embryo grows

On or about the fifth day of development, the blastocyst attaches to the blood-rich lining of the uterus during a process called *implantation*. Part of the blastocyst grows to become the *embryo* (the baby in the first eight weeks of development), and the other part becomes the *placenta* (the organ that implants into the uterus to provide oxygen and nourishment to the fetus and eliminate its waste products).

From the blastocyst, the embryo develops into three differ-ent tissue layers: the endoderm, mesoderm, and ectoderm. These three layers ultimately give rise to all of the structures of the body and are initially organized into a flat disk. Around the beginning of the fourth week of embryonic development, the flat disk begins to fold and form a cylinder. At this point, the embryo begins to take on the form of the general body plan,

with a mouth region and an anal region. Between weeks four and eight, all of the organ systems that you find in an adult will be forming. After the eighth week of your pregnancy, the developing embryo is referred to as a *fetus*. Amazingly, by this time almost all the baby's major organs and structures are already formed. The remaining 32 weeks allow the fetus's structures to grow and mature. On the other hand, the brain, although also formed very early, isn't mature at birth; rather it continues to develop into early childhood.

Your baby grows within the *amniotic sac* in the uterus. The amniotic sac is full of clear fluid, known as *amniotic fluid*. This water balloon-like structure actually comprises two thin layers of membrane called the *chorion* and *amnion* (which together are known as the *membranes*). When people talk about water "breaking," they're referring to the rupturing of those membranes that line the uterus's inner walls. The baby "swims" in this fluid and is attached to the placenta by the umbilical cord. Figure 5-2 shows a diagram of an early pregnancy, including a developing fetus and the *cervix,* which is the uterus's opening. The cervix opens up, or *dilates,* when you're in labor.

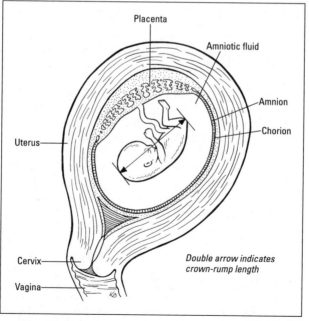

Placenta

Amniotic fluid

Amnion

Chorion

Uterus

Cervix

Vagina

*Double arrow indicates
crown-rump length*

Kathryn Born, MA

Figure 5-2: An early pregnancy.

The placenta begins to form soon after the embryo implants in the uterus. Maternal and fetal blood vessels lie very close to one another inside the placenta, which allows various substances (such as nutrients, oxygen, and waste) to transfer back and forth. The mother's blood and the baby's blood are in close contact, but they don't actually mix.

The placenta grows like a tree, forming branches that in turn divide into smaller and smaller ones. The tiniest buds of the placenta are called the *chorionic villi,* and it's within these villi that small fetal blood vessels form. About three weeks after fertilization, these blood vessels join to form the baby's circulatory system, and the heart begins to beat.

When we refer to weeks, we mean menstrual weeks, which means weeks from the last menstrual period, not weeks from conception. So at eight weeks, the baby is really six weeks from conception.

By the end of the eighth week, arms, legs, fingers, and toes begin to form. In fact, the embryo begins to perform small, spontaneous movements. If you have an ultrasound examination performed in the first trimester, you can see these spontaneous movements on the screen. The brain enlarges rapidly, and ears and eyes appear. The external genitalia also emerge and can be differentiated as male or female by the end of the 12th week, although sex differences are not yet detectable by ultrasound.

By the end of the 12th week, the fetus is about 4 inches long and weighs about 1 ounce. The head looks large and round, and the eyelids are fused shut. The intestines, which protruded slightly into the umbilical cord at about week 10, are by this time well inside the abdomen. Fingernails appear, and hair begins to grow on the baby's head. The kidneys start working during the third month. Between 9 and 12 weeks, the fetus begins to produce urine, which you can see within the small fetal bladder on ultrasound.

Take two: Noting how twins develop

Twins form basically in two possible ways: Either two eggs are produced (ovulated) and two sperm fertilize the eggs, or one egg is fertilized by one sperm and the embryo splits into two very early in development (early in the blastocyst stage). If two eggs are produced and fertilized, the genetic information

contained in each embryo is different from the other, just like siblings. These are called "fraternal" twins. If one egg is fertilized and splits, the resulting two embryos are genetically identical, hence the term "identical" twins.

Twins (or higher order multiples) are more common in women who undergo in vitro fertilization (IVF). This is most often because two (or more) embryos that are fertilized in a petri dish are placed back into the uterus and implant. It is still possible, however, to have identical twins when a single blastocyst is transferred back into the uterus and splits into two embryos later.

Adapting to How Your Body Changes

Your baby isn't the only one growing and changing during your pregnancy (not that we have to remind you of that!). Your body also has to adjust, and the adjustments it makes aren't always the most pleasant and comfortable for you. Being prepared for what lies ahead can help ease your mind. So in the following sections, we let you know what is in store for you during the first trimester.

Breast changes

One of the earliest and most amazing changes in your body happens to your breasts. Even during the first month of pregnancy, most women notice that their breasts grow considerably larger and feel very tender. The nipples and *areolae* (the circular areas around the nipples) also grow bigger and may begin to darken. Breast changes are caused by the large amounts of estrogen and progesterone your body produces during pregnancy. These hormones cause the glands inside your breasts to grow and branch out, in preparation for milk production and breast-feeding after the baby is born. Blood supply to the breasts also increases markedly. You may notice large, bluish blood vessels coursing along your breasts.

 Plan to go through several bra sizes while you're pregnant — and don't skimp on buying new bras. Good support helps reduce stretching and sagging later on. Although some women like the way they look with larger breasts, others feel more

self-conscious. Whichever way you feel, we guarantee other pregnant women feel the same way, so don't be embarrassed about it.

Fatigue

During the first trimester, you're likely to feel overwhelming fatigue. This fatigue may be a side effect of all the physical changes your body is experiencing, including the dramatic rise in hormone levels. Rest assured your exhaustion will probably go away somewhere around the 12th to 14th week of your pregnancy. As your fatigue lessens, you'll probably feel more energetic and almost normal, until about 30 to 34 weeks into your pregnancy, when you may tire out again. In the meantime, remember that fatigue is nature's way of telling you to get more rest. If you can, try to catch a short nap during the day and go to bed earlier than usual at night.

Any-time-of-day sickness

For some women, the nausea that can strike during the first trimester is worse in the mornings, maybe because the stomach is empty at that time of day. But ask anyone who's had morning sickness, also known as nausea and vomiting of pregnancy (NVP), and she'll tell you it can hit any time. It often starts during the fifth or sixth week (that is, three to four weeks after you miss your period — we describe how doctors calculate the timing of pregnancy in Chapter 2) and goes away, or at least becomes much less severe, by the end of the 11th or 12th week. It can last longer, and in fact about 10 percent of women have symptoms up to 16 weeks! If you are carrying twins or more, don't be surprised if the NVP is worse than expected, because the higher hormone levels make the nausea even more extreme. Fortunately, there are things you can do to ameliorate your symptoms.

If you're experiencing nausea, we sympathize. Even when nausea doesn't actually cause you to vomit, it can be extremely uncomfortable and truly debilitating. Certain odors — from foods, perfumes, or musty places — can make it worse. Look in the nearby sidebar, "Ways to keep nausea at bay," for recommendations on how to minimize morning sickness. If your queasiness gets out of control — if you experience weight loss, if you find that you can't keep down food or liquids, or if you feel dizzy or faint — call your doctor.

Ways to keep nausea at bay

Unfortunately, we can't tell you how to make your nausea totally disappear. But you can try a few things to make it better. Here are some suggestions:

✔ Eat small, frequent meals, so that your stomach is never empty.

✔ Don't worry too much about adhering to a balanced diet initially; just eat whatever appeals to you during this relatively short period of time.

✔ Avoid perfume counters, active kitchens, smelly taxicabs, barnyards, or other places where odors may be strong.

✔ If your prenatal vitamins make the symptoms worse, try taking them at night just before you go to bed. If you find that they are still causing a problem, skipping them for a few days is okay, particularly if you're taking an omega-3 supplement in addition to your prenatal.

✔ Keep crackers by your bedside — some women find that eating them before getting out of bed in the morning helps to decrease the nausea.

✔ Ginger (in the form of tea or tablets, for example) may help some women.

✔ You may notice that your nausea worsens when you brush your teeth. Switching toothpaste brands and avoiding vigorous brushing may help.

✔ Try eating dry toast, saltines, whole-wheat crackers, potatoes, and other bland, easy-to-digest carbohydrates.

✔ If you're bothered by the accumulation of saliva in your mouth, sucking on lemon drop candies may be helpful.

✔ Acupressure wristbands, sold in drugstores and health food stores, give some women relief.

✔ Relaxation exercises and even hypnosis work for some women.

If you're really bothered by the nausea, talk to your doctor about over-the-counter or prescription medications. Your doctor may suggest or prescribe one of the following:

✔ **Vitamin B6:** Some evidence suggests that 50 milligrams of vitamin B6 three times a day can reduce nausea.

A combination of vitamin B6 and the antihistamine doxylamine (Unisom — one pill at nighttime; check before you buy because some generics substitute a different

medication) may also be helpful. This combination is similar to the medication Benedictin, which was removed from the market due to completely unsubstantiated claims of an increase in birth defects. Although Benedictin still isn't available, scientists no longer believe it's *teratogenic* (causes birth defects). Talk to your doctor about trying vitamin B6, with or without doxylamine. Remember that doxylamine is marketed as a sleep aid, so it will most likely make you drowsy.

✔ **Diclegis:** A new FDA-approved prescription medicine (pregnancy category A), Diclegis (doxylamine succinate, 10 mg, and pyridoxine hydrochloride, 10mg) can help provide relief from NVP. It is basically the old Benedictin, but revamped with improved benefits. It has a delayed-release formulation and a dosing schedule that helps you control symptoms throughout the day. Diclegis should be taken on a regular basis and not "as needed." The combination of ingredients in Diclegis has been commercially available as the active ingredients in another medication called Diclectin for more than 30 years in Canada, so it has an excellent safety record. The main side effect of this medication is drowsiness, so avoid taking it while operating heavy machinery, driving, or other situations in which drowsiness can cause a problem. Taking it with some pain medications like oxycodone, which we already know causes central nervous depression and respiratory depression, can make these problems even worse than they are with the oxycodone alone.

✔ **Ondansetron (Zofran):** Some women find relief for extreme nausea with or without vomiting from this prescription medication. Although ondansetron hasn't been extensively studied in pregnancy, we know of no reports of an increase in birth defects associated with this medication.

✔ **Metoclopramide (Reglan):** Your doctor can actually administer this drug by continuous infusion under the skin through a device known as a subcutaneous pump. This is advantageous for those women who can't even swallow a pill because they're so nauseous.

Occasionally, the nausea and vomiting are so severe that you develop a condition called *hyperemesis gravidarum.* The symptoms include dehydration and weight loss. If you develop hyperemesis gravidarum, you may need to be given fluids and medications intravenously.

If you're less than six weeks pregnant and experiencing NVP, you can take folic acid alone instead of your prenatal vitamin. Folic acid is the main supplement that you need early in your pregnancy, and it's much less likely to upset your stomach than the multivitamin you normally take during pregnancy. Check with your doctor for the correct dose for you.

You may hear some women say that morning sickness is a sign that you're experiencing a "normal" pregnancy, but that claim is a myth — and so is the reverse. If you're not having morning sickness, or if it suddenly disappears, don't worry that your pregnancy isn't normal; just enjoy your good fortune. Similarly, you may hear that the severity of your queasiness indicates whether you're having a girl or a boy. But that's also a myth, so don't buy those pink or blue outfits just yet (and turn to Chapter 2 for more myths about determining the sex of your bundle of joy).

Above all, don't compound the problem by worrying about it. The nausea is harmless — to you and the baby. Your optimal weight gain for the first three months is only 2 pounds. Even losing weight probably isn't a big problem.

Bloating

Well before the baby is big enough to stretch out your stomach, your belt may begin to feel uncomfortable and your belly may look bloated and distended. This side effect of the hormone shift starts happening as soon as you conceive. *Progesterone,* one of the two key pregnancy hormones, causes you to retain water. Plus, it slows down the bowels, causing them to enlarge and thus increase the size of the abdomen. *Estrogen,* the other key pregnancy hormone, causes your uterus to enlarge, which also makes your abdomen feel bigger. This effect is often more pronounced in second or third pregnancies because the first pregnancy causes your abdominal muscles to relax to a greater degree.

Frequent urination

From early on in your pregnancy, you may feel as if you're spending your whole life in the restroom. During pregnancy, you need to urinate more frequently for a variety of reasons. At the beginning of your pregnancy, your uterus is inside your pelvis. But toward the end of your first trimester (at around

12 weeks), your uterus expands enough to rise up into your abdominal cavity. Your enlarging uterus may compress your bladder, which both decreases its capacity and increases the feeling that you need to urinate. Also, your blood volume rises markedly during pregnancy, and that means the rate at which your kidneys produce urine also increases.

You can't do much about your need to urinate frequently, except use common sense. Before going out for long (or even short) trips, empty your bladder so that you don't find yourself needing facilities when none are available. Drink plenty of fluids during pregnancy to avoid dehydration, but try to drink more during the day and less in the evening so that you aren't up all night going to the bathroom. Coffee and tea contain caffeine (a *diuretic,* which increases the flow of urine) and may aggravate the situation, so try decreasing the amount of caffeine you consume. (For more information about caffeine, see Chapter 4.)

If you find yourself urinating even more than your pregnancy norm or if you feel any discomfort or burning or notice blood during urination, talk to your practitioner. When you're pregnant, bacteria in your urine are more likely than usual to cause a urinary tract infection (see Chapter 15).

Headaches

Many pregnant women notice that they get headaches more often than they used to. These headaches may be the result of nausea, fatigue, hunger, the normal physiologic decrease in blood pressure that starts to occur at this time, tension, or even depression. Simple pain relievers like acetaminophen (for example, Tylenol) or ibuprofen (such as Motrin or Advil), in recommended doses, are often the best treatment for headaches, including migraines. Some women find that a little caffeine can also alleviate symptoms of a headache. In fact, some women find relief from occasional headaches by taking a combination of acetaminophen and caffeine (such as Excedrin Tension Headache). Although this combination is fine to take once in a while, don't use it on a regular basis because each tablet contains 65 mg of caffeine and the package recommends two tablets every 6 hours — that's a whopping 520 milligrams of caffeine per day and way beyond the 200 mg recommended maximum for pregnant women (see Chapter 4). This much caffeine, taken on a regular basis, could potentially cause problems with your baby's growth, or, if consumed early in pregnancy may increase your risk for miscarriage.

Food and rest can usually cure headaches that are caused by nausea, fatigue, or hunger. So try eating and getting some extra sleep. If neither of those tactics works, something else is probably causing your headaches.

If over-the-counter medications don't relieve your headaches, talk with your practitioner about taking a mild tranquilizer or anti-migraine medication. Base your decision on whether to use migraine medications on the severity of your problem. If your headaches are chronic or recurrent, you may be better off taking medications, despite their potential effects on your fetus, because feeling bad all the time is likely more harmful to you baby's development than any potential risks from the various medications available. As always, consult with your practitioner before taking these medications.

Avoid taking regular doses of aspirin unless recommended by your practitioner, because adult doses of aspirin can affect platelet function (important in blood clotting).

If your headaches are severe and unremitting, you may need a thorough medical evaluation or a referral to a neurologist. Later on in pregnancy, a headache may signal the onset of a condition called preeclampsia (which we cover in Chapter 14). In that case, your headache may be accompanied by swelling of your hands and feet and by high blood pressure. If you suffer a severe headache in the late second or third trimester, call your practitioner.

Constipation

About half of all pregnant women complain of constipation. When you're pregnant, you may become constipated because the large amount of progesterone circulating in your blood-stream slows the activity of your digestive tract. The iron in prenatal vitamins may make matters worse. Try these suggestions to deal with the problem:

> ✔ **Eat plenty of high-fiber foods.** Bran cereals, fruits, and vegetables all are good sources of fiber. Some women find it helpful to eat some popcorn, but choose the low-fat kind, without all the butter and added oil. Check the fiber content on package labels and choose foods with higher fiber content.

✔ **Drink plenty of water.** Staying well hydrated helps keep food and waste moving through the digestive tract. Some juices (especially prune juice) may help, while others (such as apple juice) may only exacerbate the problem.

✔ **Take stool softeners.** A stool softener, such as Colace (docusate sodium), isn't a laxative — it just keeps the stool soft. Stool softeners are safe during pregnancy, and you may take them two to three times a day. Avoid laxatives because they can cause abdominal cramping and, occasionally, uterine contractions. For any person, pregnant or not, chronic laxative use should be avoided. If you're extremely constipated, though, and aren't at risk for preterm labor, you may want to talk to your practitioner about the short-term use of a very mild laxative, like a glycerin suppository or milk of magnesia.

✔ MiraLAX (Polyethylene Glycol 3350): MiraLAX is a great natural way of relieving constipation and most women find it very effective. Constipation may occur when stool moves slowly through the colon, which could allow too much water to be removed. This can make the stool hard, dry, and difficult to pass. The active ingredient in MiraLAX, Polyethylene Glycol 3350, works by replenishing the water to your digestive system, which helps naturally cause a bowel movement. This water both increases the frequency of bowel movements and softens the stool, making it easier to pass. The other good news is that it generally doesn't have some of the uncomfortable side effects of more potent laxatives, such as cramping, gas, and bloating.

✔ **Exercise as regularly as you can.** Exercise helps constipation, so enjoy some safe exercise (even if it's only walking).

Cramps

You may feel a vague, menstrual-like cramping sensation during the first trimester. This is a very common symptom, so don't worry. The cramping is probably related to the uterus growing and enlarging.

If you experience cramping along with vaginal bleeding, give your practitioner a call. Although the majority of women who experience bleeding and cramping go on to have perfectly normal pregnancies, sometimes these two symptoms together are associated with miscarriage. Cramping alone, without bleeding, is unlikely to be a problem.

Going to Your First Prenatal Appointment

After the at-home pregnancy test reveals the news, set up an appointment with a practitioner. Make visits to your practitioner a regular part of your pregnancy, not only to ensure your health, but also to ensure your baby's health. Your first prenatal visit may be your first meeting with the practitioner who will guide you through your pregnancy. (If you don't already have a practitioner selected, see Chapter 1 for information on the kinds of care available and tips for choosing a health-care provider.) Or you may have a long-standing relationship with an OB/GYN or family-practice doctor with whom you've already discussed many of the topics that are typically covered at an initial prenatal visit.

If possible, bring the father-to-be for this initial visit. His family medical history and ethnic roots are important, too. If the father is not part of the picture, bring your life partner or anyone else who may be helping you through the pregnancy process to the appointment. That person should have a chance to ask questions, address concerns, and find out what to expect in the coming months.

Your first prenatal visit usually lasts 30 to 40 minutes or more because your doctor has so much information to provide and so many topics to discuss. Subsequent visits are usually much shorter, sometimes only 5 to 10 minutes long. The frequency of your visits depends on your particular needs and any special risk factors you may have, but in general they're about every four weeks during the first trimester. At these visits, the nurse or practitioner checks your urine, blood pressure, and weight, and the baby's heartbeat.

Understanding the consultation

During your first visit, your practitioner discusses with you your medical and obstetrical history. She asks about various aspects of your physical health, as well as elements of your lifestyle that may affect your pregnancy.

Lifestyle

Your practitioner asks about your occupation to find out whether your job is sedentary or active, whether you spend your days standing or lifting heavy objects, or whether you work nights or long shifts. She also asks you about your general lifestyle — for example, smoking, heavy alcohol use, dietary restrictions, and exercise patterns.

Date of your last menstrual period

Your practitioner questions you about the start date of your last menstrual period to determine your due date. (For more information on calculating your due date, see Chapter 1.) If you don't know exactly when your last period began, try to remember the exact date of conception. If you're unsure about either of these dates, your practitioner may want to check on how far along you are by scheduling an ultrasound exam.

Obstetrical and gynecological history

Your provider will ask you about your obstetrical and gyne-cological history, including any prior pregnancies and any experiences with fibroid tumors, vaginal infections, and other gynecological problems. Your history can help determine how best to manage this pregnancy. For example, if you have a his-tory of preterm labor (see Chapter 14) or gestational diabetes (Chapter 15), knowing that history prepares your practitioner for the possibility that it may happen again.

Pregnancy after infertility treatment

If you conceived with infertility treatments, inform your prac-titioner of this during your first prenatal visit because it brings up several points that need to be addressed. Most of the impact of infertility treatment on pregnancy outcomes is related to the higher incidence of multi-fetal pregnancies — twins and more. In general, children born to couples who have gone through in vitro fertilization (IVF) are as healthy as those who were con-ceived spontaneously. Recently, some controversy has cropped up in medical literature about an increase in certain birth defects in children born after IVF, as well as an increase in certain chro-mosomal abnormalities after intracytoplasmic sperm injection (ICSI). Although some studies suggest the incidence may be slightly higher, other studies document no increase at all.

Medical problems

Your practitioner asks you about any medical problems you have had and any surgeries you have undergone, including

problems that aren't gynecological in nature. Certain medical conditions may affect pregnancy, and others don't. She also asks you about any allergies to medications you may have. Tell your practitioner so she can know everything about you and your health.

Family medical histories

The family medical histories of both you and the baby's father are important for two reasons. First, your practitioner can identify pregnancy-related conditions that can recur from generation to generation, like having twins or exceptionally large babies. The other reason is to identify serious problems within your family that your baby can inherit. Blood tests can screen for some of these problems, such as cystic fibrosis.

Other available genetic screening tests include:

✓ **Fragile X:** Fragile X syndrome is the most common inherited form of mental retardation. The mental retardation can vary from learning disabilities to severe disabilities. Fragile X syndrome is also the most common known cause of autism, or autistic-like tendencies. While the syndrome is quite rare (affecting 1 in 3,600 males and 1 in 4,000 to 6,000 females), about 1 in 250 women carry what's called a *premutation*. The genetics of this disease are quite complicated, but the disorder is caused by expansion of a repeated DNA sequence, known as *CGG repeats*. The number of CGG repeats varies among different people and is categorized into four groups: unaffected (less than 45 repeats), intermediate or gray zone (45-54 repeats), premutation (55-200 repeats), and full mutation (more than 200 repeats). The number of repeats can expand in a fetus, and so based on the number of repeats a parent carries, genetic testing by CVS (chorionic villus sampling) or amniocentesis is recommended. A woman carrying an intermediate number of repeats is unlikely to transmit a full mutation to her fetus, while a woman carrying a permutation can expand in the fetus to a full mutation. While many practitioners recommend screening all women for fragile X, the American College of Obstetrics and Gynecology guidelines suggest screening only those women with a family history of fragile X syndrome or undiagnosed mental retardation, developmental delay, autism, or ovarian insufficiency. Certainly, talk with your doctor or healthcare provider if you are interested in fragile X screening.

✔ **Spinal Muscular Atrophy (SMA):** Spinal Muscular Atrophy (SMA) is an autosomal recessive neurodegenerative disorder that occurs due to degeneration of nerve cells in the spinal cord. The disease is caused by mutations in a gene known as SMN1 (survival motor neuron gene 1). The incidence of SMA is not very common (1 in 10,000 live births), although it is thought to be the most common genetic cause of infant death. The chance of being a carrier of this disorder is 1 in 40 to 1 in 60. Currently, couples with a family history of SMA are being offered carrier screening, although many obstetricians offer routine screening. In fact, the American College of Medical Genetics has recently recommended offering carrier testing to all couples, regardless of race or ethnicity.

✔ **Expanded Carrier Screening for other genetic diseases:** Several companies have come out with tests to screen for over 100 different genetic disorders (including the ones that are mentioned in the following section for certain ethnic groups). Almost all are autosomal recessive, meaning that you and your partner would have to be carriers for there to be a 1 in 4 chance of the fetus inheriting the disease. One such company is called the Counsyl panel. You may want to discuss the option for screening with your healthcare provider, as the test has to be ordered by a healthcare professional.

Ethnic roots

Even if you and your partner have family histories that are free of any known genetic disorders, your ethnic backgrounds are important because some genetic disorders occur more frequently in one ethnicity than others. Jewish people of Eastern European descent, for example, are ten times more likely than others to carry the rare gene for *Tay-Sachs,* a disease of the nervous system that is usually fatal in early childhood. French Canadians and Cajuns (from Louisiana) also have a higher-than-normal risk of carrying this gene. Most of the time, a simple blood test can determine whether you're a carrier of this disease.

Tay-Sachs is inherited in what's known as a *recessive* manner, which means that both parents would need to be carriers to place the baby at risk for having the disease. Being a carrier doesn't mean that you *have* Tay-Sachs, only that you carry a gene for it. Most genetic counselors recommend that both members of a couple undergo the blood tests for carrier status because it often takes several weeks to find out the results. If one member of a couple is tested only after the other is found

to be a carrier, the whole process can take a long time, perhaps even too long to leave time for certain prenatal diagnostic tests (like CVS — chorionic villus sampling — or amniocentesis, which we describe later in this chapter and in Chapter 6).

Although Tay-Sachs and some other conditions are found more frequently among the Jewish population, individuals from other ethnic groups can still be carriers, but that is much less common. For this reason, even if only one member of a couple is Jewish, both should still be tested, if possible. Although at this time only Tay-Sachs, cystic fibrosis, Canavan disease, and familial dysautonomia testing is recommended by the American College of Obstetricians and Gynecologists, here is a list of genetic disorders for which screening is available to couples of Jewish descent:

- Tay-Sachs
- Cystic fibrosis
- Canavan
- Familial dysautonomia
- Gaucher
- Neimann-Pick
- Mucolipidosis IV
- Fanconi anemia

- Bloom syndrome
- Familial hyperinsulinemia
- Lipoamide dehydrogenase deficiency
- Maple syrup urine disease
- Glycogen storage disease 1a
- Nemaline myopathy
- Usher syndrome

Another ethnically selective medical condition is *sickle-cell anemia,* a blood disorder that's especially prevalent among people with African or Hispanic ancestors. This condition, too, is recessive, so both members of a couple must be carriers for the baby to be at risk of inheriting the disease.

People whose ancestors come from Italy, Greece, and other Mediterranean countries are at elevated risk of having — and passing to their children — genes for the blood disorder *beta-thalassemia,* also known as *Mediterranean anemia* or *Cooley's anemia.* Among Asians, the analogous blood problem is *alpha-thalassemia.* Both of these disorders produce abnormalities in hemoglobin (the protein in red blood cells that holds onto oxygen) and therefore result in varying degrees of anemia. Like Tay-Sachs and sickle-cell anemia, both parents have to carry the gene in order for their baby to be at risk of having the disease.

Screening for cystic fibrosis

Cystic fibrosis (CF) is one of the most common genetic diseases in the United States, with an incidence of about 1 in 3,500. CF is also a recessive condition, like Tay-Sachs (see the previous "Ethnic roots" section). More than 1,700 different genetic mutations have been associated with CF. It is more common among the non-Hispanic white population compared with other racial and ethnic groups. Because it may be difficult to categorize someone as being a particular racial or ethnic group due to varied backgrounds, obstetricians and geneticists recommend that CF screening, through a blood test, be offered to all pregnant couples. Screening for the 23 most common mutations will pick up 49 to 94 percent of carriers of cystic fibrosis, depending on the ethnic background. (For example, it detects 94 percent of carriers among the Ashkenazi Jewish population, 88 percent of carriers among the Northern European Caucasian population, 64 percent of carriers among the American Hispanic population, and 49 percent of carriers among the Asian American population.) Speak to your doctor about CF screening during your first prenatal visit.

The risks of inheritable diseases overlap from one ethnic or geographic group to another. Genes get passed around among the various populations whenever the parents are from different ethnic groups. But you can roughly gauge whether your ancestry puts you at an elevated risk of carrying genes for certain diseases.

Some people don't know very much about their ethnic background or family medical history, perhaps because they were adopted or haven't had much contact with their biological families. If this is your situation, don't worry. Keep in mind that the chances of both you and your partner carrying a gene for a particular disorder are extremely low.

Considering the physical exam

At your first prenatal visit, your practitioner examines your head, neck, breasts, heart, lungs, abdomen, and extremities. She also performs an internal exam (see Figure 5-3). During this exam, your practitioner evaluates your uterus, cervix, and ovaries, and performs, if due, a Pap test (cervix cancer and pre-cancer screening). The recommendations for cervical cancer screening have changed over the last few years.

No screening is needed for women under age 21. For women age 21–29, a Pap test is recommended every three years. The recommendation for women age 30–65 is a Pap test plus human papillomavirus (HPV) testing every five years, or a Pap test only every three years.

Be sure to inform your physician if you feel you also should be tested for the possibility of sexually transmitted diseases, because the Pap test doesn't screen for all of them.

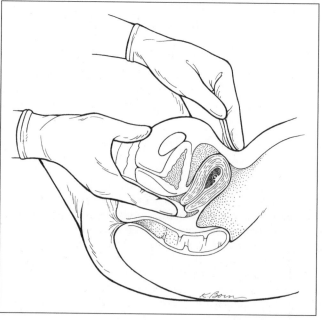

Kathryn Born, MA

Figure 5-3: A typical pelvic exam.

After the exam, you and your practitioner will discuss the overall plan for your pregnancy and talk about any possible problems. You can also discuss what medications you can take while you're pregnant, when you should call for help, and what tests you can expect to undergo throughout your pregnancy.

Eyeing the standard tests

Brace yourself: You're probably going to be stuck with a needle and have to pee in a cup during your first prenatal visit. Here's a look at the standard procedures, including blood and urine tests.

Get ready for the prick: Blood tests

On your first prenatal visit, your practitioner will draw your blood for a bunch of standard tests to check your general health, as well as to make sure you are immune to certain infections. The following tests are routine:

✔ **A standard test for blood type, Rh factor, and antibody status.** The blood type refers to whether your blood is type A, B, AB, or O and whether you're Rh-positive or Rh-negative. The antibody test is designed to tell whether special blood-group antibodies to certain antigens (like the Rh antigen) are present. (See Chapter 14 for more about the Rh factor and the implications of blood incompatibilities.)

✔ **Complete blood count (CBC).** This test checks for *anemia,* which refers to a low blood count. It also checks your *platelet count* (a component of blood important in clotting).

✔ **VDRL or RPR.** These tests check for *syphilis,* a sexually transmitted disease. They're very accurate, but sometimes they produce a false positive result if the patient has other conditions, such as lupus or antiphospholipid antibody syndrome (see Chapter 15). However, these kinds of false positive results are usually weakly positive. These tests are nonspecific, so in order to confirm the diagnosis of syphilis, another, more specific blood test should be performed. Because it's essential that syphilis be adequately treated, make sure you receive a test. In fact, most states require it. Unfortunately, the incidence of syphilis is on the rise in the United States.

✔ **Hepatitis B.** This test checks for evidence of the hepatitis viruses. These viruses come in several different types, and the hepatitis B virus is one that can be present without producing actual symptoms. In fact, some women are diagnosed only during a blood test, such as the one performed during pregnancy.

✔ **Rubella.** Your practitioner also checks for immunity to *rubella* (also called *German measles*). Most women have been vaccinated against rubella or, because they have had the illness in the past, their blood carries antibodies, which is why the risk of contracting German measles during pregnancy is so rare. Most practitioners test to see that the mother is immune to rubella during the very first prenatal visit. Any woman who isn't immune is counseled to be careful to avoid contact with anyone who has

the illness. A practitioner also advises these women to get vaccinated against rubella soon after they deliver, so that they aren't susceptible in subsequent pregnancies.

✓ **HIV.** Some states require that healthcare providers routinely ask whether you want to be checked for HIV, the virus that causes AIDS. Because medication is available to reduce the risk of transmission to the baby, as well as to slow disease progression in the mother, being aware of your HIV status is very important. A doctor can usually perform this test at the same time as the other prenatal blood tests.

Doctors sometimes need to perform other tests during your first prenatal visit. These additional tests include the following:

✓ **Glucose screen.** You usually get this test around 24 to 28 weeks, but your doctor may administer it in the first trimester if you're at a high risk of developing *gestational diabetes.* Check out Chapter 6 for the details of how the testing is done, and Chapter 15 to find out why treating gestational diabetes is important.

✓ **Varicella.** Your doctor may conduct this test to check for immunity to *varicella* (chickenpox). If you're unsure whether or not you've had chickenpox or you know that you haven't had it, let your practitioner know so that you can be tested for immunity. For more detailed information on varicella, see Chapter 15.

✓ **Toxoplasmosis.** Sometimes a doctor administers a test in order to check for immunity to *toxoplasmosis,* which is a type of parasitic infection. In the United States, testing for toxoplasmosis isn't considered routine unless you're at a higher risk for contracting it. For example, if you have an outdoor cat and you're the one who changes the litter box, your practitioner is likely to send off a test to check for past or recent exposure. If you're in France, where the incidence of toxoplasmosis is much higher, your practitioner will probably recommend that you be tested. See Chapter 15 for more information on toxoplasmosis.

✓ **Cytomegalovirus (CMV).** Testing for CMV, a common childhood infection, isn't routine during pregnancy. However, if you have a lot of contact with school-age children who may have the infection, your practitioner may suggest you have this test. As with toxoplasmosis, the blood test looks for evidence of past or recent infection. See Chapter 15 for more details on CMV.

✔ **Vitamin D.** Vitamin D deficiency is more common in pregnancy than previously thought. In fact, it is quite common in certain high-risk groups, including vegetarians, women who have limited sun exposure, and ethnic minorities. Babies born to vitamin D-deficient moms are also at risk of vitamin D deficiency. When severe, this can lead to problems in the development of the bones in the newborns. For pregnant women at risk for vitamin D deficiency, a simple blood test for 25-OH-D can be used to indicate vitamin D status. Although an optimal level is not known, some believe the level should be above 20–32 ng/ml. If you do find that you are vitamin D-deficient, your provider may recommend a supplement with 1,000 to 2,000 international units per day (in addition to your prenatal multivitamin), which is safe and helpful.

✔ **Lead screening.** Prenatal lead exposure has been linked to a variety of adverse outcomes for mom and baby. Recently, the Centers for Disease Control and Prevention (CDC) and the American College of Obstetricians and Gynecologists (ACOG) have addressed the issue of screening for elevated lead levels in maternal blood. While they do not recommend routine screening, they do suggest evaluating pregnant women for risk factors and testing those women at high risk. Some risk factors for lead exposure include the following:

- Recent emigration from a place where lead contamination is high

- Living near a high source of lead, such as land mines or battery recycling plants

- Being in close contact with someone who works with lead

- Eating nonfood substances (*pica* is a disorder where individuals eat non-nutritive substances), such as soil or paint containing lead or glazed ceramic pottery

- Using home remedies or certain therapeutic herbs traditionally used by East Indian, Indian, Middle Eastern, West Asian, and Hispanic cultures that may be contaminated with lead

- Having a history of previous lead exposure or living with someone identified as having an elevated lead level

For women with levels of 5 mg/dL or higher, the source of lead exposure should be found and they should be counseled and re-tested. If you are found to have a very high level, you need to speak with your doctor about treatment. A diet containing adequate amounts of calcium, iron, zinc, and vitamins C, D, and E is also known to help decrease lead absorption.

Take a quick trip to the bathroom: Urine tests

Each time you visit your practitioner during your pregnancy, including the first prenatal visit, you're asked to give a sample of urine. Your practitioner uses the urine sample to check for the presence of glucose (for a possible sign of diabetes) and protein (for evidence of preeclampsia).

Sneak the first look at your baby: Ultrasound

An ultrasound uses sound waves to create a picture of the uterus and the baby inside it. Ultrasound examinations don't involve radiation, and the procedure is safe for both you and your baby. Your practitioner may suggest that you undergo a first-trimester ultrasound exam. Often, this ultrasound is performed transvaginally, which means that a special ultrasound probe is inserted into the vagina. The advantage to this technique is that the probe, or transducer, is closer to the fetus, so a much clearer view is attained than with a standard transabdominal ultrasound examination.

 Some women worry that a probe inserted into the vagina could harm the baby. Although understandable, you don't need to worry. The probe is completely safe.

The following are evaluated during a first-trimester ultrasound exam:

- ✔ **The accuracy of your due date:** An ultrasound can show whether the fetus is any larger or smaller than the date of your last menstrual period would suggest. If the *crown-rump measurement* (which measures the fetus from the crown of the head to the rump; refer to Figure 5-2) is more than three or four days off your due date, your doctor may change your due date. An ultrasound in the first trimester is actually more accurate than a later ultrasound in confirming or establishing your due date.

✔ **Fetal viability:** By five to six weeks into your pregnancy, an ultrasound can detect a fetal heartbeat. After a fetal heartbeat has been identified, the risk of miscarriage drops significantly (to about 3 percent). Prior to five weeks, the fetus itself may not be visible; instead, the ultrasound may show only the gestational sac.

✔ **Fetal abnormalities:** Although a complete ultrasound examination to detect structural abnormalities in the fetus usually isn't performed until about 20 weeks, some problems may already be visible by 11 to 12 weeks. Much of the brain, spine, limbs, abdomen, and urinary tract structures can be seen with a transvaginal ultrasound. In addition, the presence of a thickening behind the neck of the fetus (known as *increased nuchal translucency*) may help to indicate an added risk for certain genetic or chromosomal conditions (see Chapter 6).

✔ **Fetal number:** An ultrasound shows whether you're carrying more than one fetus. In addition, the appearance of the membrane separating the babies, as well as the placental locations, helps to indicate whether the babies share one placenta or have separate placentas. We go into greater detail about this topic in Chapter 13.

✔ **The condition of your ovaries:** An ultrasound can reveal abnormalities or cysts in your ovaries. Sometimes an ultrasound shows a small cyst, called a *corpus luteal cyst,* which forms at the site where the egg was released. Over the course of three or four months, it gradually goes away. Two other types of cysts, called *dermoid cysts* and *simple cysts,* are unrelated to the pregnancy and may be found incidentally during an ultrasound exam. Whether removal of these types of cysts is necessary and when they should be removed depends on the size of the cyst and any symptoms you may be having.

✔ **The presence of fibroid tumors:** Also called *fibroids,* these are benign overgrowths of the muscle of the uterus. We go into more details about these in Chapter 15.

✔ **Location of the pregnancy:** Occasionally, the pregnancy may be located outside the uterus, which is called an *ectopic pregnancy* (see the "Ectopic pregnancy" section later in this chapter for more information).

Considering Options for Detecting Genetic Abnormalities in the First Trimester

With the explosion of genetic technology, there is a whole menu of options for detecting genetic abnormalities in your baby and many of them can be done in the first trimester. The options fall mainly into two categories: screening tests and diagnostic tests. A screening test will take bits of information about the developing fetus that can be collected and used to estimate the probability that your baby has certain genetic abnormalities and is usually expressed as a ratio (1/100, 1/1,000, 1/10,000, and so on). The bits of information can be substances produced by the placenta that can be measured in the mother's blood, measurements on an ultrasound, or fragments of fetal DNA that circulate in mom's bloodstream. A diagnostic test utilizes tiny pieces of placental tissue (chorionic villus sampling, or CVS), fetal skin cells that have flaked off the surface of the baby (amniocentesis), or fetal lymphocytes (fetal blood sampling) to directly look at the tissue to see if the genetic makeup is normal or abnormal. The screening tests available in the first trimester are the First Trimester Screen (utilizing components from the maternal blood and measurement of the nuchal translucency on the back of the baby's neck by ultrasound).

The diagnostic tests involve testing the developing baby's chromosomes. Chromosomes carry the genetic information (DNA) that determines what a person is like. People normally have 46 chromosomes — 23 inherited from their mother and 23 from their father (see Figure 5-4). The 23 from each side are paired inside the nucleus of each human cell. Twenty-two of these pairs are what's known as *autosomes,* which are the chromosomes that aren't sex-related. The 23rd pair of chromosomes are the sex chromosomes, which can be either XX (girl) or XY (boy).

A woman has two X chromosomes, so she can only give an X chromosome to her offspring. A man has one X and one Y chromosome and can therefore give either to his offspring. As you can see, the man determines the baby's sex, so you know who is to blame if you don't get the little girl or little boy you were hoping for!

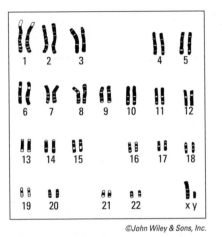

©John Wiley & Sons, Inc.

Figure 5-4: A typical set of human chromosomes.

Certain abnormalities in chromosome number or structure can lead to problems in the baby. For example, *Down syndrome,* one of the more common chromosomal abnormalities associated with severe mental retardation, may occur if the fetus has an extra copy of chromosome 21. (The condition is also known as Trisomy 21, because the fetus has three copies of chromosome number 21.) Amniocentesis, CVS, and other tests detect such abnormalities in chromosome number and structure by yielding an enlarged picture of the individual chromosomes called a *karyotype* (refer to Figure 5-4). In addition, if a couple has a known risk for carrying a child with a genetic disease that runs in that couple's family or ethnic group (Tay-Sachs or cystic fibrosis, for example), your practitioner also can use the material obtained during these procedures to test for such diseases. However, unless a couple is specifically at risk for one of these rare genetic disorders, your practitioner won't routinely administer this testing; the chromosomes are checked only for number and structure.

Looking at age

In the past, women who were going to be age 35 or older at their due date were offered the chance to undergo prenatal diagnosis to check the fetal chromosomes. Thirty-five was chosen as the target age because a woman's risk of having a baby with a chromosomal abnormality increases significantly after she reaches that age. It was also the age at which the risk of miscarriage from the procedure itself was equal to

the actual chances that the fetus would have a chromosomal abnormality. However, although the risk of a chromosome abnormality is much less for women under the age of 35, most babies with Down syndrome are born to women under the age of 35 simply because they have more babies as a group than women older than 35. The cutoff age of 35 is somewhat arbitrary and not followed in all countries. In Great Britain, for example, women are offered prenatal chromosomal testing at age 37 or after. Once nuchal translucency testing became available, the American College of Obstetricians and Gynecologists recommended that doctors stop using age to determine who should have a diagnostic test. The current practice is to offer every woman the same thing and allow her to choose which test or tests she wants to undergo.

Even among women at risk for a chromosomal problem, some choose not to be tested, either because they don't want to run any risk of miscarriage associated with the test or because of their personal beliefs about terminating a pregnancy.

Even if pregnancy termination isn't something you would consider, prior knowledge of a fetus's abnormalities can give you time to make preparations for a child that may have special needs.

Chorionic villus sampling

Chorionic villi are tiny, budlike pieces of tissue that make up the placenta. Because they develop from cells arising out of the fertilized egg, they have the same chromosomes and genetic makeup as the developing fetus. By checking a sample of chorionic villi, the laboratory can see whether or not the chromosomes are normal in number and structure, determine the fetal sex, and test for some specific diseases (if the fetus may be at risk for these diseases).

Your doctor performs a chorionic villus sampling (CVS) by withdrawing placental tissue (containing chorionic villi) either through a hollow needle inserted through the abdomen *(transabdominal CVS)* or through a flexible catheter inserted through the cervix *(transcervical CVS,* see Figure 5-5), depending on where the placenta is located within the uterus and the uterus's general shape and position. Your doctor uses ultrasound equipment as a guide as she performs the procedure. She then examines the tissue under a microscope, and the cells are cultured in a laboratory.

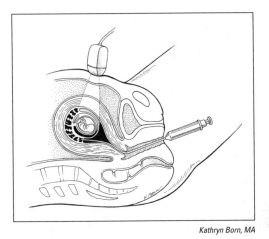

Kathryn Born, MA

Figure 5-5: In transcervical CVS, your doctor uses a flexible catheter inserted into the cervix to withdraw a tiny amount of placental tissue, using ultrasound as a guide.

Like amniocentesis, CVS raises the risk of miscarriage slightly — about 1/1000. Neither CVS method is more risky than the other. The person performing the test should have plenty of experience doing the procedure; experience helps reduce the risk of miscarriage.

CVS results are typically available in seven to ten days. The main advantage that CVS has over amniocentesis is that it can provide information earlier in the pregnancy. This time factor may be important to some women who feel that termination is an option if severe abnormalities are present.

Unlike amniocentesis, CVS can't measure AFP (*alpha-fetoprotein;* see Chapter 6 for more). However, your practitioner can take this measurement from maternal blood drawn at 15 to 18 weeks into the pregnancy.

If you undergo CVS and are Rh-negative, you should receive an injection of Rh-immune globulin (Rhophylac or Rhogam are examples) following the procedure to prevent you from developing rH disease (see Chapter 14).

Non-invasive screening in the first trimester

CVS and early amniocentesis (which is no longer recommended due to concerns about causing birth defects) are the only tests that can give definitive information about fetal chromosomes during the first trimester. There are two screening tests now available in the first trimester.

The First Trimester Screen uses a combination of a special ultrasound measurement, called *nuchal translucency*, and two substances found in mom's blood. Eighty to 90 percent of fetuses with Down syndrome may be detected through this type of screening. These first-trimester screening tests are usually performed between the approximate gestational ages of 10 weeks and 4 days to 13 weeks and 6 days. Here's how they work:

✔ **Nuchal translucency (NT):** This test uses ultrasound to measure a special area behind the fetal neck. Only physicians specially trained in the procedure should conduct a nuchal translucency test. When measurements of nuchal translucency are combined with blood screening tests, the accuracy of these tests is probably increased.

✔ **Serum screening:** Tests that check the levels of PAPP-A, a substance produced by the placenta, and hCG, a hormone in the mother's blood, may help screen for Down syndrome in the first trimester. Usually this blood test is drawn around the same time that the ultrasound to measure the nuchal translucency is performed.

The equation to calculate your risk ratio for Down syndrome takes into account the NT, the two blood components mentioned previously, a measurement of the length of the embryo called the "crown to rump" length (CRL), and your age at your expected due date. The results come as a risk ratio — like 1/310. If your chances of having a Down syndrome baby are high after the test, then your doctor will recommend that you have a diagnostic test. CVS can be done in the first trimester, but for amniocentesis, you have to wait until the second trimester. If your results are good (for example, if they show that you have a low risk for Down syndrome), you may want to wait until the second trimester and have a Quad Test (see Chapter 6). The results of this test will be integrated with the First Trimester Screen to even further refine your risk for Down syndrome. Doing it this way will detect almost 96-98% of fetuses with Down syndrome.

The newest way of screening for Down syndrome is called NIPS, or Non-invasive prenatal screening. For this procedure, a sample of blood is drawn from mom and sent to the lab where tiny fragments of the baby's

(continued)

(continued)

DNA (which are normally present in small quantities in mom's blood) are isolated and analyzed. This method can detect about 98-99% of babies with Down syndrome. The sample of blood can be drawn and sent anytime during pregnancy, but it's best to do it in the first trimester so that you can get the results back in time to make reproductive choices that are right for you. You can also predict the gender with this test and it will also detect many cases of trisomy 13 and 18 (similar disorders to Down syndrome but different chromosomes are involved) — but not at the same detection rate as for Down syndrome.

The original studies on NIPS were done in high-risk women (women over the age of 35, with a family history of chromosomal abnormalities, or with high risk First Trimester Screen results) so that's whom the test was recommended for. Recently, however, data is emerging suggesting that NIPS may be useful in low risk women also.

Recognizing Causes for Concern

In each trimester, a few things may, in some cases, go less than smoothly. The following sections describe some of the things that can happen during the first trimester of your pregnancy and what they may mean to you.

Bleeding

Early in pregnancy, around the time of your missed period, experiencing a little bleeding from the vagina isn't uncommon. The amount of bleeding is usually less than what you would expect with a period and lasts for only one or two days. This is called *implantation bleeding,* and it happens when the fertilized egg attaches to the uterus's lining. Bleeding due to implantation isn't a cause for concern, but many women may be confused by it and mistake it for their period.

Bleeding also may occur later in the first trimester, but it doesn't necessarily indicate a miscarriage. About one-third of women experience bleeding during the first trimester, and the majority of them go on to have perfectly healthy babies. Bleeding is especially common in women carrying more than one fetus — and again, most go on to have normal pregnancies. Bright red bleeding usually indicates active bleeding, while dark staining usually indicates old blood that is making its way out from the cervix and vagina. Most of the time, an

ultrasound exam doesn't show any evidence of the source of the bleeding. However, sometimes a collection of blood, known as a *subchorionic* or *retroplacental hemorrhage* or *collection,* is visible and indicates an area of bleeding from behind the placenta. It usually takes several weeks for this blood to be reabsorbed. During this time, some dark blood continues to pass out through the cervix and vagina.

In some cases, bleeding can be the first sign of an impending miscarriage (see the next section for more information). In this case, the bleeding often accompanies abdominal cramping. However, keep in mind that the vast majority of women who experience bleeding go on to have a completely normal pregnancy.

If you notice some bleeding, let your practitioner know. If the bleeding is a small amount and not associated with a lot of abdominal cramping, it isn't an emergency. However, if you're bleeding very heavily (much more than a period), call your practitioner as soon as you can. She may want to do an ultrasound and perform a pelvic exam to investigate the cause of the bleeding and see whether the pregnancy is still viable and located inside the uterus. Most of the time, your practitioner can do very little about the bleeding. Some doctors may suggest that you rest at home for a few days and avoid exercise and sex. No scientific data supports these instructions, but given that no really good alternatives exist, they certainly don't hurt.

Miscarriage

The great majority of pregnancies proceed normally. But about one in five ends in early miscarriage, often before a woman even knows she's pregnant. If a miscarriage occurs early in a pregnancy, you may mistake it for a regular menstrual period. About half the time, chromosomal abnormalities in the embryo cause the miscarriage. In another 20 percent of cases, the embryo may have structural defects that are too small to be detectable by ultrasound or pathological examination. *Note:* Having one miscarriage doesn't mean that you have an increased chance of it happening again. Also, no routine everyday activities can cause a miscarriage.

Miscarriage may lead to cramping and bleeding. You may feel abdominal pains that are stronger than menstrual cramps, and you may pass fetal and placental tissue. In cases where all the tissue is passed, your practitioner doesn't need to do anything

else. Often, though, some tissue remains in your uterus, and you may need medication to encourage its passing or have a D&C *(dilation and curettage)* procedure, designed to empty the uterus. Your doctor dilates, or gently opens, the cervix with surgical instruments and then empties the remaining contents of the uterus with a suction device and/or a scraping of the uterus. A D&C can be performed either in the doctor's office or in an operating suite, depending on the doctor, the gestational age, and any other important medical problems.

Sometimes, you may have no overt signs of miscarriage. Your practitioner may discover during a routine prenatal visit that the fetus is no longer alive, which is known as a *missed abortion.* If you have a missed abortion very early in your pregnancy, a D&C may not be necessary. But if it happens later in the first trimester, you may need to have a D&C to reduce the risk of heavy bleeding or incomplete passage of tissue. Depending on your obstetrical history and your desire to try to determine the cause of the miscarriage, you may decide to have the tissue sent for genetic analysis (to find out whether the chromosomes were normal or abnormal). Because half of all miscarriages are due to chromosomal abnormalities, it may be useful to find out whether this was the cause.

 Unfortunately, most miscarriages can't be prevented. Many, if not most, of them may simply be nature's way of handling an abnormal pregnancy. However, having a miscarriage doesn't mean that you can't have a perfectly normal pregnancy in the future. In fact, even in women who have had two consecutive miscarriages, the chances are very good (about 70 percent) that the next pregnancy will be successful without any special treatment.

 Any woman who experiences two or three consecutive miscarriages *may* have some underlying condition that can be identified and possibly treated. She should have a complete physical examination and undergo special tests to look for causes. Some women who have even one miscarriage may want to be examined. If you miscarry, discuss with your practitioner the possibility of undergoing certain tests or sending fetal or placental tissue to a laboratory for chromosomal analysis.

Ectopic pregnancy

An *ectopic pregnancy* occurs when the fertilized egg implants outside the uterus — in one of the fallopian tubes, the ovary, the abdomen, or the cervix. An ectopic pregnancy is a serious

threat to the mother's health. Fortunately, ultrasound has advanced to the point that it can detect ectopic pregnancies very early.

Signs of an ectopic pregnancy that you may notice include vaginal bleeding, abdominal pain, pelvic pain, dizziness, and feeling faint. You may not have any symptoms, in which case your doctor identifies the condition during an ultrasound. Your doctor can treat the problem in one of several ways, depending on the location of the embryo or fetus, how far along the pregnancy is, and the particular symptoms you are experiencing. Unfortunately, a doctor can't move the embryo or fetus to the uterus so that the pregnancy can continue as normal.

For Partners: Reacting to the News

"Honey, I think I'm pregnant!" You hear the words that millions of other partners before you have heard and you feel pure joy and excitement. Well, you probably also feel some concern, even fear, for the future. Rest assured that these feelings are completely normal. You may be concerned about how parenthood may change your relationship with your partner, or change your life in general. You may worry that you and your partner won't be able to support a family financially, or that you won't be a good parent. Just keep in mind that your partner's feelings about having a baby aren't all that different. She's probably having a few worries herself. So talk to her about what you're both feeling.

A woman's role in pregnancy is undoubtedly pivotal, but, biologically speaking, she can't do it alone. If you're the dad, your part is vital, too, right from the start. Your sperm's DNA provides half the baby's total DNA. And your share of DNA determines the baby's sex. If you donate an X chromosome, it's a girl; if you hand in a Y, it's a boy. (A woman's egg always contains an X chromosome.)

Supporting the mother during pregnancy is very important. Just as pregnancy is a time of tremendous change in a woman's body, so is it a time of tremendous emotional change for both the partner and mother, and it's a time of transition for

you as a couple — a transition to parenthood. Recognizing this fact can make it easier for you to become comfortable with the whole process and play your role as well as possible.

After both of you get over the initial surprise, you're faced with the realities of pregnancy during the first trimester. Your partner is likely to feel exceptionally tired and may need to urinate with remarkable frequency. Chances are she also has morning sickness (see the earlier section, "Any-time-of-day sickness"). You can be supportive by doing the following:

✔ **Assume more of the day-to-day responsibilities of running the household.** (Yes, that means cleaning the house, doing some laundry, washing the dishes, and even cooking.)

✔ **Give her the extra time she needs to rest.** A catnap here and there can make a world of difference, but sometimes she may need to hibernate for a few hours when the fatigue gets really rough.

✔ **Be aware of what a drag it can be to be nauseated all the time.** Don't get too upset if she can't stand to be around steak (your favorite) or some other food.

✔ **Go out of your way to help her.** If she asks you to run out for more pickles and ketchup at midnight (Joanne's favorite first-trimester snack), just smile and ask, "Whole or slices?" "Dill or gherkins?"

✔ **Try to make room in your schedule to accompany your partner to her first prenatal visit to her practitioner.** Your participation is important not only because it tele-graphs your support, but also because you may need to answer questions about your family medical history. In addition, you probably have questions to ask the practitioner.

You can make life easier for both of you. Studies clearly show that pregnancy, labor, and delivery are associated with fewer complications when the partner is involved and supportive.

Chapter 6

The Second Trimester

*T*he second trimester, which encompasses the three months between weeks 13 and 26, is often the most enjoyable part of pregnancy. The feelings of nausea and fatigue so common during the first trimester are usually gone, and you feel more energetic and comfortable. The second trimester is a very exciting time because you can feel the baby moving within you and you're finally starting to show. During the second trimester, blood tests, prenatal tests, and ultrasound (sonogram) can confirm that the baby is healthy and growing normally. And many women find they can finally grasp the concept that they'll soon be having a baby. The second trimester is often the time you start sharing the exciting news with family, friends, and co-workers.

Discovering How Your Baby Is Developing

Your baby grows rapidly during the second trimester, as you can see in Figure 6-1. The fetus measures about 3 inches (8 centimeters) long at 13 weeks. By 26 weeks, it's about 14 inches (35 centimeters) and weighs about 2¼ pounds (1,022 grams). Somewhere between weeks 14 and 16, the limbs begin to elongate and start to look like arms and legs. Coordinated arm and leg movements are observable on ultrasound, too. Between 18 and 22 weeks, you may begin to feel fetal movements, although they don't necessarily occur regularly throughout the day.

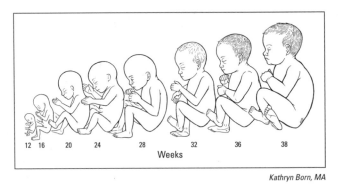

Figure 6-1: Notice that during the second trimester (13–26 weeks), your baby grows and develops at an astounding rate.

The baby's head, which was large in relation to the body during the first trimester, becomes more proportional as the body catches up. The bones solidify and are recognizable on ultrasound. Early in the second trimester, the fetus looks something like an alien (think E.T.), but by 26 weeks, it looks much more like a human baby.

The fetus also performs many recognizable activities. It not only moves, but also undergoes regular periods of sleeping and wakefulness and can hear and swallow. Lung development increases markedly between 20 and 25 weeks. By 24 weeks, lung cells begin to secrete *surfactant,* a chemical substance that enables the lungs to stay expanded. Between 26 and 28 weeks, the eyes — which had been fused shut — open, and hair (called *lanugo*) appears on the head and body. Fat deposits form under the skin, and the central nervous system matures dramatically.

At 23 to 24 weeks, the fetus is considered *viable,* which means that if it were born at this time, it would have a chance of surviving in a center with a neonatal unit experienced in caring for very premature babies. A premature baby born at 28 weeks (nearly three months early) and cared for in an intensive care unit has an excellent chance of survival.

Most mothers begin to feel their babies move at about this time. Knowing for sure when you first feel your baby moving inside you is difficult. Many women sense fluttering movements (called *quickening*) at about 16 to 20 weeks. Not every woman can tell that sensation is actually the baby moving. Some think it's just gas (and maybe you *did* eat too much

chili) — but most likely, it's the baby. Around 20 to 22 weeks, the fetal movements are much easier to identify, but they still aren't consistent. Over the course of the next four weeks, they fall into a more regular pattern.

Different babies have different movement patterns. You may notice your baby tends to move more at night — perhaps to prepare you for all the sleepless nights you'll have after he is born! Or you may simply be more aware of the baby's movements at night because you're more sedentary at that time. If this is your second (or third or fourth . . .) child, you may start to feel movements a couple of weeks earlier.

Clothing yourself in maternity garb

Thank goodness the fashion industry has recognized that women continue to care about looking chic and professional when they're pregnant — which doesn't necessarily mean wearing those choir-boy blouses with big bows at the neck. Many women look forward to shopping for maternity clothes, while others aim to stay in their usual clothes for as long as possible. Keep in mind that you're only going to need maternity clothes for a few months, and they're not cheap. Here are a few suggestions:

✔ Don't plan too far ahead; buy clothes only as you need them. Anticipating how big you'll become and whether you'll carry the baby high up in your belly or down low is difficult. When you do shop, buy clothes that fit comfortably but have enough room to accommodate further growth.

✔ Don't be shy about accepting hand-me-downs. Women rarely wear out their maternity clothes.

Your friends are probably happy to see their clothes get more use.

✔ Look for consignment shops, secondhand stores, and garage sales. They're good places to find inexpensive maternity clothes.

✔ If you have trouble finding maternity clothes in your style, remember that you can often go a long way through your pregnancy in regular leggings and big shirts or sweaters. (Joanne never had to buy any maternity clothes at all.)

✔ Perhaps the most important items to buy are comfortable shoes and roomier bras. Both shoe size and bra size can increase during pregnancy.

✔ You don't have to wear special maternity underwear — unless you find it especially comfortable. Many kinds of regular underwear, especially the bikini kind, fit well under a bulging belly.

If you haven't felt your baby move at all by 22 weeks, let your practitioner know. He may recommend an ultrasound, especially if you haven't had one already, to check the baby. A common explanation for not feeling the baby's movements is that the placenta is implanted on the anterior (front) wall of the uterus between the baby and your skin. The placenta acts as a cushion and delays the time when you first feel movements.

After 26 to 28 weeks, if you stop feeling the baby move as much as usual, call your practitioner. By 28 weeks, you should feel movement at least six times an hour after you eat dinner. If you aren't sure whether the baby is moving normally, lie down on your left side and count the movements. If the baby moves — any movement counts — at least six times in an hour, be reassured that the baby is okay. On the other hand, if you feel that the baby's movements are still less than they should be, call your practitioner.

Understanding Your Changing Body

By 12 weeks, your uterus begins to rise out of your pelvis. Your practitioner can feel the top of the uterus through your abdominal wall. By 20 weeks, the top of your uterus reaches the level of your navel. Then each week, your uterus grows by about one centimeter (½ inch). Your doctor may run a tape measure from your pubic bone to the top of your uterus to measure the *fundal height* (see Chapter 3) to see that your uterus and the baby are growing appropriately. Many women begin to show at 16 weeks, although looking pregnant varies a great deal. Some women look pregnant at 12 weeks; others aren't obvious until 28 weeks.

Many of the changes you experience have little to do with your belly's size. Rather, they involve your baby's development and your body's continuing adaptation to pregnancy. You may experience some, none, or all the symptoms in this section.

Forgetfulness and clumsiness

Until she was pregnant, Joanne never would have believed that misplacing keys, bumping into furniture, and dropping things could be real side effects of pregnancy. We don't know

of any medical explanation for these effects, but some women do feel they're more scatterbrained and clumsy. If it happens to you, don't worry. You're not losing your mind. Look at it this way: Now you have an excuse for having forgotten your best friend's birthday. And rest assured you'll go back to being your brilliant, coordinated self after your baby is born.

Gas

You may find that you develop the annoying and embarrassing tendency to burp and pass gas at inopportune times during this trimester. (Now you can duel it out with your husband.) If it's any consolation, you're not the first pregnant woman to run into this problem. Unfortunately, though, you can do very little about it — besides getting a dog to blame it on. Try to avoid becoming constipated (see Chapter 5) because that can make things worse. Also avoid eating large meals that may leave you feeling bloated and uncomfortable or foods that you know make the problem even worse.

Hair and nail growth

While you're pregnant, your fingernails and toenails may become stronger than they've ever been before and grow at an unprecedented rate. Manicures are safe when done in a reputable, clean salon and often relieve stress, so sit back and enjoy your beautiful nails!

Pregnancy also speeds up hair growth. Unfortunately, some women find hair also begins growing in unusual places — on their face or stomach, for example. Waxing, plucking, or shaving the unwanted hair is safe, but hair removal creams (depilatories) contain chemicals that haven't been extensively studied. Because safer alternatives are readily available, we suggest avoiding these creams. Take comfort in the likelihood that the unwanted hair will disappear after your baby is born.

Heartburn

Heartburn — the burning sensation you feel when stomach acids rise into your esophagus — is common during pregnancy. Heartburn has two basic causes (neither of which

validates the myth that heartburn means your baby will have a lot of hair). First, the high level of progesterone your body is producing can slow digestion and relax the sphincter muscle between the esophagus and the stomach, which normally prevents the upward movement of stomach acids. Second, as the uterus grows, it presses upward on the stomach, which can push stomach acids into the esophagus. (See Figure 6-2.)

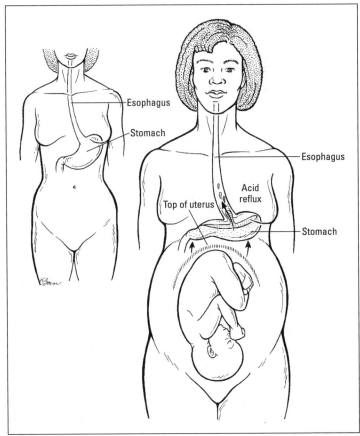

Esophagus

Stomach

Esophagus

Acid reflux

Top of uterus

Stomach

Kathryn Born, MA

Figure 6-2: As your baby grows, your uterus expands, pushing upward on your stomach and esophagus, sometimes leading to heartburn.

You may get relief from heartburn by following these suggestions:

✔ Eat small, frequent meals rather than large ones.

✔ Carry an antacid when you're away from home.

✔ Carry a package of dry crackers to munch on when you feel heartburn. They may neutralize the gas.

✔ Avoid spicy, fatty, and greasy foods.

✔ Avoid large amounts of soda, caffeine, and coffee.

✔ Avoid eating just before bedtime, because heartburn occurs most readily when you lie down. Also, try sleeping with your head elevated on several pillows.

✔ If your heartburn becomes intolerable, talk to your doctor about taking a prescription treatment. Many effective heartburn treatments are considered safe for use during pregnancy. The use of famotidine (Pepsid), ranitidine (Zantac), and omeprazole (Prilosec/Nexium) in the first trimester has been studied, and researchers found no increased risk for birth defects, preterm labor, or problems with fetal growth. (The first trimester is the period of greatest risk, so medications proven safe for use in the first trimester are presumably safe in the second trimester, too.)

Lower abdominal/groin pain

Between 18 and 24 weeks, you may feel a sharp pain or a dull ache near your groin on either or both sides. When you move quickly or stand, you may notice it worsen, and it may fade if you lie down. This pain is called *round ligament pain*. The round ligaments are bands of fibrous tissue on each side of the uterus that attach the top of the uterus to the labia. The pain occurs because as the uterus grows, the ligaments stretch. The pain can be quite uncomfortable and sometimes can stop you in your tracks, but it's normal. The good news is that it usually goes away — or at least lessens considerably — after 24 weeks.

Sometime in the middle of the second trimester (the exact time varies), you may start to feel mild, short-lived contractions or cramps. These are referred to as *Braxton-Hicks contractions* and

are nothing to worry about. They often are more noticeable when you're walking or physically active and then go away when you get off your feet. If they become uncomfortable and regular (more than six in an hour), call your practitioner.

Nasal congestion

The increased blood flow that occurs during pregnancy can also cause stuffiness and some swelling of the mucous membranes inside your nose. This, in turn, can lead to postnasal drip and, ultimately, a chronic cough. Nasal saline drops may provide some relief and are perfectly safe to use during pregnancy. Keeping the air in your home or office well humidified also helps. Nasal sprays and decongestants work, too, but avoid using these medications for more than a few days at a time. You (or your partner, especially) may notice that suddenly you're snoring like never before! This common symptom again relates to the increase in nasal congestion. Our advice? Buy your partner a good set of earplugs!

Nosebleeds and bleeding gums

Because of the higher volume of blood coursing through your body to support your pregnancy, you may experience some bleeding from small blood vessels in your nose and gums. This bleeding usually stops by itself, but you can help by applying slight pressure to the point of bleeding. If bleeding becomes particularly heavy or frequent, call your doctor.

Using a softer toothbrush may help to minimize bleeding when you brush your teeth.

Skin changes

The hormones coursing through your body at soaring levels may make strange things happen to your skin. These changes, illustrated in Figure 6-3, don't occur in all women, and if they do happen to you, rest assured they usually fade away after the baby is born.

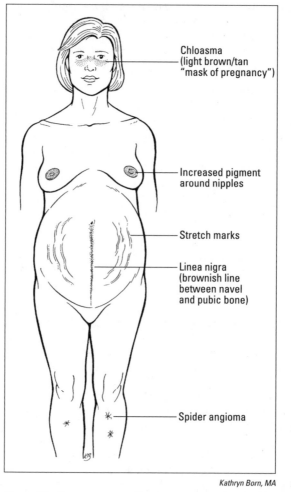

Chloasma
(light brown/tan
"mask of pregnancy")

Increased pigment
around nipples

Stretch marks

Linea nigra
(brownish line
between navel
and pubic bone)

Spider angioma

Kathryn Born, MA

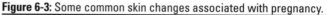

Figure 6-3: Some common skin changes associated with pregnancy.

✔ You may notice a dark line, called the *linea nigra,* on your lower abdomen running from your pubic bone up to your navel. This line may be more noticeable in women with relatively dark skin. Fair-skinned women often don't develop this line at all.

✔ The skin on your face may also darken in a masklike distribution around your cheeks, nose, and eyes. This darkening is called *chloasma* or the *mask of pregnancy.* Sun exposure makes it even darker. Use a facial cream with sun block to minimize the effects of the sun on chloasma.

✔ Red spots, called *spider angiomas,* may suddenly appear anywhere on your body. Press on them, and they probably turn white. These spots are concentrations of blood vessels caused by the high level of estrogen in your body. They'll probably disappear after delivery.

✔ Some women notice a reddish coloring on the palms of their hands. Known as *palmar erythema,* this coloring is another estrogen effect, and it, too, will go away.

✔ *Skin tags* (small, benign skin growths) are also a common occurrence, although it isn't totally clear why they develop. Fortunately, they, too, fade away or disappear after pregnancy. Because they're likely to resolve in time, you don't need to rush to the dermatologist to have them removed, unless they're really bothersome.

Checking In: Prenatal Visits

In the second trimester, you're likely to see your practitioner about once every four weeks. At each visit, he checks your weight, your blood pressure, your urine, and the fetal heart rate. You may want to bring up any questions you have about fetal movement, childbirth classes, your weight gain, and any unusual symptoms or discomforts you may have.

As your baby grows and changes, so does the range and scope of possible prenatal tests. In the second trimester, you will likely undergo a blood test or two, and an ultrasound for a general scan of your baby's anatomy, growth, and well-being. At this point, you can also find out the sex of your baby. Amniocentesis may also be performed in the second trimester. This section outlines the different tests you may undergo.

Second-trimester blood tests

The following blood tests usually yield normal results, but if yours are at all unusual, you may need further testing — an ultrasound examination, perhaps. But keep in mind that further testing doesn't necessarily mean that anything is wrong — only that your practitioner is being careful to ensure that everything is okay.

Alpha-fetoprotein screen

MSAFP stands for *maternal serum alpha-fetoprotein,* a protein made by the fetus that also circulates in the mother's bloodstream. Doctors use a simple blood test to check the level of MSAFP, usually sometime between 15 and 18 weeks. The test result is affected by weight, race, and preexisting diabetes, so it has to be adjusted for those factors. An elevated MSAFP is expressed as more than 2.0 or 2.5 *multiples of the median,* or MOMs, for women carrying only one baby and more than 4.0 or 4.5 MOMs for mothers of twins. (In triplets and quadruplets, the measurement hasn't been well studied.)

Abnormal MSAFP can usually indicate whether a pregnancy is at risk for certain complications and *may* indicate

- ✔ Underestimation of the fetus's age (how far along you are)

- ✔ The presence of twins or more

- ✔ Bleeding that may have occurred earlier in the pregnancy

- ✔ Neural tube defects (spina bifida, anencephaly, and others — see the following sidebar, "Understanding neural tube defects")

- ✔ Abdominal wall defects (protrusion of the fetus's abdominal contents through a defect in the abdominal wall)

- ✔ Rh disease (see Chapter 14) or other conditions associated with *fetal edema* (abnormal fluid collection in the fetus)

- ✔ Increased risk for low birth weight, preeclampsia, or other complications (see Chapter 14)

- ✔ A rare fetal kidney condition known as *congenital nephrosis*

- ✔ Fetal death

- ✔ Other fetal abnormalities

Remember that the MSAFP test is only a screening test. Most women with an elevated MSAFP have a normal fetus and continue to have a completely normal pregnancy. Only about 5 percent of women with a positive maternal serum screen actually have a fetus with a neural tube defect. On the other hand, the test isn't perfect, and therefore it can't identify all abnormal fetuses. To reduce the risk of getting a false positive result (that is, an abnormal test result but a normal fetus), a

positive test should be repeated (especially if it's only mildly elevated or under 3.0 MOMs), and an ultrasound should be performed to confirm the fetus's age. If a test comes back elevated a second time or if it's greater than 3.0 MOMs on the first screen, a detailed ultrasound exam should be done to look for any detectable abnormalities.

Understanding neural tube defects

The baby's central nervous system begins as a flat sheet of cells that rolls up into a tube as it matures. The front of the tube, which closes at about day 23 of life, becomes the brain. The other end of the tube, which closes at about day 28 of life, becomes the lower end of the spinal cord. If either end fails to close for some reason (nobody knows why it sometimes doesn't), a neural tube defect occurs. The most common neural tube defects are *spina bifida* (an opening in the spine), *anencephaly* (absence of the skull), and *encephalocele* (an opening in the skull). These defects cause abnormalities in the nervous system such as paralysis, extra fluid in the brain, or mental retardation. Fetuses with anencephaly usually don't survive more than a few days after birth.

This all sounds pretty scary, but fortunately, these defects are rare. We discuss these defects because screening programs are available in most countries to help identify those fetuses that may have one of these defects, and because you can follow recommendations to reduce the likelihood of having a baby with a neural tube defect — by taking folic acid before you conceive, for example, and by getting your blood sugar under control if you have diabetes.

In the United States, a neural tube defect occurs about once in every 1,000 babies born. The incidence in the United Kingdom is higher: 4 to 8 cases in every 1,000 babies. In Japan, the incidence is quite low, at about 1 case per 2,000 babies. No one knows exactly why the incidence varies among countries, but it has something to do with the interaction between the environment and one's genetic makeup. If you or your baby's father has a family history of neural tube defects, let your practitioner know at your first visit, because that slightly raises your risk of having a baby with a neural tube defect, and you can discuss your options for prenatal diagnosis (ultrasound or amniocentesis). Also, if you had a previous pregnancy in which a neural tube defect was diagnosed or if you have a family history of this condition, increase the amount of folic acid you take at the beginning of pregnancy to 4 mg per day. The earlier in pregnancy you start taking it, the better it is at preventing neural tube defects.

If you have two elevated MSAFP tests, a very high single test, or a questionable ultrasound for spine and head defects, you may want to have an amniocentesis to check the level of AFP in the amniotic fluid (see the "Testing with amniocentesis" section later in this chapter). Your practitioner can also check the amniotic fluid for a substance called *acetylcholinesterase,* which is present if the fetus has an open neural tube defect (see the previous "Understanding neural tube defects" sidebar). In most cases, the amniotic fluid AFP is negative and the pregnancy continues normally. Some studies suggest, however, that women who have an abnormal MSAFP and then a normal amniotic fluid AFP *may* be at risk for preterm delivery, low birth-weight babies, or hypertension. If you fit the pattern, your doctor may suggest that you and your baby be closely observed, either with ultrasound or with other tests of fetal well-being, such as non-stress tests (see Chapter 7). Specific protocols for fetal monitoring vary from doctor to doctor.

The quadruple test for Down syndrome

Another test that can be performed with the same sample of blood that's used for the MSAFP during the second trimester is a screening test for Down syndrome — the most common chromosomal abnormality in babies. This test can also help identify women at risk of having babies with other chromosomal abnormalities, like *Trisomy 18* or *Trisomy 13* (an extra copy of either the number 18 or 13 chromosome). These particular chromosomal abnormalities are associated with severe birth defects, and are often not compatible with life.

Your practitioner performs this test by measuring four substances in the blood:

- ✔ MSAFP
- ✔ hCG (human chorionic gonadotropin)
- ✔ Estriol (a form of estrogen)
- ✔ Inhibin A (a substance secreted by the placenta)

Your practitioner uses the results of these tests to calculate risk for Down syndrome. In women under the age of 35, the test detects Down syndrome in about 80 percent of the cases where it's present. (In other words, if 100 women carrying fetuses with Down syndrome had the test, the condition would be diagnosed in about 80 of them.) This test is only a screening, so even if the result is abnormal, the fetus is normal in the

majority of cases. If your test is abnormal, your practitioner will discuss with you the possibility of having an amniocentesis to check the baby's chromosomes. The quad test often combined with the first-trimester tests described earlier (see Chapter 5) to improve the detection of Down syndrome.

 Unlike the screen for neural tube defects, which yields a high MSAFP and is often repeated when abnormal, the screens for Down syndrome should *not* be repeated, because doing so will only provide a less accurate result.

Cell-free fetal DNA

If abnormalities are suspected on your baby's ultrasound, your doctor may recommend sending off a sample of your blood to check the baby's chromosomes. This test examines the cell-free fetal DNA that circulates in your blood and is the same test that was discussed in Chapter 5.

Glucose screen

The *glucose screen* is a test to identify women who may have gestational diabetes. Your practitioner conducts the test by first having you drink a super-sweet-tasting glucose mixture (it tastes like flat soda) and then, exactly one hour later, drawing a sample of blood. He checks this sample for the level of glucose (sugar). High levels indicate that you're at risk for gestational diabetes. We discuss why treating gestational diabetes is important in Chapter 15.

The one-hour screening test is usually performed between 24 and 28 weeks, though some doctors do it twice — once early in the pregnancy and again at 24 to 28 weeks. About 25 percent of obstetricians test only those women who are at risk for gestational diabetes. The risk factors, which follow, are broad, and about 50 percent of all pregnant women have one of them:

- Maternal age greater than 25 years
- Previous birth of a large infant
- Previous unexplained fetal death
- Previous pregnancy with gestational diabetes
- Strong family history of diabetes
- Obesity

If your initial glucose screening test is abnormal, you don't necessarily have gestational diabetes. (Remember, it's only a screening test.) Only about 5 percent of pregnant women actually develop gestational diabetes (although 15 percent may screen positive). Your practitioner will recommend another test that tells whether gestational diabetes is really present. This three-hour test involves drawing blood after you fast overnight, having you drink a different glucose mixture, and then drawing blood three more times, at one, two, and three hours later. Some practitioners recommend eating an extra helping of pasta or rice for the three days before the test (called *carbohydrate loading*) in order to get your body ready for the test.

A test is considered *positive* — or abnormal — if two (or more) of the four blood levels are in the abnormal range. If you test positive for gestational diabetes, your doctor will put you on a special diet and check your glucose levels throughout the remainder of your pregnancy. If you have elevated glucose levels despite adhering to this special diet, you may need to be on insulin or an oral medication to keep your sugars well controlled. (See Chapter 15 for more on this topic.)

Complete blood count (CBC)

Many obstetricians check a complete blood count at the same time that they do your glucose test in order to see whether you've developed significant *anemia* (iron deficiency) or a variety of other less-common problems. Anemia is common during pregnancy, and some women need to take extra iron. A CBC also gives your physician a *platelet count,* which is a blood factor that helps with clotting.

"Looking" at sound waves: Ultrasound

An *ultrasound* (also referred to as a *sonogram*) exam is an incredibly useful tool that allows you and your doctor to see the baby inside your uterus. A device called a *transducer* emits sound waves. The sound waves are reflected off the fetus and converted into an image that appears on a monitor. (See sonogram photos in Chapter 19.) You can see almost all the structures in the fetus's body, and you can see the fetus moving around and performing all its normal activities — kicking, waving, and so on. The best time to view the baby's anatomy is around 18 to 22 weeks.

An ultrasound exam doesn't hurt. Your practitioner spreads gel or lotion over your abdomen, and then moves the transducer around through the gel (see Figure 6-4). A full bladder isn't necessary because the amniotic fluid surrounding the fetus provides the liquid needed to transmit the sound waves to create a clear or detailed picture. Picture quality varies, depending on maternal fat, scar tissue, and the fetus's position.

A doctor (an obstetrician, a perinatologist, or a radiologist) or an ultrasound technologist may perform the ultrasound. Sometimes a technologist does a preliminary exam, and the doctor comes in later to check on images or review the printed pictures.

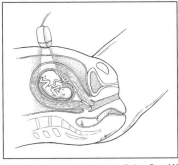

Kathryn Born, MA

Figure 6-4: An ultrasound test being performed during the second trimester.

What an ultrasound can reveal

Ultrasound is like a checkup for the fetus. It can provide information about the following:

- ✔ Number of babies
- ✔ Gestational age
- ✔ Rate of fetal growth
- ✔ Fetal position, movement, and breathing exercises (the fetus moves its chest and abdomen as if it were breathing air)
- ✔ Fetal heart rate

✔ Amount of amniotic fluid

✔ Location of placenta

✔ General fetal anatomy, including the identification of some birth defects

✔ The baby's sex (after 15 to 16 weeks), although depending on the position of the fetus, the sex may be difficult to visualize

Typically, the examiner measures the fetus first and then studies its anatomy. The extent and degree of detail of the exam varies from woman to woman and doctor to doctor. A detailed ultrasound can examine these structures:

✔ Arms and legs

✔ Bladder

✔ Brain and skull

✔ Face

✔ Genitalia

✔ Heart, chest cavity, and diaphragm

✔ Kidneys

✔ Spine

✔ Stomach, abdominal cavity, and abdominal wall

Expectant mothers ask . . .

Q: "Is ultrasound safe?"

A: The technology has been in widespread use for more than 40 years, and overwhelmingly most studies show no harmful consequences for the baby or mom. In addition, the information provided by an ultrasound examination has been shown to have many health benefits. For example, certain conditions (such as bladder outlet obstruction) may be treated during the pregnancy, and diagnosis of others (such as a congenital heart defect) allow for careful planning for delivery. Detection of problems with fetal growth or amniotic fluid volume lets your doctor know that close surveillance of the pregnancy may be indicated.

Reasons for having an ultrasound

Whether and how often you need an ultrasound depends on your particular risk factors, your doctor's preferences, and your insurance coverage. Some doctors recommend that all women have an ultrasound exam at about 20 weeks; others feel that it's unnecessary if your risks for having problems are low. Multiple ultrasound examinations may be needed if any of the following conditions arise:

- ✔ You're carrying twins or more.

- ✔ Your doctor suspects that the baby is too small or too large for its age.

- ✔ Your doctor suspects that you have too little or too much amniotic fluid.

- ✔ You're at risk for preterm labor or incompetent cervix (see later in this chapter and Chapter 14).

- ✔ You have diabetes, hypertension, or other underlying medical conditions (see Chapter 15).

- ✔ You're bleeding.

- ✔ Your doctor wants to do a *biophysical profile,* which is an assessment of fetal well-being that looks at movement, breathing exercises, amniotic fluid volume, and fetal tone (ability to flex the muscles).

3-D and 4-D ultrasound

Most perinatal ultrasound centers now have special machines with the capability of showing three-dimensional images of the fetus, known as 3-D ultrasound. 4-D ultrasound is similar, but instead of seeing a still (static) 3-D picture, you can see the fetus move. These high-tech ultrasound machines aren't available everywhere, and no medical data has shown that a 3-D or 4-D ultrasound is better at detecting problems than the usual 2-D image. However, you may see certain features in the fetus better, such as the face, hands, and feet. Also, many women experience a real bonding with the fetus, seeing it three-dimensionally. If a 3-D or 4-D ultrasound is available, you may enjoy and benefit from the experience. If not, don't feel bad — you'll have the baby — all four dimensions of it — in real life soon enough.

Recently, doctors have also used ultrasound to get an accurate measurement of the *cervix* (the uterus's opening) in women at risk for preterm delivery or incompetent cervix. Your practitioner places a transducer in the vagina to measure the cervix's length and check the appearance of the lower part of the uterus.

Testing with amniocentesis

Amniocentesis is a test that is performed by inserting a thin, hollow needle into the amniotic fluid and then withdrawing some of the fluid through the needle into a syringe (see Figure 6-5). The amniotic fluid can then be tested in a variety of ways. If your practitioner performs a *genetic amniocentesis* — a check of fetal chromosomes — he usually conducts it at 15 to 20 weeks. Your practitioner may perform amniocentesis for other reasons, like checking for lung maturity in the baby, at any time later in the pregnancy.

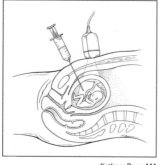

Kathryn Born, MA

Figure 6-5: An amniocentesis procedure.

During the amniocentesis procedure, you lie flat on your back on top of a table. Your doctor cleans your abdomen with an iodine solution. Using ultrasound to locate an area of amniotic fluid that is away from the baby, your doctor inserts a thin needle through your abdomen and uterus into the amniotic sac. After withdrawing enough amniotic fluid (usually about 15 to 20 cc, or 1 to 2 tablespoons), he removes the needle.

A common misconception is that the needle is inserted through the navel. The exact point of insertion depends on where the fetus, the placenta, and the amniotic sac are located within the

uterus. You may have heard that the amniocentesis needle is exceptionally long, and you may be afraid of long needles. But the needle's length, which enables it to reach the amniotic sac, doesn't make it painful. A needle's thickness determines how uncomfortable it is, and an amniocentesis needle is very thin.

The procedure typically lasts no longer than one to two minutes, but it may seem like an eternity to an anxious woman. It's mildly uncomfortable but not terribly painful. Many women feel a slight, brief cramping sensation as the needle goes into the uterus and then a weird pulling sensation as the fluid is withdrawn through the needle. Some women worry about moving too much during an amniocentesis. This usually isn't a problem. If you really are flinching or moving too much, your doctor will let you know. Also, it's a common misconception that the risk of an amniocentesis is that the needle may hurt the baby. You don't really need to worry that the needle will hurt the baby. Your doctor will place the needle in a place well away from the baby. Sometimes, however, a fetus may actually move towards the needle, but this doesn't cause any harm. Your doctor will simply reposition the needle in a safe place and wait for the baby to stop moving.

Having an amniocentesis performed isn't altogether pain-free, but most women report that it isn't as bad as they expected it to be. Afterward, your doctor may advise you to rest and avoid strenuous activity and sex for one to two days. Most women cramp a bit the day of the procedure, which is expected and normal.

A genetic amniocentesis primarily tests to see that 23 chromosome pairs are present and that their structure is normal. It doesn't routinely test for all possible genetic diseases or birth defects. The amniotic fluid cells must be incubated before your doctor can read the results of a genetic amniocentesis. Results are usually available in one to two weeks.

If prenatal blood studies show that you're Rh-negative, your doctor will give you an injection of Rh-D immune globulin (Rhogam and Rhophylac are two examples currently on the market), which helps prevent Rh sensitization.

Risks and side effects of amniocentesis

Not all patients have these symptoms or problems after an amniocentesis, but remember that they can occur:

✔ **Cramping:** Some women experience cramping for several hours after the procedure. The best treatment for this cramping is rest. Some practitioners recommend a single glass of wine to help ease the discomfort.

✔ **Spotting:** This may last one to two days.

✔ **Amniotic fluid leak:** A leakage of 1 to 2 teaspoons of fluid through the vagina occurs in 1 to 2 percent of patients. In the great majority of these cases, the membrane seals over within 48 hours. Leakage stops and the pregnancy continues normally. If you experience a large amount of leakage or persistent leakage, call your doctor.

✔ **Fetal injury:** Injury to the fetus is extremely rare, given the use of ultrasound guidance.

✔ **Miscarriage:** Although amniocentesis is considered very safe, it's still invasive and is associated with a small risk of pregnancy loss. Recent studies have shown that the risk of pregnancy loss after amniocentesis is much less than the 0.5 percent risk previously quoted and is probably closer to about 1 in 1,000.

Your decision to undergo the procedure must weigh both risks and benefits, which vary according to the individual. For example, a 40-year-old woman with a history of infertility may not want to undergo any test that carries an increased risk of miscarriage, even though she stands a higher risk of carrying a fetus with a chromosomal abnormality. On the other hand, a 32-year-old maternal-fetal medicine specialist who sees patients with a multitude of problems every day — we're thinking of Joanne during her first pregnancy — may opt to undergo an amniocentesis even though her risk of having a fetus with a chromosomal abnormality is relatively low — lower, in fact, than her risk of miscarriage because of the test. The peace of mind may be worth the small increased risk of miscarriage.

An amniocentesis performed later in the pregnancy — later than 20 weeks — doesn't carry the same increased risk of miscarriage. It carries only a very small risk of infection, rupture of membranes (breaking the water), or onset of labor.

Reasons for having an amniocentesis

Your practitioner may recommend a genetic amniocentesis for the following conditions or situations:

✔ Your age is 35 or more at your due date (even though the recommendations have changed, as mentioned earlier, some practitioners still recommend amniocentesis for all women over the age of 35). This age recommendation also depends on the number of babies you're carrying. For example, if you're carrying twins, your practitioner may offer an amniocentesis at age 33.

✔ You had an elevated MSAFP (see the "Alpha-fetoprotein screen" section earlier in this chapter).

✔ You had abnormal results from Down syndrome screening (during either your first or second trimester).

✔ Your ultrasound exam was abnormal, indicating, for example, poor fetal growth or suspected structural abnormalities.

✔ You had a previous child or previous pregnancy with a chromosomal abnormality.

✔ You're at risk of having a baby with a certain genetic disease.

✔ You and your partner have concerns and want to confirm that the chromosomes are normal.

Your practitioner may perform amniocentesis for other reasons:

✔ **Preterm labor:** An infection within the amniotic fluid may be a cause of preterm labor. Your practitioner can send the fluid to a lab for tests to look for any such infection. If an infection is present, your doctor may want to deliver your baby right away to minimize harm to you and the baby.

✔ **Other infections:** Some patients may find that they're at risk of developing infections such as toxoplasmosis, CMV (cytomegalovirus), or parvovirus (see Chapter 15). The amniotic fluid can be tested for evidence of such problems in patients at risk.

✔ **Rh sensitization:** Patients with Rh sensitization are sometimes monitored with a test known as *delta OD-450*, in which the amniotic fluid is examined for evidence of broken-down fetal red blood cells. However, currently, most doctors perform a special type of Doppler ultrasound called an MCA (middle cerebral artery) Doppler (see the "Doppler studies" section later in this chapter) to monitor the baby for this, but in case MCA Dopplers are not available in your area, amniocentesis to check the delta OD-450 will be used. See Chapter 14.

✔ **Lung maturity studies:** Sometimes your doctor needs to find out whether the fetus's lungs are mature enough for the baby to be delivered. Certain tests on the amniotic fluid can determine the maturity of the lungs.

Other prenatal tests and procedures

Not all the tests or procedures in this section are performed in all pregnancies — only when a specific problem is present. When needed, they are usually performed in the second or third trimester. In fact, most of these tests are rarely done and are usually done in centers that specialize in fetal medicine. They may sound scary, but we include them just to let you know what may be available if you develop a problem.

Fetal blood sampling

For fetal blood sampling — also known as *PUBS (percutaneous umbilical blood sampling)* or *cordocentesis* — a doctor withdraws fetal blood from the umbilical cord. This test lets your doctor obtain blood for rapid chromosomal diagnosis when time is critical, although testing cell-free fetal DNA in the mother's blood can also be used in this situation (see the "Cell-free fetal DNA" section earlier in this chapter). Your

doctor may perform this test in order to diagnose fetal infections, detect evidence of fetal anemia, or diagnose and treat a
condition called *nonimmune hydrops,* in which fluid accumulates abnormally in the fetus. A maternal-fetal medicine specialist performs the procedure under ultrasound guidance.
The procedure is similar to an amniocentesis, except that the
doctor directs the needle into the umbilical cord rather than
into the amniotic fluid. Risks are low but include infection,
rupture of the membranes, or fetal loss. (The risk of fetal loss
is about 1 percent.)

Some fetuses develop anemia, which can be treated *in utero*
(within the womb) with a blood transfusion directly into the
umbilical cord. Conditions that may lead to anemia include
certain infections (like parvovirus), genetic diseases, or certain blood group incompatibilities (see Chapter 14).

Fetal echocardiogram

A *fetal echocardiogram* is basically a sonogram focused on the
fetal heart. A maternal-fetal medicine specialist, a pediatric
cardiologist, or a radiologist usually performs this procedure.
You may need a fetal echo if you have a history of diabetes
or a family history of congenital heart disease, or if an ultrasound shows any signs of a heart abnormality. Sometimes
your practitioner recommends a fetal echo if he sees *any*
structural problem on ultrasound, because heart abnormalities are often associated with other birth defects.

Doppler studies

Ultrasound can be used to perform Doppler studies of fetal
and umbilical blood flow. These studies are a way of assessing blood flow to various organ systems and also within the
placenta. A Doppler study is sometimes used as a test of
well-being in fetuses with IUGR (intrauterine growth restriction). See Chapter 14 for more on IUGR. MCA Dopplers, as
mentioned in the "Reasons for having an amniocentesis" section earlier in this chapter, measure the blood flow through
a major blood vessel in the fetal brain and can detect fetuses
that may be anemic from an infection or a blood group
incompatibility.

Recognizing Causes for Concern

In this section, we talk about certain problems that can develop during the second trimester and symptoms that you should discuss with your practitioner.

Bleeding

Some women experience bleeding in the second trimester. Possible causes include a low-lying placenta *(placenta previa)*, premature labor, cervical incompetence, or placental abruption (all covered in Chapter 14). Sometimes the doctor can't find a cause. If you do experience bleeding, it doesn't necessarily mean you will have a miscarriage, but you should call your doctor. Most often he'll recommend you have an ultrasound exam and be monitored to make sure that you're not contracting. Bleeding may increase the risk for premature delivery, so your doctor may recommend that your pregnancy come under extra-close surveillance.

Fetal abnormality

Although the vast majority of pregnancies proceed normally, about 2 to 3 percent of infants are born with some abnormality. Most of these abnormalities are minor, although some do lead to significant problems for the newborn. Some are due to chromosomal problems, and others stem from abnormal development of organs and structures. For example, some newborns may have heart defects or abnormalities of the kidneys, bladder, or gastrointestinal tract. Many of these problems, though not all of them, can be diagnosed on a prenatal ultrasound exam (see the "'Looking' at sound waves: Ultrasound" section earlier in this chapter). When confronted with any such problem, the most important first step is to gather all the available information about it, so that you know what to expect and what the treatment options are. Keep in mind that even specialists may not be able to tell you everything to expect until your baby is born and they can further evaluate the situation.

Cervical insufficiency/ Incompetent Cervix

During the second trimester, usually between 16 and 24 weeks, some women develop a problem known as *cervical insufficiency* or *incompetent cervix*. The cervix opens up and dilates, even though the woman feels no contractions. This condition may lead to miscarriage. Indeed, an incompetent cervix is most often diagnosed after the miscarriage occurs and, in most cases, couldn't have been predicted. A woman who develops this condition ordinarily doesn't notice any symptoms, although sometimes she may report feeling pelvic heaviness or pressure that's out of the ordinary, or she may notice some spotting. Most women who experience cervical insufficiency do so for no identifiable reason. Others may have one of the following risk factors:

- ✔ **Cervical trauma:** Some evidence suggests that multiple *D&Cs* (dilation and curettage, see Chapter 5) or procedures called *cervical cone biopsy* or *LEEP* (in which a cone-shaped portion of the cervix is removed in the diagnosis or treatment of cervical abnormalities) can increase the risk of cervical insufficiency. A significant tear of the cervix during a prior delivery may also increase the risk for this disorder.

- ✔ **Multiple gestations:** Some obstetricians believe that carrying multiple babies, especially triplets or more, may increase the risk for cervical insufficiency. This issue is very controversial because some doctors feel strongly about putting them in, but placing a *cerclage* (a stitch in the cervix — see the explanation that follows) in all patients with triplets or more does not appear to help based on the available literature surrounding this subject. Some patients who have undergone a procedure called *multi-fetal pregnancy reduction* (see Chapter 13) may also be at increased risk for incompetent cervix, although routine cerclage placement isn't recommended for them at this time.

- ✔ **Prior history of cervical insufficiency:** After you have had a cervical insufficiency, your risk of having it again in a subsequent pregnancy is increased.

In cases in which a cervical insufficiency is diagnosed before the pregnancy is lost, attempts can be made to hold the cervix shut with a stitch, called a *cerclage,* around the cervix. The

cerclage is usually placed at 12 to 14 weeks, although it's occasionally performed as an emergency procedure later in the pregnancy. Doctors most commonly perform the procedure in the hospital under spinal or epidural anesthesia, but the woman is usually discharged later the same day.

Some women with a cerclage notice they have a heavy discharge throughout pregnancy. If you need to have a cerclage, talk to your doctor about how active you can be — whether you can have sex and how much exercise is advisable. Complications associated with emergency cerclage include infection, contractions, rupture of membranes, bleeding, and miscarriage. The same complications can occur with elective cerclage, but they're unusual.

Many doctors are now using a pessary, which is a plastic/rubber device that is inserted into the vagina to take some of the pressure off of the cervix. The device is easily inserted and removable, so it doesn't carry the same risks as a cerclage since there are no needles involved.

Knowing when to seek help

The following is a list of second-trimester symptoms that require some attention. If you experience any of them, call your practitioner:

- ✔ Bleeding

- ✔ An unusual sense of pressure or heaviness

- ✔ Regular contractions or strong cramping

- ✔ A lack of normal fetal movement

- ✔ High fever

- ✔ Severe abdominal pain

For Partners: Watching Mom Grow

"Honey, do you think I'm fat and ugly now?" You may start to hear this question during the second trimester when the mother's body really begins to change. Here's a tip: It's not a multiple-choice question. You only have one answer, and

you may as well commit it to memory so that you can answer without hesitation: "Absolutely not, honey. You're the most beautiful woman I've ever laid eyes on."

Tread lightly when making comments about your partner's belly size. Maybe you are just being observant, but it's a great way to get the cold shoulder without intending it!

Enjoy the second trimester. Often, it's the most fun part of pregnancy for both parents. Morning sickness fades away, fatigue subsides, and your partner begins to feel the baby move around inside her. Often, you, too, can feel the baby move by placing your hand on the mom's abdomen.

During this trimester, many mothers get an ultrasound exam to check the baby's anatomy. Try to go along to see the ultrasound exam (see Chapter 19); it's one of the most enjoyable prenatal tests. You get to see the baby's hands, feet, and face, and you get to watch the baby move around. For the first time, you see the living, moving, growing little human inside, and suddenly the whole enterprise seems so much more real!

By the end of the second trimester, you may begin prenatal classes (check out Chapter 7 for more information). Don't make excuses! Go with your partner! The classes are designed for both the partner and mother. During this time, you can find out how to be useful during labor and delivery. And you can also ask questions about what to anticipate — to relieve some of your own anxiety.

Chapter 7

The Third Trimester

In This Chapter

▶ Getting ready for life outside the womb — your baby will arrive soon!

▶ Dealing with the discomforts of the home stretch

▶ Knowing which tests may be administered

▶ Planning for the main event at childbirth classes

▶ Preparing to go to the hospital — and to bring your baby home

▶ Knowing when to be concerned

*Y*ou're finally ready for the third act — your pregnancy's final trimester. By now, you're probably accustomed to having a protruding belly, your morning sickness is long gone, and you've come to expect and enjoy the feeling of your baby moving around and kicking inside you. In this trimester, your baby continues to grow, and your practitioner continues to monitor you and your baby's health. You also begin making preparations for the new arrival, which may mean anything from getting ready to take a leave of absence from your job to taking childbirth classes (or otherwise finding out what to expect during labor and delivery).

Your Baby Gets Ready for Birth

At 28 weeks, your baby measures about 14 inches (about 35 cm) and weighs about 2½ pounds (about 1,135 grams). But by the end of the third trimester — at 40 weeks, your due date — it measures about 20 inches (50 cm) and weighs 6 to 8 pounds (about 2,700 to 3,600 grams) — sometimes a bit more, sometimes a bit less. The fetus spends most of the third trimester growing, adding fat, and continuing to develop various organs, especially the central nervous system. The arms and legs get chubbier, and the skin becomes thicker and smooth.

During the third trimester, your baby is less susceptible to infections and to the adverse effects of medications, but some of these agents may still affect its growth. The last two months are usually spent getting ready for the transition to life in the world outside the uterus. The changes are less dramatic than they were early on, but the maturation and growth that happen now are very important.

By 28 to 34 weeks, the fetus generally assumes a head-down position (called a *vertex presentation*), like in Figure 7-1. This way, the buttocks and legs (the bulkiest parts of its body) occupy the roomiest part of the uterus — the top part. In about 4 percent of singleton pregnancies, the baby may be positioned buttocks-down (breech) or lie across the uterus (transverse). (See the "Recognizing Causes for Concern" section later in this chapter for more on breech presentation.)

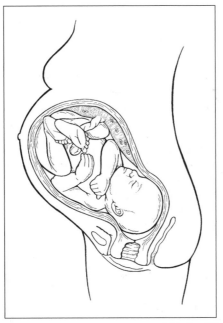

Kathryn Born, MA

Figure 7-1: How your baby may look inside your uterus during the third trimester.

By 36 weeks, growth slows, and amniotic fluid volume is at its maximum level. After this point, the amount of amniotic fluid may start to decline because blood flow to the baby's kidneys

decreases as the placenta ages, and the baby produces less urine (and therefore less amniotic fluid). In fact, most practitioners routinely check the amniotic fluid volume on ultrasound or by feeling your abdomen during the last few weeks to make sure that a normal amount remains.

Movin' and shakin': Fetal movements

Look down at your belly during times of fetal activity during the third trimester, and it may appear that an alien from outer space is doing an aerobic dance inside you. Although fetal movements don't actually diminish as your due date approaches, the timing and quality of the movements change. Toward the end of pregnancy, fetal movements may feel less like jabs and more like tumbles or rolls, and you notice longer periods of quiet between movements. The fetus is adapting to a more newborn-like pattern, taking longer naps and having longer active cycles.

 If you don't sense a normal amount of activity, let your practitioner know. A good general rule is that you should feel about six movements in one hour after dinner, while resting. Any movement, no matter how subtle, counts. Some women find that they go for periods of feeling less fetal movement, but then the movements pick up again and are normal. This is very common and isn't a reason to be concerned. However, if you notice a pattern of diminishing fetal movements or you feel absolutely no fetal movements over several hours (despite resting or eating), give your practitioner a call right away.

If you have certain risk factors or if you need specific guidelines to track the adequacy of fetal movements, your practitioner may suggest that you keep a diary to chart fetal movement, starting at 28 weeks. You can track fetal movements in several different ways. One way is to lie down on your left side after dinner to count fetal movements, and write down how long it takes to count ten movements. Another way of doing the test is to count fetal movements while lying down for an hour each day (it doesn't have to be the same hour every day) and to plot the number of movements on a chart given to you by your practitioner. With this method, you can see the pattern of the baby's movements throughout the day.

Flexing the breathing muscles

Fetuses undergo what are called *rhythmic breathing move-ments* from 10 weeks onward, although these movements are much more frequent in the third trimester. The fetus doesn't actually breathe, but its chest, abdominal wall, and diaphragm move in a pattern that is characteristic of breathing. You don't notice these movements, but a doctor can observe them with ultrasound. These movements are signs that the baby is faring well. During the third trimester, the amount of time a fetus spends performing the breathing movements increases, espe-cially after meals.

Hiccupping in utero

At times, you may feel a quick, rhythmic pattern of fetal move-ments, occurring every few seconds. These movements are most likely hiccups. Some women feel fetal hiccups several times throughout the day; others sense them only rarely. Occa-sionally you may actually see the baby hiccupping during an ultrasound exam. These hiccups are completely normal. They may feel strange, but standing on your head and drinking water, which we hear is a great cure, probably isn't your best option now.

Keeping Up with Your Changing Body

As the baby grows, so does your belly! Although big is beauti-ful, it can become uncomfortable. You may notice that your uterus pushes up on your ribs, and sometimes you notice kick-ing in one spot in particular — that is probably where the baby's extremities are, either feet or arms. If you're pregnant with twins or more, the discomforts are, of course, even more pronounced. Women with twins may feel one baby move more than the other, which is usually related to the babies' positions — one baby may be oriented with the arms and legs facing out and the other with them facing in. Whether you are carrying one, two, or more babies, you notice that moving around like you used to becomes more and more difficult as you get bigger.

If you find rising after lying on your back is difficult and no one is around to help, try turning on your side first and then pushing yourself up to a sitting position (see Figure 7-2).

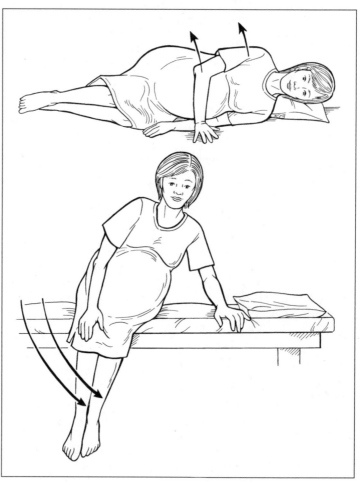

Kathryn Born, MA

Figure 7-2: Make it easy on your back: Before trying to get up from lying down, roll over to your side and then push yourself up while swinging your legs down.

Accidents and falls

Being pregnant may make you more cautious about taking obvious risks, but it doesn't prevent you from stumbling or otherwise having an occasional mishap. If you do fall, don't worry. Chances are good that the baby remains well protected in your uterus and within its sac of amniotic fluid, which is an excellent natural cushion. But just to be careful, let your practitioner know. She may want you to come in to check that the baby is fine.

A pregnant woman knows no strangers

You may find that your belly has suddenly become public property. Perfect strangers feel compelled to put their hands on your abdomen and tell you how pleased they are that you're about to have a baby! Although some women find this kind of behavior caring and supportive, others find it annoying, embarrassing, and uncomfortable. Politely telling people not to touch your belly if they're making the move is okay.

Many people consider it perfectly polite to also comment on your appearance. They may tell you that you look too fat or too thin; that you're carrying too wide or all in your buttocks. They may say that this or that is a sign that the baby is a boy or a girl. "Whoa, you must be about ready to pop!" they may exclaim, or "My goodness, you're enormous!" Try, if you can, *not* to pay attention to what they say. Indeed, the very best piece of advice we can offer is to not let other people drive you crazy. They may have the best of intentions, but they rarely realize how their words sound to you.

We tell our patients all the time to talk to us if they have concerns. So don't hesitate to ask your doctor or other healthcare provider if what you hear worries you. But also remember what you know: If someone tells you that you look too small, tell her your practitioner measures you at each visit to make sure that you're okay growth-wise. Also remember that if you had an ultrasound exam recently and the size of your fetus was perfectly appropriate, you have nothing to worry about. Your practitioner can always reassure you that your belly is measuring perfectly normal.

Many women feel compelled to tell you all the horror stories of their own pregnancies — or all the pregnancy horror stories they've ever heard. If you pay too much attention, you'll only suffer anxiety and needless worry. Just tell the person politely that you'd really prefer not to hear her story (unless, of course, you don't mind these stories).

If, after your fall, you suffer severe abdominal pain, contractions, bleeding, or leakage of amniotic fluid, or if you notice a decrease in fetal movements, call your practitioner immediately or go to the hospital where you receive care. If the fall or injury involves a direct blow to your uterus (for example, the steering wheel hits your belly in a car accident), your practitioner will probably want to monitor your baby for a while.

Braxton-Hicks contractions

In the late second trimester or beginning of the third trimester, your uterus may, from time to time, become momentarily hard or feel as though it's balling up. Most likely, you're experiencing *Braxton-Hicks contractions.* They're not the kind of contractions you have in labor; they're more like practice ones.

Braxton-Hicks contractions are usually painless, but at times they may be uncomfortable, and they may occur with more frequency when you are active and subside when you rest. Women who have already had children tend to notice more Braxton-Hicks contractions. You may have a hard time distinguishing Braxton-Hicks contractions from fetal movements, especially if this is your first pregnancy. Other times, Braxton-Hicks contractions can become uncomfortable and progress to false labor.

 If you're less than 36 weeks along and you experience contractions that are persistent, regular, and increasingly painful, call your doctor to make sure that you're not in premature labor.

Carpal tunnel syndrome

If you feel numbness, tingling, or pain in your fingers and wrist, you're probably experiencing *carpal tunnel syndrome.* It occurs when swelling in the wrist puts pressure on the *median nerve,* which runs through the *carpal tunnel* from the wrist to the hand. It can happen in one or both hands, and the pain may be worse at night or upon awakening. Carpal tunnel syndrome is more common in women who are pregnant than in those who aren't because of the swelling that goes along with pregnancy.

If carpal tunnel syndrome becomes persistent or bothersome, discuss it with your practitioner. Wrist splints, available at some drugstores or surgical supply stores, can relieve the

problem. Try not to be discouraged if it doesn't seem to get better during pregnancy, though, because it usually improves (often dramatically fast) after delivery.

Fatigue

DON'T WORRY The fatigue you felt early in your pregnancy may return in the third trimester. You may feel as if you're just slowing down. You're tired all the time, you're carrying around more weight, you're not very comfortable much of the time, and you may feel that you can't accomplish everything you need to. Women may find their second or third pregnancies more tiring than the first because they have to care for one or more older children.

Try to be realistic about what you can do, and don't feel guilty about what you can't get done. No one wants you to be Superwoman. Take time for yourself and get as much rest as you can. Delegate tasks. Whenever possible, let other people help with household chores and other responsibilities. Do whatever you can to take advantage of the quiet times. Rest as much as you can now, because after delivery, the work really picks up!

Feeling the baby "drop"

During the month before delivery, a woman may notice that her belly feels lower and that suddenly it's easier to breathe. This feeling is because the baby has *dropped,* or descended lower into the pelvis. This movement is also called *lightening.* It typically happens two to three weeks before delivery in women who are having their first child. Those who have had children before may not drop until they're in labor.

When dropping happens, you may find that you're suddenly much more comfortable. Your uterus doesn't press up on your diaphragm or stomach as much as it used to, so breathing is easier, and heartburn may improve. At the same time, however, you may feel more pressure in your vaginal area — many women feel heaviness there. Some women report feeling strange, sharp twinges as the baby's head moves and exerts pressure on the bladder and pelvic floor. Having the baby "drop" doesn't predict when labor will happen.

You may not notice that you have dropped. During your prenatal visit, your doctor may be able to tell by an external or
internal exam how low the baby's head is and whether it's
engaged. The fetal head is engaged when it has reached the
level of the *ischial spines,* which are bony landmarks in your
pelvis that can be felt during an internal exam (see Figure 7-3).

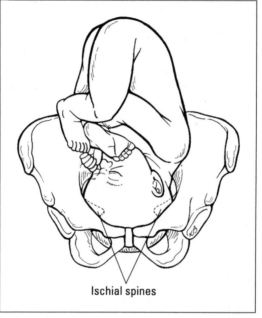

Ischial spines

Kathryn Born, MA

Figure 7-3: The baby's head reaches the bony ischial spines in your pelvis
and is engaged.

When the fetal head is at this level, it's at *zero station.* Most
practitioners divide the pelvis into descending stations from –5
to +5 (although some use –3 to +3). Often at the beginning
of labor, the head may be at –4 or –5 station (fairly high —
sometimes called *floating,* because the fetal head is still floating in the amniotic cavity). Labor proceeds until the head
descends all the way to +5, when delivery is about to begin.

If the baby's head is engaged prior to labor, you're more likely
to deliver vaginally, although obviously there are no guarantees. Similarly, although a floating (unengaged) head isn't
every obstetrician's dream, it doesn't mean that you won't
have a completely normal delivery.

If you're having your second child or more, the baby's head may not engage until well into labor.

Hemorrhoids

No one wants to talk about them, but *hemorrhoids* — dilated, swollen veins around the rectum — are a common problem for pregnant women. They're essentially varicose veins of the rectum (we talk about varicose veins later in this section). The enlarging uterus causes hemorrhoids by pressing on major blood vessels, which leads to pooling of blood, and ultimately makes the veins enlarge and swell. Progesterone relaxes the veins, allowing the swelling to increase. Constipation makes hemorrhoids worse. Straining and pushing hard during bowel movements puts added pressure on the blood vessels, causing them to enlarge and possibly protrude from the rectum.

Hemorrhoids sometimes bleed. This bleeding doesn't harm the pregnancy, but if it becomes frequent, talk to your doctor and possibly see a colorectal specialist or general surgeon. If hemorrhoids become very painful, you may want to discuss whether treatment is necessary. Meanwhile, you can try the following:

- ✔ **Avoid constipation (see Chapter 5).** Straining to push out hard stool can make hemorrhoids worse.

- ✔ **Exercise.** Activity increases bowel motility, so the stool doesn't get too hard.

- ✔ **Get off your feet when you can.** Doing so alleviates extra pressure on your veins.

- ✔ **Try over-the-counter topical medications, such as Preparation H or Anusol, or a steroid cream.** Many women find some relief with these medications.

- ✔ **Take warm baths two to three times a day.** Soaking in warm water can help relieve the muscle spasms that most often cause the pain.

- ✔ **Use over-the-counter hemorrhoidal pads (such as Tucks) or witch hazel pads to clean and medicate the area.** These pads often provide a cooling, soothing relief.

Pushing during the second stage of labor can make hemorrhoids worse or make them appear where they weren't before. But, most of the time, hemorrhoids go away after delivery.

Insomnia

During the last few months of pregnancy, many women find sleeping difficult. Finding a comfortable position when you're eight months along isn't easy. You feel a little like a beached whale. Getting up five times a night to go to the bathroom doesn't make things any easier. However, you may find relief in the following:

> ✔ **Drink warm milk with honey before bedtime.** Warming the milk releases *tryptophan,* a naturally occurring amino acid that makes you sleepy; the honey causes you to produce insulin, which also makes you drowsy. Leave the honey out, however, if you have gestational diabetes (see Chapter 15).

> ✔ **Exercise during the day.** Activity helps to tire you out, which means you'll fall asleep sooner.

> ✔ **Go to bed a little later than usual.** You'll spend less time *trying* to fall asleep.

> ✔ **Limit your liquid intake after 6 p.m.** Don't limit it to the point that you become dehydrated, however.

> ✔ **Invest in a body pillow.** You can tuck it around your body in various places, making it easier to find a comfortable position. You can get a body pillow in almost any department store.

> ✔ **Take a warm, relaxing bath before going to bed.** Many women say a bath helps make them feel sleepy.

Pregnancy rashes and itches

Pregnant women are subject to the same rashes that nonpregnant women get. One rash is unique to pregnancy, however: *Pruritic Urticarial Papules of Pregnancy,* or PUPP. It sounds scary, but it's really more of a nuisance than anything else because it can cause some intense itching. It occurs more often during a first pregnancy and in women having twins or more (the more fetuses, the greater the likelihood).

PUPP tends to occur late in pregnancy and is characterized by hives or red patches that first appear in the stretch marks on your abdomen. These patches can spread to other areas on the abdomen and to the legs, arms, chest, and back. They

almost never spread to the face. (Thank heaven for small favors.) The good news is that the condition poses no risk to the baby. But if you develop this rash, your doctor may recommend that you have some blood tests to make sure you don't have other conditions that can be associated with itching.

The only surefire way to make PUPP go away is to deliver. Some women tell us that the itching goes away within hours of giving birth. If delivery is still weeks away, it sometimes helps to bathe in a solution of colloidal oatmeal (Aveeno makes a good one). Skin lotions containing Benadryl can also help, but these products can sometimes dry the skin, which only makes the itching worse. Some women get relief from taking Benadryl orally, but check with your doctor before doing so. Finally, in very severe cases (which are rare), the doctor may prescribe a short-term course of steroids or other medications.

Even if you don't have a rash, you may notice that you itch a lot, especially where stretch marks develop. This itching is very common and usually is caused by the stretching of your skin as the baby gets bigger.

Up to 2 percent of pregnant women develop *cholestasis of pregnancy,* which is a condition where an increase of bile acids in the blood causes the itching. If the itching is mild, you can treat it with skin moisturizers, topical anti-itching medications, or oral antihistamines such as Benadryl (but remember to talk to your doctor first before taking). If the itching is severe, your doctor may recommend oral medications that help to clear the bile acids from the bloodstream. Some studies have suggested that the baby should be monitored with non-stress tests (see the "Non-stress test (NST)" section later in this chapter) when the mother has this condition, because it is associated with an increased risk of complications. The itching goes away shortly after delivery, but the condition may recur in future pregnancies.

Preparing for breast-feeding

If you plan on breast-feeding, you may want to take steps to toughen the skin around your nipples, which can help prevent them from cracking and becoming painful and sore when you're breast-feeding. You can try very gently rubbing

or massaging your nipples between your fingers, exposing them to air, rubbing them gently with a washcloth, or wearing a nursing bra with the flaps down so that your nipples rub against your clothes. Creams and oils work against toughening, so don't use them on your nipples.

 Some women worry that they don't have the right type of breasts for breast-feeding, but no breast type is right or wrong. Breasts both large and small can produce adequate milk. Some women with retracted or inverted nipples can make breast-feeding easier by massaging their nipples so that they protrude more (see Chapter 12). Some maternity or baby stores sell special breast shells that use suction to help the nipples come out.

Many women notice from early on in pregnancy that their breasts occasionally secrete a yellowish discharge. This discharge is *colostrum,* and it's what the newborn baby sucks out and swallows in the first few days of life before actual milk comes in. Colostrum has a higher protein and lower fat content than milk; most importantly, it contains antibodies from your immune system that help protect your baby against certain infections until her own immune system matures and can take over.

 Don't worry if you don't produce any visible colostrum during pregnancy; not producing colostrum in no way means that you won't produce adequate milk. Each woman is different; some leak from the breasts during pregnancy, and some don't. Even if it isn't obvious, your baby will still get colostrum the first few times she breast-feeds.

Sciatica

Some women experience pain extending from their lower back to their buttocks and down one leg or the other. This pain or, less commonly, numbness, is known as *sciatica,* because it's due to pressure on the sciatic nerve, a major nerve that branches from your back, through your pelvis, to your hips, and down your legs. You can relieve mild cases of sciatica with bed rest (shift from side to side to find the most comfortable position), warm baths, or heating pads applied to the painful areas. If you develop a severe case, you may need prolonged bed rest or special exercises. Ask your doctor.

Shortness of breath

You may find that as pregnancy proceeds, you become increasingly short of breath. The hormone progesterone affects your central breathing center and may cause these feelings of breathlessness. Furthermore, as your enlarging uterus presses upward on your diaphragm, your lungs have less room to expand normally. (When Joanne was pregnant with her second child, she used to be so short of breath that the only books she could read to her daughter were ones with very short sentences. Dr. Seuss had to sit on the shelf until after she delivered.)

In most cases, shortness of breath is perfectly normal. But if it comes on very suddenly or if it comes with chest pain, call your doctor.

Stretch marks

Stretch marks are an almost inevitable part of pregnancy, though some women do manage to avoid them. Your skin stretches to accommodate the enlarging uterus and weight gain, causing the stretch marks. Some women probably also have some genetic predisposition for stretch marks. The marks typically appear as pinkish-red streaks along the abdomen and breasts, but they fade to silvery gray or white several months after delivery. Their exact color depends on your skin tone — they appear browner on dark-skinned women, for example.

No cream or ointment is completely effective in preventing stretch marks, although products continue to enter the market. Many people think that rubbing vitamin E oil on the belly helps prevent stretch marks or helps them fade faster, but the effectiveness of vitamin E has never been proven scientifically. Your best bet is to avoid excessive weight gain and to exercise regularly to maintain muscle tone, which eases the pressure of the uterus on the overlying skin.

Recently, some dermatologists have started offering a special laser procedure that may be helpful in reducing stretch marks after delivery. Also, some advise using a cream containing retinoic acid to treat stretch marks after delivery. However, don't use these creams during pregnancy; also, you shouldn't use some of them when you're breast-feeding. If your stretch marks are particularly noticeable, consult a dermatologist a few months after your pregnancy is over.

Swelling

Swelling (also called *edema*) of the hands and legs is very common in the third trimester. It most often occurs after you've been on your feet for a while, but it can happen throughout the day. Swelling tends to be even more common in warm weather.

Contrary to popular wisdom, no evidence indicates that lowering your salt intake or drinking a lot of water prevents swelling or makes it go away.

Although swelling is a normal symptom of pregnancy, it can occasionally be a sign of preeclampsia (see Chapter 14). If you notice a sudden increase in the amount of swelling or a sudden, large weight gain — 5 pounds or more in a week — or if the swelling is associated with significant headache or right-sided abdominal pain, call your practitioner immediately.

For ordinary swelling, try the following:

- ✔ Keep your legs elevated whenever possible.

- ✔ Stay in a cool environment.

- ✔ Wear supportive pantyhose or stockings that aren't tight around your knees.

- ✔ When in bed, don't lie flat on your back; try to lie on your side.

Urinary stress incontinence

Leaking a little urine when you cough, laugh, or sneeze isn't unusual when you're pregnant. This kind of *urinary stress incontinence* occurs because your growing uterus is putting pressure on your bladder. Relaxation of the pelvic floor muscles increases the problem during the late second and third trimesters. And sometimes the baby may give the bladder a swift kick and cause it to leak urine. *Kegel exercises* — in which you repeatedly contract the pelvic floor muscles as if you're trying very hard not to urinate — can prevent or markedly reduce the problem (see Chapter 11). Some women continue to experience a little stress incontinence even after delivery, but it usually goes away after about 6 to 12 months.

If you had a particularly difficult labor, where you pushed for a long time, or had a very large baby, the stress incontinence may not completely go away. Give it at least six months to see whether it goes away. After that, talk to your doctor about how to proceed.

Varicose veins

You may notice that a small road map has suddenly appeared on your lower legs (and sometimes the vulvar area). These marks are dilated veins, referred to as *varicose veins*. The pressure of the uterus on major blood vessels — the *inferior vena cava* (the vein that returns blood to the heart) and the pelvic veins, in particular — causes them. Pregnancy also causes the muscle tissue inside your veins to relax and your blood volume to increase, and these conditions add to the problem. Women with light skin or with a family history of varicose veins are particularly susceptible. Very often, the bluish-purple highways fade after delivery, but sometimes they don't disappear completely. They're most often painless, but occasionally they may be associated with discomfort, achiness, or pain.

In rare instances, a blood clot develops in the superficial veins of the legs. This condition, called *superficial thrombophlebitis,* isn't a serious problem; it's often successfully treated with rest, leg elevation, warm compresses, and special stockings. A clot that forms in the deep veins of the leg is more serious (see Chapter 15 for a discussion of *deep vein thrombosis*).

You can't prevent varicose veins — you can't fight heredity — but you can reduce their number and severity by following these tips:

- ✔ Avoid standing for prolonged periods of time.

- ✔ Avoid wearing clothes that are very tight around one part of your leg, like socks with tight elastic; which has a tourniquet-like effect.

- ✔ If you must be relatively stationary, move your legs around from time to time to stimulate circulation.

- ✔ Keep your legs elevated whenever you can.

- ✔ Wear support stockings or talk to your doctor about a prescription for special elastic stockings.

Hitting the Home Stretch: Prenatal Visits in the Third Trimester

Between 28 and 36 weeks, your practitioner probably wants to see you every two to three weeks, and then weekly as you close in on delivery. She takes the usual measurements: blood pressure, weight, fetal heart rate, fundal height, and urine tests. These visits are a good time to discuss issues related to labor and delivery with your practitioner.

If you don't deliver by your due date, your practitioner may want to start performing non-stress tests (see the "Non-stress test (NST)" section later in this chapter for details). These tests assess fetal well-being. After 40 to 41 weeks, placental function and amniotic fluid may decline, and ensuring that both remain adequate to support the pregnancy is important. By 42 weeks, many practitioners recommend inducing labor (see Chapter 8) because the risk of problems for the baby rises significantly after that time.

As your pregnancy winds down, your practitioner may perform certain tests to make sure that your baby is as healthy as possible. Some tests, like Group B strep cultures (see the following section), are done so that measures can be taken to avoid certain problems. Other tests, like a non-stress test or a biophysical profile, are performed to ensure fetal well-being.

Taking Group B strep cultures

The only routine test that may be performed during one of your final prenatal visits is a culture for *Group B strep,* bacteria commonly found in the vagina and rectum. The Centers for Disease Control and Prevention (CDC) and the American College of Obstetricians and Gynecologists now recommend that all women be routinely screened for Group B strep at around 36 weeks gestation. About 15 to 20 percent of women harbor this organism. If the culture is positive at 36 weeks, your doctor will recommend that you receive antibiotics during labor to reduce the risk of transmitting the bacteria to the baby. Treating the bacteria any earlier doesn't help, because it can come back by the time you're in labor.

Currently, no tests that yield immediate results are available, so you can't test for Group B strep at the time of labor; it must be done in advance.

Gauging lung maturity

If you're planning a repeat cesarean delivery (meaning that you had one in an earlier pregnancy) or an elective induction at less than 39 weeks, some practitioners may recommend that you have an amniocentesis to establish that the fetus's lungs are mature and ready to function. Over the past few years, there has been a movement across the country to stop performing elective deliveries before 39 weeks because newer studies have shown that these place newborns at increased risks for problems in the newborn period, so the need for fetal lung maturity amnioceneses is declining. The American College of Obstetricians and Gynecologists and the March of Dimes both strongly discourage such deliveries.

The most commonly performed test for lung maturity is called L/S ratio, which measures the ratio of *lecithin* to *sphingomyelin* (both are substances found in the amniotic fluid). If the L/S ratio is 2.0 or greater or if PG (*phosphatidyl glycerol,* a substance produced by mature lung cells) is present in the amniotic fluid, the baby's lungs are considered mature.

Assessing your baby's current health

At certain times, your practitioner may suggest that you undergo tests for the baby. These tests, also referred to as *antepartum fetal surveillance,* check the baby's well-being. Your practitioner can perform these tests at any time after about 24 to 26 weeks if cause for concern exists, or after 41 weeks if you haven't delivered. Several different tests can be used, which we describe in the following sections.

Non-stress test (NST)

Non-stress testing consists of measuring the fetal heart rate, fetal movement, and uterine activity using a special monitoring machine. Your practitioner hooks you up to this device, which picks up uterine contractions and the baby's heart rate and generates a tracing of both. The NST is similar to the

device used during labor to monitor the fetal heart rate and contractions. You also receive a button to press each time you perceive fetal movement. The monitoring goes on for about 20 to 40 minutes. The doctor then looks at the tracing for signs of *accelerations,* or increases, in the fetal heart rate. If accelerations are present and occur often enough, the test is considered *reactive,* and the fetus is thought to be healthy and should continue to be so for three to seven days. (The fetus is healthy in more than 99 percent of cases.) If the accelerations aren't adequate (that is, the test is *nonreactive*), you still have no cause for alarm. In 80 percent of cases, the fetus is fine and probably just in sleep cycle, but further evaluation is needed.

Your practitioner may perform this test (which is usually repeated once or twice a week) for a variety of reasons, particularly when

- ✔ You are past your due date.
- ✔ The baby is not growing properly.
- ✔ You have a decreased volume of amniotic fluid.
- ✔ Your blood pressure is high.
- ✔ You have diabetes.
- ✔ You notice decreased fetal movement.

Contraction stress test (CST)

The contraction stress test is similar to a non-stress test except that the fetal heart is timed in relation to uterine contractions. The contractions sometimes occur by themselves, but more often are brought on with low doses of oxytocin (Pitocin) or by nipple stimulation.

Don't stimulate your nipples at home to bring on contractions. Perform nipple stimulation only under your doctor's supervision, because you doctor wants to monitor you and make sure that the uterus doesn't contract too much.

Three good contractions in a ten-minute period need to be present in order for the test to be interpreted. If the fetal heart rate doesn't drop after the contractions, the test is considered *negative,* and the baby is thought to be fine for at least one more week. If the test is *positive* (the fetal heart rate does drop after the contractions) or suspicious, your practitioner investigates the situation further. Proper management

depends on your particular situation. A CST is performed if the results of the non-stress test are inconclusive, or if your doctor wants additional testing of fetal well-being.

A CST shouldn't be performed under certain circumstances, such as if the mother has placenta previa (see Chapter 14) or if she's at risk of preterm delivery.

Biophysical profile (BPP)

A biophysical profile, which combines ultrasound with a non-stress test, may be performed instead of the NST alone, or in addition to the NST if further testing is warranted. Which test is performed (NST or BPP) is often just a matter of physician preference.

The BPP evaluates the following:

- ✔ Fetal movements, observed by ultrasound

- ✔ Fetal body tone, observed by ultrasound

- ✔ Fetal breathing movements for 30 seconds in a row (chest motions that mimic breathing), observed by ultrasound

- ✔ Quantity of amniotic fluid, observed by ultrasound

- ✔ Non-stress test (see "Non-stress test," earlier in this section)

The baby receives 2 points for each parameter that's normal. A perfect score is 10 out of 10. Babies who score 8 out of 10 or better are considered okay. A score of 6 out of 10 is probably fine but usually calls for follow-up testing. A score of less than 6 out of 10 needs further evaluation.

Vibracoustic stimulation

Your doctor may perform a vibracoustic stimulation test during a non-stress test. During the test, the fetus's response to stimulation by sound or vibrations is observed. The practitioner "buzzes" the mother's belly with a vibrating device, which causes a transmission of sound or vibrations to the fetus. Normally, the fetal heart rate accelerates when the fetus is stimulated in this way. Vibracoustic stimulation can often cut down the time necessary to perform a non-stress test, because you see accelerations in the heart rate more quickly. It is often performed if the NST is still not reactive after 20 to 30 minutes.

Doppler velocimetry

A doctor performs a Doppler velocimetry test only in certain situations — if certain fetal problems exist (like intrauterine growth restriction — see Chapter 14), for example, or if you have high blood pressure. Basically, with this test, your doctor performs a special type of ultrasound exam that assesses the blood flow through the umbilical cord.

Preparing for Labor

Toward the end of your third trimester, you're likely to think more about delivery and anticipate what that's going to be like. Many of our patients want to know when their labor may start and whether they can do anything to influence the timing or to bring it on sooner. In this section, we help you plan your labor, provide some insight on some classes you can take to get ready for labor, discuss what you can tell your doctor if you want a cesarean section, and give you some pointers on how to prepare yourself as labor nears.

Making a birth plan

A *birth plan* is a statement of your preferences for how you want to manage your labor and delivery. It's about educating yourself about your options and feelings, rather than making hard and fast — "I absolutely will/won't" decisions. It involves sorting through things like where you want to deliver, whom you want to have with you during the process, and how you want to manage any pain you may experience. It can be something you simply sort out in your mind and convey verbally, or it can be something you put in writing. No matter how you develop your plan, make sure you discuss your wishes with your provider well in advance of the big day because obstetric practices vary widely by provider and hospital. For example, some hospitals have rules about fetal heart monitoring during labor. The most important part of a birth plan — be it written or verbal — is to provide a platform that fosters an open discussion between you and your provider about your preferences wherever there is a choice.

If you put your plan in writing, we encourage you not to make it a manifesto that attempts to anticipate any and every possibility that can occur with labor and delivery. Keeping it short and

sweet not only saves paper, but also makes it easier for your providers to carry out given the unpredictability of the whole process. If your birth plan includes having an on-demand cesarean delivery, check out the "Asking for a c-section on demand" section later in this chapter.

Check out an online birth plan worksheet at `www.babycenter.com/calculators-birthplan`.

Going back to school: Classes to take

In order to prepare yourself for labor, you may want to consider taking some birthing classes to find out about breathing, relaxation, and massage techniques that help alleviate the fear, anxiety, and pain associated with labor. Today, a great majority of first-time expectant parents attend childbirth classes. Childbirth education has dramatically changed the average woman's experience of labor and delivery. Today's birthing experience is a far cry from the middle part of the last century, when women were knocked out with anesthesia for the delivery and the expectant father's only job was to pace around the waiting room like Ricky Ricardo anticipating the arrival of Little Ricky.

As you look toward your labor, you need to have a basic understanding of the different types of birthing methods in order to determine which classes may be right for you. The following is a primer on different birthing methods:

- ✔ **Lamaze:** Developed in the 1940s by Dr. Fernand Lamaze, a French obstetrician, this birthing method is probably the best known. Lamaze focuses on deep breathing techniques and other exercises aimed at distracting you from the pain associated with childbirth. For more info, go to `www.lamaze.org`.

- ✔ **Bradley:** Developed in the 1940s by an American obstetrician named Dr. Robert Bradley, this method focuses on a "natural" (drug-free) childbirth. This method involves training in deep breathing and other techniques to control the pain of labor and uses a coach. Check out `www.bradleybirth.com`.

✔ **Leboyer:** The cornerstone of this method is to minimize the shock for the baby of transitioning from inside the uterus to outside. It involves being born in a dimly lit room and immediate bonding with mom. Although there is no specific website devoted to this method, you can read the original text of Dr. Leboyer's book at `http://ebookbrowsee.net/birth-without-violence-leboyer-pdf-d123360765`.

✔ **Alexander:** This method focuses on intensive conditioning of your body to promote balance, flexibility, and coordination, thereby enhancing comfort during labor. Find out more at `www.alexandertechnique.com/articles2/pregnancy`.

✔ **HypnoBirthing:** The origins of this technique were originally described by Dr. Grantly Dick-Read, an English obstetrician, in 1944 in a book called *Childbirth without Fear*. (Keith still has the copy of this book his mom used when she was preparing for his birth!) The focus of this method is to use hypnosis to break the "fear-tension-pain" cycle, thereby making labor easier. For more information, go to `http://hypnobirthing.com`.

If you decide to take a class, make sure the one you choose provides reliable and accurate information. Ask your healthcare provider for recommendations, or ask friends who have already attended classes.

Being prepared: Infant CPR

No one wants to think about the possibility of finding your newborn unresponsive or having difficulty breathing, but the truth is that being prepared definitely helps pull your baby through these scary situations. Hence, infant and child CPR are recommended to all parents and childcare providers.

Infant CPR is a technique that all parents should be familiar with. Many people think it requires intensive training to master, but the American Heart Association has simplified the training so that almost anyone can do it with a minimum of effort. In fact, check out `www.americanheart.org`. In the upper-right corner of the home page, search for "Infant CPR Anytime" for information about a valuable 20-minute training session for parents and family members.

Most contemporary childbirth education classes teach a combination of some of these techniques. The greatest benefit of childbirth classes is probably the opportunity they provide to find out what to anticipate during labor, because a little information goes a long way in reducing anxiety and fear about the big event. Other benefits to the classes include

- ✓ **Bringing your partner into the process of pregnancy.** If attending your prenatal visits isn't always possible for your partner, a class may be the best time for your partner to find out about what's ahead and to ask questions.

- ✓ **Meeting other parents-to-be.** You may make friends and, ultimately, find playmates for your child.

- ✓ **Touring the hospital or childbirth center where you plan to deliver.** Seeing where it's all going to happen is often very helpful. (If your class doesn't include a tour, ask your practitioner to arrange one.)

You don't have to believe everything you hear at a childbirth class. If you plan to use medication or anesthesia to reduce the pain of labor and the instructor warns you that all such medications are evil, don't be bullied into accepting her point of view. You gain no advantage for being a martyr during labor. Just find out in class whatever you can that may be helpful and take the rest in stride. Ultimately, it's your labor, and you need to do what makes you feel comfortable.

Childbirth education isn't for everyone. Some women feel that becoming fully informed about what's ahead only adds to their nervousness — and that's a valid concern. Every woman should make her own decision about whether to attend childbirth classes. Also, if for some reason you deliver before you finish your classes, don't be overly concerned. Most nurses in labor and delivery are trained to show you the techniques you need to know during labor.

Asking for a c-section on demand

Cesarean section on demand (also known as a *cesarean delivery on maternal request*) is having a cesarean delivery just because the mom asks for it, even though no medical or obstetrical reasons for a cesarean exist. If you want to have a c-section on demand, make sure you discuss your wishes with your doctor well in advance of your delivery. She'll talk to you in depth about the risks and benefits of doing this to help you

make an informed decision. If you plan on having lots of children, having a c-section on demand probably isn't a good idea because the risks for some problems increase with each subsequent cesarean delivery.

Over the past ten years or so, having a c-section on demand has become increasingly more popular. In fact, statistics show that about 2.5 percent of all deliveries in the United States each year are by c-section on demand.

The potential benefits of this mode of delivery are a lower risk of postpartum bleeding or hemorrhage (see Chapter 11) and a lower risk of urinary incontinence. The latter has been shown to be true in the first year after delivery, but after that time, the risk of this problem is equal between moms who deliver vaginally and those who have c-section on demand.

The downsides to c-section on demand are a longer stay in the hospital, transient breathing problems for the baby, and higher risks in your subsequent pregnancies for problems like uterine rupture (see the information in Chapter 13 on TOLAC and VBAC) and an adherent placenta (also known as *placenta accrete*).

Timing labor

"When am I going to have this baby?" We hear this question very frequently as the due date approaches. We wish we had a foolproof way of knowing, but not even a crystal ball works. Sometimes a woman whose cervix is long and closed goes into labor within 12 hours of an internal exam, yet other women can walk around for weeks with a cervix dilated to 3 centimeters! Some uncertain signs that something may happen include loss of the *mucous plug* (not really a plug, but thick mucus produced in the cervix), *bloody show* (an unfortunately named and blood-tinged mucous discharge), increasing frequency of Braxton-Hicks contractions, and diarrhea. But nothing is a sure sign. Loss of the mucous plug or bloody show may occur hours, days, or weeks before labor, or in some cases, not at all. This unpredictability may add to your anxiety, but it also makes the whole process more exciting.

Women have tried all kinds of tricks (Chinese food, enemas, sex, and raspberry tea, to name a few) to induce labor on their own, but nothing — short of medical induction — really has been proven to work.

Vigorously rubbing or massaging the nipples can cause contractions, but it shouldn't be performed at home because it can lead to hyperstimulation of the uterus (that is, too-frequent contractions), which isn't healthy for you or your baby. It's not a sure thing, in any case, because as soon as you stop the nipple stimulation, the contractions usually also stop.

Using perineal massage

In the past few years, *perineal massage* has generated a great deal of interest. This process involves using an oil or cream on the *perineum* (the area between the vagina and the rectum) and massaging the area in preparation for childbirth. Although studies suggest that this practice decreases the need for *episiotomies* (cutting the perineum to allow room for the baby to pass during childbirth — see Chapter 11) or lacerations, the number of cases in which it has made a clear difference isn't very large. There's no harm in trying it, though. If you think perineal massage may help and it's comfortable for you, go right ahead.

Getting Ready to Head to the Hospital

You're so close to delivery now that it's a good idea to make sure you're ready to walk out the door and head for the hospital. You probably won't want to stop to pack a suitcase at the last minute, nor will you have time to stop off at the store to shop for a car seat. Getting these must-do items off your pre-delivery checklist now will free you up to concentrate on the important things, like that 437th daily trip to the bathroom.

Packing your suitcase

Many women find it comforting to know that their bag is packed for the trip to the hospital or birthing center. Having your bag ready allows you to concentrate on watching for signs of labor and helps keep you from worrying about being prepared.

You may want to have a few things on hand while you're in labor, including the following:

- ✔ **A camera.** Don't forget to charge the batteries and get extra memory cards.

- ✔ **A cell phone or calling card.** Bring along your address book with home, work, and cell numbers.

- ✔ **Insurance information.** Don't forget your card. (This one is actually a "must bring.")

- ✔ **Socks.** Your feet will probably get cold, so plan ahead.

- ✔ **Glasses.** They may be less trouble than contact lenses during labor.

- ✔ **A snack for your partner or coach.** You don't want your partner to leave you for a trip to the hospital cafeteria.

- ✔ **Hard candies or lollipops.** You may have to go for some time without eating or drinking.

- ✔ **Something your partner can use to massage your back during labor.** Some people find that a tennis ball, a narrow paint roller, or a lightweight rolling pin works well.

- ✔ **A CD or MP3 player, if you find music relaxing.** Don't forget to bring your favorite CDs.

- ✔ **Change for parking meters, telephones, or vending machines.** You never know when someone may need some quarters (hopefully not your practitioner).

After delivery, some additional items can help make your life easier, more comfortable, or more fun:

- ✔ A post-delivery snack for yourself

- ✔ Champagne for a post-delivery toast, if you like

- ✔ Modern, stick-on sanitary napkins

- ✔ Sturdy cotton underwear that you won't mind staining

- ✔ A bathrobe and nightgown

- ✔ Toiletries

- ✔ Extra-large shoes that will accommodate your swollen feet

   ✔ Loose, comfortable clothes to go home in

   ✔ Clothes for your baby — or babies! — to go home in

   ✔ An infant car seat

Determining who's coming to the hospital

The vast majority of cultures have specific childbirth rituals that involve the presence of other women attending to a woman's labor. In recent times, the trend has shifted toward involving the baby's father or your partner, family members, close friends, or hired labor support. So before the time comes to head to the hospital, take a moment and think about whom you want to accompany you.

These days, many hospitals allow more than one family member or friend in the labor and delivery room to offer continuous labor support. You may want to consider having some of the following people in your room during delivery:

   ✔ **The baby's father or your partner:** This is an obvious choice.

   ✔ **Your parents:** Some women choose to have one or both of their parents with them.

   ✔ **Your sister or a close friend:** Either may provide the support you need.

   ✔ **A doula:** Some women choose to hire a doula to provide support. A *doula* is a woman with extensive experience with birth who provides emotional and physical support throughout labor. The following are some doula referral organizations that you may find helpful:

   • Doulas of North America (DONA); phone 888-788-DONA; Web site www.dona.org

   • Association of Labor Assistants and Childbirth Educators (ALACE); phone 888-222-5223; Web site www.alace.org

Continuous labor support refers to the constant, nonmedical care given to a woman in labor. It involves emotional support and encouragement to both the patient and her partner, attention to physical comforts (massage, assistance with

positioning and grooming) and, often, providing information and explanation for various procedures and events. Advantages to continuous labor support may include a shorter labor, less need for a cesarean section, less need for pain relief, and a more positive childbirth experience.

Some women with other children may want them to be present during the delivery to share the full family experience. However, you should consider the maturity of the children (or other family members) and whether it would be an emotionally satisfying or unnerving situation for them. Although many labors proceed completely smoothly and without any complications, others may be stressful or more difficult. Keep this in mind when you are considering whom to bring with you to the delivery.

Choosing — and using — a car seat

Buying a car seat for your baby is one of the most important, but confusing, purchases you'll make. You have many choices, so staying informed about what to look for is important. Basically, you can choose from two types available for newborns:

- ✔ **Infant-only seat:** Designed for babies who are under 1 year of age or weigh less than 20 pounds, this car seat is smaller and more lightweight than the alternative and should be used only in a rear-facing position. (A seat that faces the rear is essential for newborns, because it supports the child's back, neck, and head during a car accident.) This type of seat is also more convenient because it's lightweight and can also be used as an infant carrier, feeding chair, or rocker.

- ✔ **Convertible or infant-toddler seat:** Car seats of this type are usually larger than infant-only car seats. You use them in a rear-facing position until your baby reaches 1 year of age or about 20 pounds. (Check your state's car seat laws to make sure you are up-to-date.) Some models have weight limits as high as 30 to 32 pounds for rear-facing use. The advantage of this type of seat is that you make only one purchase instead of buying both an infant seat and then a convertible seat after the age of 1.

When shopping, look for a model that is simple to use. Also, pay attention to price — the higher-priced seats aren't necessarily better. If you choose a convertible seat, try it out in your car to make sure it fits both backward and forward before you throw away the receipt. Also, check out whether the car seat is easy to install — you shouldn't need to be a mechanical engineer to properly install your baby's car seat.

The following considerations are also important when choosing a car seat:

- ✔ A five-point safety harness with straps that adjust from the front
- ✔ Plenty of head and neck support
- ✔ An easy-to-clean seat

After you've made your selection, you may want to practice buckling the seat into your car before taking your baby out for her first ride. Remember that your baby should ride in a semi-reclined position (at about a 45-degree angle), with the straps snugly against her body.

If you want to cover your baby, buckle the harness first, and then put a blanket over her — a blanket under the harness, or even a bulky clothing garment like a snowsuit, may make the harness too loose.

If your baby is a preemie, ask your doctor if the baby needs to be tested in her car seat before discharge. Premature babies are at a greater risk for periods of *apnea* (absent breathing) or depressed heart rate in a car seat. You may need to use rolled-up towels or diapers on either side of the baby's head to help keep her head and neck from slumping.

Recognizing Causes for Concern

During the final weeks and months of pregnancy, you see your practitioner more often than before. Still, certain questions and problems may arise between visits. Everything starts to heat up during the later stages of the third trimester, with both the baby and your body preparing for delivery. Here are some of the key things that may lead you to call your doctor.

Bleeding

If you experience any significant bleeding, let your practitioner know immediately. Some third-trimester bleeding is harmless to you and your baby, but sometimes it can have serious implications. Getting evaluated to be sure everything is fine makes sense. Possible causes of third-trimester bleeding include

- ✔ **Preterm labor:** This is defined as having contractions and changes in the cervix before you're 37 weeks along.

- ✔ **Inflammation or irritation of the cervix or the harmless bleeding of a superficial blood vessel on the cervix:** Either of these can occur after intercourse or after a pelvic exam.

- ✔ **Placenta previa or a low-lying placenta:** See Chapter 14.

- ✔ **Placental separation or abruption:** See Chapter 14.

- ✔ **Bloody show:** This show is usually less than the amount of blood you would see during a normal menstrual period, and it's often mixed with mucus. See Chapter 8.

Breech presentation

A baby is in a so-called *breech* position when its buttocks or legs are down, closest to the cervix. Breech presentation happens in 3 to 4 percent of all singleton deliveries. A woman's risk of having a breech baby decreases the further along she goes in her pregnancy. (The incidence is 24 percent at 18 to 22 weeks but only 8 percent at 28 to 30 weeks. By 34 weeks, it's down to 7 percent, and by 38 to 40 weeks, 3 percent.) If your doctor determines your baby is in a breech position during your third trimester, she will discuss your options, including vaginal breech delivery (which is rarely done these days), external cephalic version, or cesarean section. See Chapter 14 for details about breech presentation.

Decreased amniotic fluid volume

The medical term for decreased amniotic fluid volume is *oligohydramnios*. (It also used to be called *dry birth*.) It may be found on a routine ultrasound, or your doctor may suspect it just by

feeling your uterus. This condition can occur in association with intrauterine growth restriction (see the later section "Fetal growth problems"), preterm rupture of the membranes, or other conditions, or the cause may not be identifiable. Usually, a mild decrease in amniotic fluid isn't a major cause for concern; however, your practitioner begins to monitor you more closely — with non-stress tests and ultrasound exams — to make sure no problem arises. If you're very close to your due date, your practitioner may want to deliver the baby. On the other hand, if you're only 30 weeks along, the best option may be increased rest and close observation. Of course, the management of the problem also depends on its cause. See Chapter 14 for more details about problems with amniotic fluid.

Decreased fetal movement

If you're not feeling the amount of fetal movement you're accustomed to, let your doctor know. Fetal movement is one of the most important things to pay attention to as you near your due date (see the "Movin' and shakin': Fetal movements" section earlier in this chapter).

Fetal growth problems

You may find out at a routine prenatal visit that your practitioner thinks your uterus is measuring either too big or too small. This finding isn't cause for immediate alarm. Often in this situation, your practitioner suggests that you have an ultrasound exam to get a better idea of how big the baby is. Ultrasound is used to measure parts of the baby — the head's size, the abdomen's circumference, and the thighbone's length. Your practitioner then plugs these measurements into a mathematical equation that gives the estimated fetal weight (EFW). That estimate is then entered on a curve plotting the baby's age in weeks against weight (see Figure 7-4), which represents the average growth of thousands of fetuses at each gestational age.

Your practitioner can check to see where your baby's weight falls on the curve and thus tell which percentile the baby is in. If the baby's weight is anywhere between the 10th and the 90th percentiles, the weight is considered normal. Remember, not every baby is at the 50th percentile, so the 20th percentile is still normal and no reason to worry.

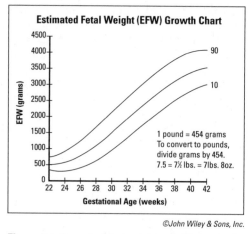

Figure 7-4: Average fetal weights at different points during pregnancy.

Keep in mind that although ultrasound is an excellent tool for assessing fetal growth, it isn't perfect. Judging the baby's weight by an ultrasound exam isn't the same as putting the baby on a scale. Weight estimates can vary by as much as 10 to 20 percent in the third trimester due to variations in body composition. So if your baby is outside the normal range, don't worry.

If your baby measures very large *(macrosomia)*, your practitioner may suggest you have another glucose screen to check for gestational diabetes (see Chapter 15). If your baby measures especially small *(intrauterine growth restriction)*, your doctor may suggest you be followed more closely — that you undergo non-stress tests and repeat ultrasound exams to keep an eye on fetal growth. We go into problems with fetal growth and how to manage them in greater detail in Chapter 14.

Leaking amniotic fluid

If you notice your underwear is wet, several explanations are possible. It may be a little urine, vaginal discharge, the release of the mucous plug in the cervix, or actual leakage of amniotic fluid (also known as *rupture of the membranes*). Often, you can tell what it is by examining the fluid. Mucous discharge tends to be thick and globby, whereas vaginal discharge is whitish and smooth. Urine has a characteristic odor and doesn't flow continuously without your effort. Amniotic fluid, on the other

hand, is normally clear and watery and often is lost in spurts. Sometimes you have a big gush of water when membranes rupture, but if the membrane has only a small hole, the leakage may be scant.

If you leak what you think may be amniotic fluid, call your practitioner right away or go in to your hospital for evaluation. If you aren't preterm and the amniotic fluid is clear, leaking fluid isn't an emergency; however, most practitioners want you to let them know so that they can tell you what to do. If the fluid is bloody or greenish-brown, be sure to let your practitioner know. Greenish fluid may mean the baby has had a bowel movement (meconium) inside the uterus. Most of the time, such an event doesn't indicate a problem, but sometimes it means the baby is being stressed. Your practitioner makes sure the baby is okay by monitoring the baby's heartbeat (usually by performing a non-stress test).

Preeclampsia

Preeclampsia, in which high blood pressure is associated with the spilling of protein into the urine and sometimes swelling *(edema)* in the hands, face, and legs, is a condition unique to pregnancy. Preeclampsia (also called *toxemia* or *pregnancy-induced hypertension*) isn't uncommon; it occurs in 6 to 8 percent of all pregnancies. It can range from being very mild to being a serious medical condition. Chapter 14 provides you with the signs and symptoms of preeclampsia.

Preeclampsia usually comes on gradually. Your practitioner may at first notice only a slight elevation in your blood pressure. She may then tell you to rest more, to lie on your side as much as possible, and to come in for more frequent visits. But occasionally, preeclampsia happens suddenly.

Preterm labor

The strict technical definition of preterm labor is when a woman begins to have contractions and changes in her cervix before she's 37 weeks along. Many women have contractions but no cervical change — in which case it isn't real preterm labor. However, in order to find out whether your cervix is changing, you need to be examined. In addition, your practitioner determines how often you're contracting by placing you on

a uterine contraction monitor (like the one used to perform a non-stress test — see the "Non-stress test [NST]" section earlier in this chapter).

The contractions associated with preterm labor are regular, persistent, and often uncomfortable. They usually start out feeling like bad menstrual cramps. (Braxton-Hicks contractions, in contrast, aren't regular or persistent, and they usually aren't uncomfortable.) Preterm labor may also be associated with increased mucous discharge, bleeding, or leakage of amniotic fluid. Diagnosing preterm labor as early as possible is important. Medications aimed at arresting premature labor work best if the cervix is dilated less than 3 centimeters. If labor occurs after 35 weeks, your practitioner probably won't try to stop your contractions except in rare circumstances (such as poorly controlled diabetes).

If you find that you're having regular, uncomfortable, persistent contractions (more than five or six in an hour) and you're not yet 35 to 36 weeks pregnant, call your practitioner. The only way to tell whether you're experiencing real preterm labor is to be examined. Also, if you think your membranes have ruptured (your water has broken) or if you're having any bleeding, call your practitioner right away. See Chapter 14 for more detailed coverage on preterm labor.

When the baby is late

For nearly 40 weeks, you think that your baby is going to come on a certain date. But in fact, only about 5 percent of women actually deliver on their due date. Eighty-two percent deliver between 37 and 42 weeks, which used to be considered "full-term." Five-and-a-half percent fall into the latter category and the rest (12.5%) are preterm deliveries. At one time, what were thought to be postterm pregnancies were often simply a reflection of incorrectly estimated due dates. But today, with the widespread use of ultrasound, the due dates are pretty accurate. An ultrasound performed during the first trimester is especially accurate, usually within three to four days. A third-trimester ultrasound, in contrast, may be off by two to three weeks.

Many practitioners advise that labor be induced if the pregnancy reaches 42 weeks. If your pregnancy goes on any longer, the baby is likely to still be fine, but greater health risks are possible. See Chapter 8 for details.

Considering umbilical cord blood collection

Umbilical cord blood is sometimes saved because it contains stem cells, the kind of cells that can be used to treat a variety of blood disorders, such as some that may develop later in the child's life, like severe anemia. The decision of whether to donate cord blood is a personal one and based on many factors. The cost involved and your feelings about how important this is to your family play a role in the decision-making process.

If you do decide to donate, you can utilize either of two different types of banks to store cord blood:

✔ **Public banks:** Public banks store blood from a variety of individuals at no cost to those who choose to donate. These banks amass thousands upon thousands of cord blood specimens, thus maximizing the chances of a tissue "match" for anyone who might need it. Given that these samples are available to the public, the children who donate them lose control of the cells after they donate the cells.

✔ **Private banks:** Private banks, on the other hand, charge the donor (or her family) an up-front fee to process the cells and a yearly fee to store the cells. The cells stay in the bank until the donor or a family member needs them. Research has shown the likelihood of the donor or a family member actually needing the cells is about 1 in 2,700.

Not all hospitals have the facilities to collect umbilical cord blood for public banks. If you decide not to donate or can't afford to, you shouldn't feel the least bit guilty. Some people feel that investing the money that you would have spent on cord blood storage can provide more of a potential benefit to your child than the stem cells. Considering your options well before delivery is important. If you opt for a private bank, you'll need to complete the paperwork, get the collection kit from the company, and take it with you when you go in to deliver. You should also inform your provider that you want to have the cord blood collected so that she'll be prepared at the time of delivery.

For Partners — Getting Down to the Wire

Your partner may begin to feel uncomfortable because of all the changes in her body — and because of her sheer size. Many women have trouble sleeping late in pregnancy, which only makes it harder for them to tolerate their discomfort. As you did during the first and second trimesters, take on more of the day-to-day household duties and give your partner the time she needs to rest. Consider treating her to a day at her favorite salon, or send her out for something else that makes her feel special. She deserves to feel good about herself and the changes her body is going through. And things will go easier for both of you if you can find a way to help her accept her pregnant body, relax, and take things a little easier.

Later in the third trimester, naturally, both of you start to focus on labor and delivery. You may have a million questions: Will the baby be okay? Do I really want to be in the delivery room? How will my partner tolerate labor? How will I tolerate labor? Will I get queasy during the delivery? Psychologically, childbirth can be a real challenge for the partner. You care about the course of events very much, but you're clearly not in the driver's seat, and this situation may make you feel anxious.

At the same time, imminent parenthood faces you head-on. And the onset of this new responsibility may cause still more anxiety and more questions: Will I be able to provide for my family? Will I be a good parent? Can I figure out how to change a diaper? How will I know how to handle a fragile newborn? These questions are all normal. Again, they're probably very similar to the questions running through your partner's head. Communication is everything. Most couples find they can talk each other through their respective panic attacks.

Part III
The Big Event: Labor, Delivery, and Recovery

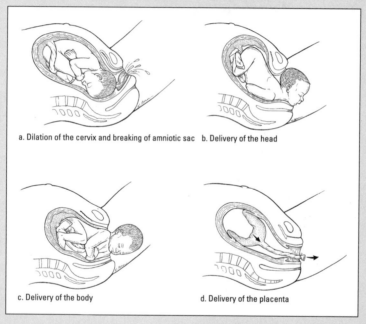

a. Dilation of the cervix and breaking of amniotic sac   b. Delivery of the head

c. Delivery of the body   d. Delivery of the placenta

Kathryn Born, MA

Find out how skin-to-skin contact is becoming an increasingly popular post-delivery process in a bonus article at www.dummies.com/extras/pregnancy.

In this part . . .

- ✔ Learn how to recognize labor signs and find out what to expect during each of the three stages of labor.

- ✔ The big moment is just about here. Discover the different ways of giving delivery and what you can expect right after delivery occurs.

- ✔ Your new baby is here! Newborn babies all look different, find out what to expect about your baby's appearance. Also, understand what the hospital's role is in these early days and prepare for the pediatrician's first visit.

- ✔ Now that your body belongs to you again, find out what you can expect with postpartum changes and resuming normal activities.

- ✔ Choosing bottle-feeding or breast-feeding (or a combination of both) is a big decision. We guide you through the benefits of each.

Chapter 8

Honey, I Think I'm in Labor!

● ●

In This Chapter

▶ Determining whether you're in labor

▶ Looking at the three stages of labor

▶ Managing the pain of childbirth

▶ Checking out alternative birthing methods

● ●

Despite the incredible advances that have been made in science and medicine, no one really knows what causes labor to begin. Labor may be triggered by a combination of stimuli generated by the mother, the baby, and the placenta. Or labor may begin because of rising levels of steroid-like substances in the mother or other biochemical substances produced by the baby. Because we don't know exactly how labor starts, we also can't pinpoint exactly when it will occur.

This chapter helps you recognize the signs of labor and tells you what to expect at each of the three stages of labor. It also addresses such important issues as labor induction, pain management, the monitoring of your baby's health, and alternative birthing methods.

Knowing When Labor Is Real — and When It Isn't

Being unsure whether you're really in labor is actually fairly common. Even a woman expecting her third or fourth child doesn't always know when she's genuinely in labor. This section helps you better identify your own labor (but you still may find yourself calling your practitioner several times or even making many trips to the hospital or birthing center, only to find out that what you think is labor really isn't).

You may experience some of the early symptoms of labor before labor actually begins. Rather than indicating that you're in labor, the following symptoms suggest that labor may occur fairly soon. Some women experience these labor-like symptoms for days or weeks, and others experience them only for several hours. Most of the time, going into labor isn't as dramatic as it's portrayed on sitcoms (picture Lucy saying, "Ricky, this is it!"). Women very rarely lack the time they need to get to the hospital before they deliver.

If you think you're in active labor, don't run to the hospital right away. Instead, telephone your practitioner first.

Noticing changes before labor begins

As you near the end of your pregnancy, you may recognize certain changes as your body prepares for the big event. You may notice all these symptoms, or you may not notice any of them. Sometimes the changes begin weeks before labor starts, and sometimes they begin only days before:

- **Bloody show:** No, the bloody show isn't the newest horror flick by Wes Craven. As changes in your cervix take place, you may expel some mucous discharge mixed with blood from your vagina. The blood comes from small, broken capillaries in your cervix.

- **Diarrhea:** Usually a few days before labor, your body releases *prostaglandins,* which are substances that help the uterus contract and may cause diarrhea.

- **Dropping and engagement:** Especially in women who are giving birth for the first time, the fetus often drops into the pelvis several weeks before labor (see Chapter 7). You may feel increased pressure on your vagina and sharp pains radiating to your vagina. You also may notice that your whole uterus is lower in your belly and that you're suddenly more comfortable and can breathe more easily.

- **Increase in Braxton-Hicks contractions:** You may notice an increase in the frequency and strength of Braxton-Hicks contractions (see Chapter 7). These contractions may become somewhat uncomfortable, even if they don't grow any stronger or more frequent. Some women experience strong Braxton-Hicks contractions for weeks before labor begins.

Expectant mothers ask . . .

Q: "I've never had a contraction, so how do I know what one feels like?"

A: A *contraction* occurs when your uterus's muscle tightens and pushes the baby toward the cervix. Usually, contractions are uncomfortable and, therefore, unmistakable. But many women worry that they won't know they're having contractions. You can tell whether you're experiencing contractions by using a quick and easy trick.

With your fingertips, touch your cheek and then your forehead. Finally, touch the top part of your abdomen, through which you can feel the top part of your uterus (the *fundus*). A relaxed uterus feels soft, like your cheek, and a contracting uterus feels hard, like your forehead. This exercise is also good to try if you think you may be in preterm labor (see Chapter 14 for more information).

✔ **Mucous discharge:** You may secrete a thick mucous discharge known as the *mucous plug*. During your pregnancy, this substance plugs your cervix, protecting your uterus from infection. As your cervix starts to thin out *(efface)* and dilate in preparation for delivery, the plug may wash out. Don't worry; losing your plug doesn't mean you're prone to infection.

Discerning false labor from true labor

Distinguishing true labor from false labor isn't always easy. But a few general characteristics can help you determine whether the symptoms you're experiencing mean you're in labor.

In general, you're in false labor if your contractions

✔ Are irregular and don't increase in frequency

✔ Disappear for any reason, but especially when you change position, walk, or rest

✔ Are not particularly uncomfortable

✔ Occur only in your lower abdomen

✔ Don't become increasingly uncomfortable

On the other hand, you're more likely to be in actual labor if your contractions

- ✔ Grow steadily more frequent, intense, and uncomfortable

- ✔ Last approximately 40 to 60 seconds

- ✔ Don't go away when you change position, walk, or rest

- ✔ Occur along with leakage of fluid (due to rupture of the membranes)

- ✔ Make normal talking difficult or impossible

- ✔ Stretch across your upper abdomen or are located in your back, radiating to your front

Sometimes the only way you can know for sure whether you're in labor is by seeing your practitioner or going to the hospital. When you arrive at the hospital, your doctor, a nurse, a midwife, or a resident physician performs a pelvic exam to determine whether you're in labor. The practitioner also may hook you up to a monitor to see how often you're contracting and to see how the fetal heart responds. Sometimes you find out right away whether you're truly in labor. But the practitioner may need to keep you under observation for several hours to see whether the situation is changing.

You're considered to be in labor if you're having regular contractions and your cervix is changing fairly rapidly — effacing, dilating, or both. Sometimes women walk around for weeks with a partially dilated or effaced cervix but aren't considered to be in labor because these changes are occurring over weeks instead of hours.

Deciding when to call your practitioner

If you think you're in labor, call your practitioner. Don't be embarrassed if he tells you you're probably *not* in labor (it happens to many women). Timing your contractions for several hours before you call, to see whether they're getting closer together, is a good idea because your practitioner can use this information to help determine whether you're in true labor. If your contractions are occurring every five to ten minutes and they're uncomfortable, definitely call. If you're less than 37 weeks and feeling persistent contractions, don't sit for hours counting their frequency — call your practitioner immediately.

Call your practitioner if any of the following apply to you:

✔ Your contractions are coming closer together, and they're becoming increasingly uncomfortable.

✔ You have ruptured membranes. Having your water break may come as a small amount of watery fluid leaking out, or it may be a big gush. If the fluid is green, brown, or red, let your practitioner know right away.

Meconium (your baby's first bowel movement) usually happens after the baby is born, but 2 to 20 percent of babies pass meconium during labor, most commonly if they're born past their due date. Passing meconium doesn't necessarily indicate anything is wrong, but it can occasionally be associated with fetal stress.

✔ You have bright red heavy bleeding (more than a heavy menstrual period) or are passing clots, in which case you should go to the hospital immediately (after calling your practitioner).

✔ You're not feeling an adequate amount of fetal movement (see Chapter 7 for more information).

✔ You have constant, severe abdominal pain with no relief between contractions.

✔ You feel a fetal part or umbilical cord in your vagina. In this case, go to the hospital right away!

Checking for labor with an internal exam

When a practitioner is trying to determine whether you're in labor, he performs an internal exam to look for several things:

✔ **Dilation:** Your cervix is closed for most of your pregnancy but may gradually start to dilate during the last couple of weeks, especially if you've had a baby before. After active labor begins, the rate of cervical dilation speeds up, and the cervix dilates to 10 centimeters by the end of the first stage of labor. Often, you're considered to be in active labor when your cervix is about 4 centimeters dilated or 100 percent effaced.

✔ **Effacement:** *Effacement* is a thinning out or shortening of the cervix, which happens during labor. Your cervix goes from being thick (uneffaced) to 100 percent effaced. See Figure 8-1.

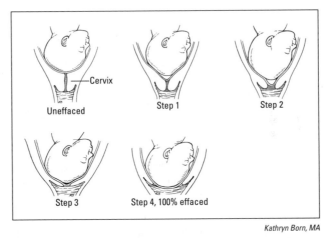

Kathryn Born, MA

Figure 8-1: During cervical effacement, the cervix progresses from an uneffaced state to 100 percent effaced and partially dilated.

✔ **Station:** When you're in labor, the practitioner uses the term *station* to describe how far your baby's head (or other presenting part) has descended in the birth canal in relation to the *ischial spines,* a bony landmark in your pelvis (see Chapter 7 for more information on station).

✔ **Position:** When labor begins, the baby typically starts out facing to the left or right side. As labor progresses, he rotates until the head assumes a facedown position so that the baby comes out looking at the floor. Occasionally, the baby rotates to the opposite position and comes out sunny-side up, looking at the ceiling.

Getting Admitted to the Hospital

Whether you're in labor, being induced, or having a cesarean delivery, you need to be admitted to the hospital's labor floor. If you're preregistered (ask your practitioner about the process), your records are already on the labor floor when you arrive, and a hospital unit number is assigned to you. When you arrive at the hospital or birthing center, you go through an admission process and are assigned to a room.

Settling into your hospital room

Although each hospital or birthing center has its own system, getting settled in usually follows this routine after you get to your room:

- ✔ A nurse asks you to change into a gown.

- ✔ A nurse asks you questions about your pregnancy, your general health, your obstetrical history, and when you last ate. If you think your bag of water has broken or you're leaking fluid, let your nurse know.

- ✔ A nurse, midwife, resident, or other practitioner performs an internal exam to see how far along in labor you are.

- ✔ Your contractions and the fetal heart rate are monitored.

- ✔ A nurse may draw your blood and start an IV *(intravenous)* line in your arm (for delivering fluids and, possibly, medications).

- ✔ You're asked to sign a consent form for routine hospital care, delivery, and possibly cesarean section. (You sign the consent form when you're admitted in case you need an emergency cesarean during labor and you don't have time to sign consent forms.) Signing a consent form doesn't mean you're limiting your care options.

You may want to hand over any valuables you have with you to your partner or another family member (or simply leave them at home).

Checking out the accommodations

Some women go through labor in the same room in which they deliver the baby, and others are moved to a different room for delivery. Most hospital rooms include some standard features, so the room you are placed in probably includes all the following:

- ✔ **Bed:** In a room used for both labor and delivery (also known as a *birthing room*), the bed is specially designed to come apart and be turned into a delivery table. Some hospitals have rooms where you labor, deliver, and even remain for your postpartum recovery. These rooms are called *LDR* (an acronym for *labor, delivery,* and *recovery*) *rooms* or *LDRP rooms* (the "P" stands for *postpartum*).

✔ **Doppler/stethoscope:** Your practitioner or nurse uses these portable tools to listen periodically to the fetal heartbeat, instead of using the continuous fetal monitor.

✔ **Fetal monitor:** This machine has two attachments, one to monitor the baby's heart rate and one to monitor your contractions. The fetal monitor generates a *fetal heart tracing*, which is a paper record of how the baby's heart rate rises and falls in relation to your contractions (see Figure 8-2).

✔ **Infant warmer:** This device has a heat lamp to keep the newborn's body temperature from dropping.

✔ **IV line:** This tube is connected to a bag of *saline* (salt water) containing a glucose mixture to keep you properly hydrated. It also provides access for medications in case you need pain control or have an emergency.

✔ **Rocking chair or recliner:** The extra chair is for your partner, your coach, or another family member.

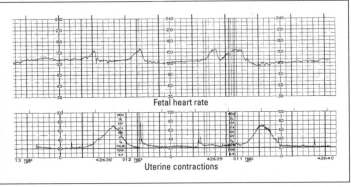

Fetal heart rate

Uterine contractions

©John Wiley & Sons, Inc.

Figure 8-2: Tracking fetal heart rate and uterine contractions.

Monitoring Your Baby

While you're in labor, your practitioner keeps an eye on your baby in a number of different ways to make sure that he is tolerating the whole process well. Most hospitals, and most practitioners, advise monitoring the baby's heart rate during

labor. Although some low-risk patients may require only intermittent monitoring, other patients are better off with continuous monitoring. Sometimes knowing whether continuous monitoring makes sense isn't possible until you're in labor and your practitioner can see how the baby is responding. The following sections outline different ways your practitioner may monitor your baby.

Fetal heart monitoring

Labor puts stress on both you and the baby. *Fetal heart monitoring* provides a way to make sure that the baby is handling the stress. Monitoring can be done through several techniques.

External monitoring

Electronic fetal heart monitoring uses either two belts or a wide, elastic band placed around the abdomen. A device attached to the belt or under the band uses an ultrasound-Doppler technique to pick up the fetal heartbeat. A second device uses a gauge to pick up the contractions. An external contraction monitor can show the frequency and duration of contractions, but it can't provide information about how strong they are. An external fetal heart monitor gives information about the fetus's response to contractions and records *variability* — that is, periodic changes in heart rate that help to determine how the baby is tolerating the labor process.

You may hear your practitioner use the following terms to describe the fetal heartbeat:

- ✔ **Normal baseline heart rate:** About 110 to 160 beats per minute.

- ✔ **Bradycardia:** A decrease in the fetal heart rate from baseline to below 110 beats per minute that lasts for more than ten minutes.

- ✔ **Tachycardia:** An increase in the fetal heart rate to above 160 beats per minute for more than ten minutes.

- ✔ **Accelerations:** Brief increases above baseline in the fetal heart rate, often after a fetal movement. Accelerations are a reassuring sign.

✔ **Decelerations:** These are intermittent decreases below the baseline fetal heart rate. The significance of decelerations depends on their frequency, how far the heart rate drops, and when they occur in relation to contractions. Decelerations are classified as early, variable, or late, according to when they occur in relation to contractions.

There tends to be a large variability in the interpretation of fetal heart rate tracings. For this reason, recently the National Institute of Child Health and Human Development created a new three-tier system for the interpretation of fetal heart rate tracings:

✔ **Category 1:** Normal tracing — predicting normal fetal acid-base status

✔ **Category 2:** Indeterminate tracing — requires closer observation and possible treatment (fluids, oxygen, change in position, and so forth)

✔ **Category 3:** Abnormal tracing — predicting abnormal fetal acid-base status at the moment

Internal monitoring

Your practitioner uses an internal fetal heart monitor when your baby needs closer observation than is possible with external monitoring. Your practitioner may be concerned about how your baby is tolerating labor, or he may simply be having difficulty picking up the heart rate externally — if, for example, you're having more than one baby. The monitor is placed during an internal exam. It's passed through the cervix via a flexible plastic tube. This procedure is no more uncomfortable than a pelvic exam. The tiny electrode is then attached to the baby's scalp.

An internal monitor for contractions (called an *internal pressure transducer,* or IPT) is sometimes used to better assess how strong the contractions are. The monitor consists of thin, flexible, fluid-filled tubing, which is inserted between the fetal head and the uterine wall during an internal exam. Sometimes, this same device is used to infuse saline into the uterus — if very little amniotic fluid is present or if the fetal heart tracing indicates the umbilical cord is being compressed.

Reassuring patterns (Category 1 tracing)

You can take heart when fetal heart monitoring indicates the following:

✔ A normal baseline heart rate of 110 to 160 beats per minute

✔ An absence of late or variable decelerations

✔ Moderate fetal heart rate variability (fluctuations of the fetal heart rate) of about 6 to 25 beats per minute above and below baseline

Other tests of fetal health

If the information from the fetal monitor raises concerns or is ambiguous, your practitioner can perform other tests to help determine how to proceed with your labor.

Labor admission test

This test involves performing electronic fetal heart rate monitoring for about 20–30 minutes upon admission to the labor and delivery floor. It is a good way of initially assessing fetal well-being, and may be helpful in quickly identifying those rare occasions where the fetus needs quick delivery.

Scalp pH

If your practitioner is concerned about how well the baby is tolerating labor, he may want to perform a *scalp pH test*. This involves sampling a small amount of the baby's blood through a little prick of his scalp and measuring the pH, which reflects how well the baby is doing during labor. This test requires that the cervix is dilated enough to access the fetal scalp. Many labor floors no longer have the machinery to perform this test because the machines require a lot of maintenance and quality control.

Scalp stimulation

Scalp stimulation is an easy test to see how the fetus is doing. The practitioner simply tickles the baby's scalp during an internal exam. If this touch causes the fetal heart rate to increase, the baby is usually doing fine.

Some practitioners, and some mothers, prefer not to monitor. But most doctors believe that monitoring is very useful and the benefits that monitoring provides outweigh any risk that monitoring may lead to an unnecessary cesarean delivery.

Fetal pulse oximetry

Another potential way of assessing fetal well-being is by measuring fetal oxygen saturation. There are a variety of ways this can be measured, including one that attaches to the fetal scalp or a probe that sits inside the mother's vagina. However, at this time there isn't good data to clarify how it improves newborn outcome beyond regular fetal heart rate monitoring.

Nudging Things Along: Labor Induction

To *induce* labor means to cause it to begin before it starts on its own. Induction may be a necessity (due to some obstetric, medical, or fetal complications) or elective (performed for the convenience of the patient or her practitioner).

Medically indicated induction

An induction is *indicated* (is a medical necessity) when the risks of continuing the pregnancy are greater — for the mother or the baby — than the risks of early delivery.

Problems with the mother's health that may warrant induction include

- ✔ Preeclampsia (see Chapter 14 for more information).

- ✔ The presence of certain diseases, such as diabetes (see Chapter 15) or cholestasis (see Chapter 7), which may improve after delivery.

- ✔ An infection in the amniotic fluid, such as chorioamnionitis.

Potential risks to the baby's health that may warrant induction include

✔ Pregnancy well past the due date. Because this can increase the risk of certain complications, most practitioners induce labor after the 41st or 42nd week.

✔ Ruptured membranes before labor has started, a situation that may place the baby at risk for developing an infection.

✔ Intrauterine growth restriction (see Chapter 14).

✔ Suspected *macrosomia* (fetus weighing more than 8 pounds, 13 ounces).

✔ Rh incompatibility with complications (see Chapter 14).

✔ Decreased amniotic fluid *(oligohydramnios).*

✔ Tests of fetal well-being indicating the fetus may not be thriving in the uterus.

Elective induction

Although some women like the idea of a planned delivery, others prefer labor to occur spontaneously. Some practitioners gladly perform elective inductions, and others are opposed to the whole concept of it. A woman may choose to undergo an elective induction for several reasons, including the following:

✔ To enable her to make arrangements for her other children, for her work or her partner's work, or for the convenience of other family members by knowing exactly which day she's going into labor

✔ To ensure that a particular physician in a group practice, with whom she has developed a special relationship, delivers her baby

✔ To deliver when the maximum number of labor floor personnel or other specialists are present if she's at risk for certain neonatal or labor complications

✔ To reduce anxiety after a history of poor pregnancy outcomes (such as a previous full-term fetal death) by delivering earlier than she naturally would

✔ To make sure she'll get to the hospital on time if she lives far away and has a history of rapid deliveries

Some studies in medical literature suggest elective induction of labor may lead to an increase in cesarean deliveries. If the cervix is neither dilated nor effaced, or if the fetal head isn't engaged in the pelvis, the risk of a cesarean delivery is probably higher. But if all conditions are favorable for induction, the risk of cesarean may not be increased at all. However, the length of time the patient spends in the hospital is likely to increase slightly when labor is induced.

If an elected induction of labor is planned, it should not be performed at less than 39 weeks along in the pregnancy. Delivery before this time should be medically indicated. If you're considering elective induction of labor, you and your partner should fully understand that you may stand a slightly increased risk of needing a cesarean delivery. If both the expectant parents and the practitioner involved understand these risks, elective induction of labor can be appropriate for personal, medical, geographical, or psychological reasons.

Inducing labor

The way in which labor is induced depends on the condition of the cervix. If your cervix isn't favorable, or *ripe* (thinned out, soft, and dilated), your practitioner may use various medications and techniques to ripen it. Occasionally, ripening alone may put you right into labor.

One of the most common agents used for cervical ripening is a form of prostaglandin that helps to soften the cervix and may cause contractions, too. A commonly used ripening agent is misoprostol, which is a prostaglandin E1 analog. It comes as a small tablet that's inserted into the vagina. An alternative is a prostaglandin E2, which comes as a vaginal insert (Cervidil). Other devices are also used that can mechanically dilate the cervix, making it more favorable for inducing labor. Laminaria are small sticks that, when inserted into the cervix, absorb water and expand the cervix. Another good alternative is a catheter, or small tube with an inflatable balloon on the end that is also inserted into the cervix and inflated. Typically once the cervix is dilated, the balloon catheter falls out.

Some recent information in medical literature indicates that the risk of uterine rupture is higher in women who have had a cesarean section in the past and are having labor induced. The risk of this potentially serious complication seems to be

highest if the patient is given a prostaglandin for induction. For this reason, many practitioners prefer not to induce with prostaglandins, and instead prefer to use a *balloon catheter,* mentioned earlier in this section.

If your cervix isn't yet ripe, you can't exactly place it on the windowsill for a couple days like Grandma did with tomatoes or peaches. If you require induction, you're likely to be admitted to the hospital in the evening and given medications to ripen the cervix at bedtime. Then your practitioner can administer *oxytocin* (a synthetic hormone similar to one that your body naturally releases during labor) to induce labor in the morning.

If your cervix is already ripe, you're likely to be admitted in the morning. Labor is then induced either by administering oxytocin intravenously or by rupturing your membranes (often called *breaking your water*). The doctor performs an *amniotomy,* or rupturing of the membranes, with a small plastic hook during an internal examination. This procedure usually isn't painful. Your practitioner then instructs your nurse to administer oxytocin (usually known by its brand name, Pitocin) through an IV, and a special pump carefully adjusts and controls the dosage. Oxytocin is a hormone that causes the uterus to contract. It can be used to start labor for induction, or speed up labor that started on its own. You begin with very little medication, and the level of medication increases at regular intervals until you have adequate contractions. Sometimes labor starts within a few hours after the induction is started, but it may take much longer. Occasionally, it may take as long as two days to really get things going.

 A common misconception is that oxytocin makes labor more painful. It doesn't. Oxytocin is similar to the hormone that your body naturally releases during labor, and it is administered in about the same doses that your body would produce to cause normal labor.

Augmenting labor

Doctors can also use oxytocin to augment labor that is already happening. If your contractions are inadequate or if labor is taking an unusually long time, your practitioner may use oxytocin to help move things along. Again, the contractions produced as a result of this augmentation are no stronger and no more painful than contractions occurring during a spontaneous labor.

Getting the Big Picture: Stages and Characteristics of Labor

Each woman's labor is, in some ways, unique. An individual woman's experience may even vary from pregnancy to pregnancy. Anyone who delivers babies knows all too well that labor can always surprise you. As doctors, we may expect a woman to deliver quickly and find that her labor takes a long time, while another woman, whom we think will take forever, may deliver very rapidly. Still, in the vast majority of pregnant women, labor progresses in a predictable pattern. It passes through easily discernible stages at a fairly standard rate.

Your practitioner can track your progress through labor by performing internal exams every few hours. How easily you progress through labor is measured by how quickly your cervix dilates and how smoothly the fetus descends downward through the pelvis and birth canal. By plotting cervical dilation and fetal station along a graph (see the "Discerning false labor from true labor" section earlier in this chapter for more information), practitioners can measure the progress of labor objectively. Your practitioner may track your progress through labor using a special graph, called a *labor curve* (see Figure 8-3), to illustrate how the labor is progressing by comparing your progress to a standard curve representing the average labor.

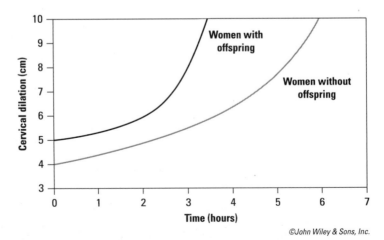

©John Wiley & Sons, Inc.

Figure 8-3: Your practitioner may use a labor curve to track your progress.

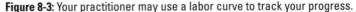

Doctors become concerned over the progress of labor if it's too slow or if the cervix stops dilating and the fetus doesn't descend. They have a shorthand system for describing the variables that determine how easily a woman makes her way through labor: the three Ps (passenger, pelvis, and power). In other words, the baby's size and position (the passenger), the pelvis's size, and the contractions' strength (the power) are all important factors. Your practitioner must pay attention to all these factors, because if labor doesn't progress normally, it may be a sign that the baby would be better off delivered with assistance — with forceps or vacuum, or by cesarean delivery.

If you're going through your first delivery, the entire labor process is likely to last between 12 and 14 hours. For deliveries after the first one, labor is usually shorter (about 8 hours). Labor is divided into three stages, described in this chapter and in Chapter 9.

The first stage

The first stage of labor occurs from the onset of true labor to full dilation of the cervix. This stage is by far the longest (taking an average of 11 hours for a first child and 7 hours for subsequent births). It is divided into three phases: the early (latent) phase, the active phase, and the transition phase. Each phase has its own unique characteristics.

Early or latent phase

During the early phase of the first stage of labor, contractions occur every 5 to 20 minutes in the beginning, and then increase in frequency until they're less than 5 minutes apart. The contractions last between 30 and 45 seconds at first, but as this phase continues, they work up to 60 to 90 seconds in length. During the early phase, your cervix gradually dilates to about 5 to 6 centimeters and becomes 100 percent effaced.

The entire early phase of the first stage of labor lasts an average of 6 to 7 hours in a first birth and 4 to 5 hours for subsequent births, although recent data shows that this may in fact be longer. Often, the exact length of labor is unpredictable because knowing when labor actually begins is difficult.

In the beginning of the early phase, your contractions may feel like menstrual cramps, with or without back pain. Your membranes may rupture, and you may have a bloody show

(see the "Noticing changes before labor begins" section earlier in this chapter). If you have been admitted to the hospital, your doctor may use a small plastic hook to rupture your membranes for you, in order to help things along.

Early on in this phase, you may be most comfortable at home. You can try resting or sleeping, or you may want to stay active. Some women find they have an overwhelming desire to clean or perform some other household chores. If you're hungry, eat a light meal (soup, juice, or toast, for example), but not a very heavy one — in case you later need anesthesia to deal with labor complications. You may want to time your contractions, but you don't need to obsess about it.

 If you start to become more uncomfortable, the contractions occur with more frequency or intensity, or your membranes rupture (your water breaks), or you have vaginal bleeding, call your practitioner or go to your hospital.

 Many women find walking around makes them more comfortable and distracts them from the pain during the early part of labor. Others prefer to rest in bed. Ask your practitioner whether your hospital has any restrictions on walking during labor.

Active phase

The active phase of the first stage of labor is usually shorter and more predictable than the early phase. For a first child, it usually lasts about 2 to 3 hours, on average. For subsequent babies, it lasts about 1½ to 2 or more hours. Contractions occur every 3 to 5 minutes in this phase, and they last about 45 to 60 seconds. Your cervix dilates from 5 or 6 centimeters to a full 10 centimeters.

You may feel increasing discomfort or pain during this phase, and maybe a backache as well. Some women experience more pain in the back than in the front, a condition known as back labor. This may be a sign that the baby is facing toward your front rather than toward your spine.

By this time, you're likely already in the hospital or birthing center. Some patients prefer to rest in bed; others would rather walk around. Do whatever makes you comfortable, unless your practitioner asks that you stay in bed to be monitored closely. Now is the time to practice the breathing and relaxation techniques you may have learned in childbirth classes.

Until recently, practitioners relied on something called a "Friedman Curve" to assess a woman's progress in labor. This was based on now "historic" data from the 1950s, when Dr. Friedman evaluated the course of labor of 500 women having their first child. Based on this original information, active labor occurred when a woman dilated to 3 to 4 centimeters and the minimum rate of cervical dilation during the active phase was 1.2 cm/hour for first births, and 1.5 cm/hour for subsequent births. More recently it seems that labor actually takes longer than previously thought. Dr. Zhang and his co-researchers evaluated data from a comprehensive study called the Consortium of Safe Labor, and looked at information on over 60,000 women with singleton pregnancies in spontaneous labor and delivering vaginally with normal newborn outcomes. This was sponsored by the National Institute of Child Health and Development (NICHD). Zhang's labor curve shows that more than half of women did not dilate at greater than 1 cm/hour until reaching 5 to 6 centimeters. It seems that the normal rate of cervical change from 3 to 6 centimeters is much slower than previously thought. After reaching 6 centimeters, cervical dilation is more rapid.

If you need pain relief, let your practitioner know (for more information on pain relief, see the "Handling Labor Pain" section later in this chapter). Your partner may help ease your pain by massaging your back, perhaps by using a tennis ball or rolling pin.

Seeing an end in sight!

In addition to intense contractions, you may notice an increase in bloody show and increased pressure, especially on your rectum, as the baby's head descends. During this last part of the first stage of labor, you may feel as if you have to have a bowel movement. Don't worry; this sensation is a good sign and indicates that the fetus is heading in the right direction.

If you feel the urge to push, let your practitioner know. You may be fully dilated, but try not to push until your practitioner tells you to do so. Pushing before you're fully dilated can slow the labor process or tear your cervix.

Try to practice breathing exercises and relaxation techniques, if they work for you. When you want pain medication or an epidural anesthetic, let your practitioner know. He decides what pain relief options are best for you based on how far along in labor you are and other factors related to you and your baby's health.

Potential problems during labor's first stage

Most women experience labor's first stage without any problems. But if a problem arises, the following information prepares you with the information you need to handle it with a clear, focused mind:

✔ **Prolonged latent phase:** The latent or early phase of labor is considered prolonged if it lasts more than 20 hours in a woman having her first child or more than 14 hours in someone who has delivered a previous child. Your practitioner may not be able to determine when labor actually starts, so knowing for sure when labor becomes prolonged isn't always easy, either.

When a practitioner determines that labor is taking too long, he responds in one of two ways. One approach is to use medication, such as a sedative, to help you relax. Labor may then subside (which means that it was false labor all along), or active labor may begin. The other approach is to try to move labor along by performing an *amniotomy* (rupturing the membranes or breaking your water) or by administering oxytocin (Pitocin). Both procedures are covered in more detail earlier in this chapter.

✔ **Protraction disorders:** Protraction disorders can occur if the cervix dilates too slowly or if the baby's head doesn't descend at a normal rate. If you're having your first baby, the upper limit of time to dilate, according to this recent data, means than it can take up to 6 hours to progress from 4 to 5 centimeters, and more than 3 hours to progress from 5 to 6 centimeters, regardless of parity. After that, the average and upper limit to dilate 1 cm/hour is shown in Table 8-1.

Table 8-1   Average and 95th percentile (extreme upper end of normal) for patients in active labor based on new Zhang labor curves

Change in Cervix	First Birth Average Hours and (95th%)	Subsequent Births Average Hours and (95th%)
From 6 to 7 cm	0.6 (2.2)	0.5 (1.9)
From 7 to 8 cm	0.5 (1.6)	0.4 (1.3)
From 8 to 9 cm	0.5 (1.4)	0.3 (1.0)
From 9 to 10 cm	0.5 (1.8)	0.3 (0.9)

Protraction disorders may be caused by *cephalopelvic disproportion,* or CPD, which is the term for a poor fit between the baby's head and the mother's birth canal. Protraction disorders may also occur because the baby's head is in an unfavorable position or because the number or intensity of contractions is inadequate. In both cases, many practitioners try administering oxytocin to improve labor progress.

✔ **Arrest disorders:** Arrest disorders occur if the cervix stops dilating or if the baby's head stops descending for more than two hours during active labor. Arrest disorders are often associated with CPD (see the preceding paragraph), but an infusion of oxytocin may solve the problem. If oxytocin doesn't alleviate the arrest disorder, you may need a cesarean section. Typically, arrest of labor is diagnosed when the cervix is at least 6 centimeters dilated and membranes are ruptured, and no cervical change occurs for at least four hours with adequate contractions, and six hours with inadequate contractions.

The second stage

Labor's second stage begins when you're fully dilated (at 10 centimeters) and ends with your baby's delivery. This part is the "pushing" stage and takes about one hour for a first child and 30 to 40 minutes for subsequent births. The second stage may be longer if you have an epidural. We describe the second stage in detail in Chapter 9.

The third stage

The third stage occurs from the time of delivery of the baby to delivery of the placenta — usually less than 20 minutes for all deliveries. We go into more detail about this stage in Chapter 9.

Handling Labor Pain

During labor's first stage, pain is caused by contractions of the uterus and dilation of the cervix. The pain may feel like severe menstrual cramps at first. But in labor's second stage, the stretching of the birth canal as the baby passes through

it adds a different kind of pain — often a feeling of great pressure on the lower pelvis or rectum. But none of this pain needs to be excruciating, thanks to well-practiced breathing and relaxation exercises and, in many cases, modern anesthesia.

Most practitioners acknowledge that even for women who have diligently attended childbirth classes, labor is inherently painful. The degree of pain — and the willingness and ability to tolerate it — varies from woman to woman. Some women choose to deal with the pain on their own or with the help of breathing and distraction techniques mastered in childbirth classes — and that's a perfectly acceptable choice. Many other women want medication to help them deal with the pain, no matter how well prepared they are.

Don't feel that you're in any way falling short of being a perfect mother or that your pregnancy isn't "natural" if you need medication to help with labor pain. We all respond to pain differently, both emotionally *and* physiologically, so even if your best friend, your sister, or your mother got through labor with little or no pain medication, you aren't weak if you choose to use it. Look at it this way: Women who are in excruciating pain usually don't breathe regularly. They also tense their muscles, and, by doing so, they may only prolong labor.

Today doctors generally administer medication in two different ways to help you deal with labor pain: *systemically* — that is, by injection either into a blood vessel (intravenously) or into a muscle (intramuscularly) — or *regionally,* with the use of an epidural or other local anesthesia.

Systemic medications

The most common medications used systemically are relatives of the narcotic morphine — drugs such as meperidine (brand name Demerol), fentanyl (Sublimaze), butorphanal (Stadol), and nalbuphine (Nubain). These medications can be given every two to four hours as needed, either intravenously or intramuscularly.

Any medication you take (even when you're not pregnant) has side effects, and pain relievers used during labor are no exception, although your doctor will do what he can to reduce these side effects, often by combining medications.

Nausea, vomiting, drowsiness, and a drop in your blood pressure are the main side effects for the mother. The degree to which the fetus or newborn is also affected depends on how close to the time of delivery the medication is given. If a large dose is given within two hours prior to delivery, the newborn may be sleepy or groggy. In rare cases, his breathing may be weak. If this problem is significant, your doctor or the baby's doctor can give a medication that immediately reverses or counteracts the pain medication. No evidence suggests that these medications, when given in appropriate doses and with proper monitoring, have any effect on the progress of labor or on the rate of cesarean deliveries.

Regional anesthetics

Systemic medications are distributed via the bloodstream to all parts of the body. Yet most of the pain of labor and delivery is concentrated in the uterus, vagina, and rectum. So regional anesthesia is sometimes used to deliver pain medication to those specific areas. Medications used in regional anesthesia can be a local anesthetic (like lidocaine), a narcotic (such as those in the preceding section), or a combination of the two. Commonly used techniques for administering regional pain relief include epidural and spinal anesthesia and caudal, saddle, and pudendal blocks. The following sections go into more detail on these techniques.

Epidural anesthesia

When it comes to relieving labor pain, there is nothing like an epidural. Epidural anesthesia is perhaps the most popular form of labor pain relief. Almost universally, women who have had it say, "Why didn't I get this earlier?" or "Why was I hesitant about this?" An anesthesiologist with special training in epidural catheter placement must administer an epidural, so epidurals may not be available in every hospital. This is definitely something you want to find out ahead of time so there are no surprises on the day (or night) of the big event!!

 With an epidural, a tiny, flexible, plastic catheter is inserted through a needle into your lower back and threaded into the space above the membrane covering the spinal cord. Before inserting the needle, the anesthesiologist numbs your skin with a local anesthetic. While the needle is going in, you may feel a brief tingling sensation in your legs, but the process really isn't painful for most women. After the catheter is in

place, medication can be sent through it to numb the nerves coming from the lower part of the spine — nerves that go to the uterus, vagina, and perineum (the area between the vagina and anus). The catheter (not the needle) stays in place throughout labor in case you need what's called a *top-up* dose of the anesthetic to get you through the rest of labor and delivery.

A major advantage of epidural anesthesia is that it uses smaller doses of pain medication. However, because your sensory nerves run very close to your motor nerves, large doses of anesthetic can temporarily affect your ability to move your legs during labor.

The amount and type of medication you need can be adjusted according to the stage of labor you're in. During the first stage, pain relief focuses on uterine contractions, but during the second (pushing) stage, pain relief focuses on the vagina and perineum, which are distended by the baby passing through. Epidurals can also make repairing a tear, or episiotomy, much more tolerable.

Years ago, anesthesiologists wouldn't give epidurals during early labor because it confined patients to their beds for the remainder of their labor. Recently, however, *walking epidurals* — the kind that allow you to walk around, because they use medications that have little or no effect on motor function — have become more popular for this often painful stage of labor. Some anesthesiologists, however, question the effectiveness of this type of epidural in relieving pain.

Epidurals can also relieve pain in cesarean deliveries, although different medications in different doses are used. In fact, epidurals are very popular for cesareans because they enable the mother to be awake during delivery and to experience her child's birth. In cases in which cesarean delivery is an emergency or when the mother has blood-clotting problems, however, an epidural may not be possible.

Doctors once thought epidurals, especially if placed too early, prolonged labor and increased the need for forceps, vacuum-assisted, or cesarean delivery. For this reason, many practitioners were reluctant to recommend epidurals to their patients. Most doctors today accept that these problems are negligible when an experienced anesthesiologist places the epidural after labor is well established, and that the benefit outweighs the risk.

Sometimes the epidural takes away the sensation you feel when your bladder is full, so you may need a catheter to empty your bladder. In some cases, the epidural may block motor nerves to the point where you have difficulty pushing. You also may experience a rapid drop in blood pressure that can lead to a temporary drop in the baby's heart rate.

A menu of epidural techniques

The method used to administer an epidural is usually determined by the anesthesiologist, based on his expertise, individual preferences, and your specific situation (such as how far along you are in labor or any medical conditions you may have). The various techniques by which an epidural can be administered include the following:

✔ **Intermittent epidural bolusdosing** was the standard way of administering epidural anesthesia for many years. With this technique, intermittent doses of local anesthesia are given through the catheter. Injections are either timed to the woman's complaints of pain or set at specific intervals. The disadvantage of this method is that often pain is felt as the medication wears off, and more intervention by the anesthesiologist is required.

✔ **Continuous epidural infusions** provide continuous infusion of pain medicine, which provides a smooth and constant relief from pain. If needed, the dosing can be changed, and extra medication can be given.

✔ **Patient-controlled epidural analgesia (PCEA)** differs from the continuous infusion method in that you are the one who controls the amount of medication given. Some anesthesiologists use this technique alone, whereas others prefer a combination of continuous infusion with the patient-controlled method.

✔ **Combined spinal-epidural analgesia** gives a dose in the spinal area for immediate pain relief (within 5 to 10 minutes) and, at the same time, places a catheter in the epidural space for continuous infusion.

✔ **Walking epidural** describes a technique of administering pain relief that does not interfere with motor function. The truth is that, for various reasons, 40 to 80 percent of women don't actually walk during labor, anyway!

Overall, pain control simply makes the whole experience of labor and delivery much more enjoyable for the mother and her partner (and the person doing the delivery, too!). We definitely favor epidurals for pain management. In fact, when she was pregnant, Joanne joked that she wanted hers placed at 35 weeks as a preventive measure, so she wouldn't feel any pain.

Spinal anesthesia

Spinal anesthesia is similar to an epidural except that the medication is injected into the space *under* the membrane covering the spinal cord, rather than above it. This technique is often used for cesarean delivery, especially when a cesarean is needed suddenly and no epidural was placed during labor. The information in the preceding section about epidurals (regarding the amount of medication needed and the risks involved) applies to spinal anesthesia, too.

Caudal and saddle blocks

Caudal and *saddle blocks* involve placing the medications very low in the spinal canal, so they affect only those pain nerves going to the vagina and perineum. These methods have a more rapid onset of pain relief, but the medication wears off sooner.

Pudendal block

Your doctor can place a *pudendal block* by injecting an anesthetic inside the vagina, in the area next to the pudendal nerves. This technique numbs part of the vagina and the perineum, but it does nothing to relieve the pain from contractions.

General anesthesia

When you have general anesthesia, you're made fully unconscious by an anesthesiologist using a variety of medications. Doctors almost never use this technique for labor anymore, and this technique is only rarely used for cesarean deliveries because it's associated with a higher risk of complications. General anesthesia obviously also causes you to sleep through your baby's delivery. But if, in a cesarean delivery, you have a clotting problem that rules out placing a needle into your spinal column or if the cesarean is an emergency and there isn't enough time to place an epidural, general anesthesia should be used.

Considering alternative forms of labor-pain management

Whereas systemic medications or various anesthetic techniques are aimed at eliminating the physical sensation of pain, alternative or non-pharmacologic methods are directed toward preventing the suffering associated with labor pain. These approaches to pain management emphasize labor pain as a normal side effect of the normal process of labor. Women are given reassurance, encouragement, and guidance to help them build self-confidence and maintain a sense of control and well-being. Many hospitals offer some of these techniques, although others require special training and may not be available in all birthing facilities:

✔ **Continuous labor support:** This refers to nonmedical care given to a laboring woman, often by a doula or trained professional (see later on in this chapter and Chapter 7 for more information).

✔ **Maternal movement and positioning:** Sometimes walking or changing positions can alleviate some of the pain associated with labor. Your caregiver or nurse may suggest different positions to try.

✔ **The Birth Ball:** The Birth Ball is a large inflated exercise ball used to help in movement and relaxation during labor. During labor, you can sit or lean against the ball, which provides stability and soft support. The ball also increases the number of positions you can find for comfort.

✔ **Touch and massage:** These techniques provide encouragement, reassurance, and a sense of love, and may be used to enhance relaxation and decrease pain.

✔ **Acupuncture and acupressure:** Acupuncture involves the placement of needles at various points on the body, whereas acupressure (or Shiatsu) refers to the placement of pressure with fingers or small beads at acupuncture points. In some studies, acupuncture use during labor was associated with more relaxation, but no difference in pain intensity.

✔ **Hypnosis:** Usually hypnosis during labor involves self-hypnosis, where the woman herself is taught to induce the hypnotic state. Studies have shown that the use of hypnosis does lead to less use of pain medication and epidural anesthesia.

(continued)

(continued)

✓ **Transcutaneous Electrical Nerve Stimulation (TENS):** This technique involves the transmission of electrical impulses from a hand-held generator to the skin through surface electrodes. During labor, the electrodes are placed near the spine, and the woman controls the intensity of the current through a dial. TENS causes a buzzing sensation that may reduce awareness of contraction pain. Most studies have not shown a real reduction in pain, but some do suggest less use of pain medication, and increased satisfaction.

✓ **Intradermal water injections:** This technique involves injecting a small amount of sterile water into four locations on the lower back. This has been shown to reduce severe back pain for 45 to 90 minutes, but it does not seem to help the abdominal pain associated with labor.

✓ **Application of heat and cold:** Often this is a matter of personal preference, as no scientific data suggests that one is better for pain relief than the other.

✓ **Music and audioanalgesia:** The idea behind this method is that music, white noise, or environmental sounds may help to decrease the perception of pain. Although not clearly beneficial for pain relief, it may help to increase pain tolerance via mood elevation, or help the woman to breathe more rhythmically (heavy metal is probably not the best choice, though!).

✓ **Aromatherapy:** The use of aromatherapy appears to be on the rise. We could only find one study looking at its effectiveness for pain relief. In that study, about half of the women felt it was helpful in reducing pain, anxiety, and nausea, while improving their sense of well-being.

Considering Alternative Birthing Methods

More and more women are expressing interest in nontraditional or alternative birthing methods, and more and more possibilities are becoming available. Certainly, the following options aren't for everyone, but knowing what's possible can be helpful.

Delivering without anesthesia

Natural childbirth usually refers to giving birth without any medications or anesthesia. (It's probably not the best terminology, because using pain medication doesn't make the birthing process unnatural.) The theory behind natural birth is that childbirth is an inherently healthy and natural process, and that women's bodies are made to handle childbirth without the need for medications.

Natural childbirth allows women to have a great deal of control over the childbirth process and their own bodies. It emphasizes having the woman choose which positions are comfortable, how mobile she wants to be, and which techniques she wants to use to be as comfortable as possible. Natural childbirth can be practiced in a hospital setting, birthing center, or even at home. Some practitioners aren't comfortable with every aspect of natural childbirth because they don't want to be limited in doing what they feel is medically necessary and important. Discuss with your practitioner what he feels comfortable with, so your delivery can be as great an experience as possible.

Giving birth at home

Home births are still relatively uncommon in the United States, with fewer than 1 percent of women choosing to deliver at home. This rate is similar to other industrialized countries, except that England has a rate of about 2.4 percent, and the Netherlands about 23 percent! Although the American College of Obstetricians and Gynecologists, in agreement with the American Academy of Pediatrics, believe that hospitals and birthing centers are the safest setting for births, they respect the right of women to make medically informed decisions about where they want to deliver. For some women, a home birth provides an ideal environment to deliver their baby. Common reasons for choosing a home birth are the desire for a low-intervention birth; a desire for control over the birth process; a desire to give birth in a familiar and comfortable environment, surrounded by family and friends; living in a rural area with lack of access to a hospital; and economic,

cultural, or religious issues. Typically, a midwife usually attends a home birth, and an obstetrician is on call in case problems arise. Home births are certainly more appropriate for women who are at very low risk for complications. Although some studies demonstrate that home births are associated with greater risks for both the mother and baby, others show that home births are at least as safe as hospital births for healthy, low-risk women.

The American College of Obstetricians and Gynecologists recently published the minimum criteria for planning a home birth, which include informed consent, a singleton pregnancy with the fetus's head down, no medical or obstetrical conditions, no contraindications to vaginal birth, and the prenatal care, labor, birth, and postpartum care administered by a licensed obstetrical caregiver. The backup hospital should also be within 15 minutes of the home. In addition, and of prime importance, is that women completely understand that while the absolute risk of home births is low, it is still associated with a two- to threefold increase in neonatal death when compared with planned hospital births.

Using a doula

A doula may be a friend, relative, or trained companion who is there to provide nonmedical continuous support during labor and delivery. Doulas often meet with prospective moms before delivery so they get to know each other. During labor, they provide both emotional support and physical support — helping to get moms into comfortable positions, massaging their back or legs, getting water or ice chips, and so forth. Some studies have shown that labors attended with doulas may actually be shorter in length, although there is no effect on cesarean delivery rates. Women who used doulas also seemed to have a slightly better overall birth experience and were more likely to rate their labor and delivery as "very good."

Some women choose doulas because they may not have someone there (like a partner or friend) who can be of emotional support. Others may be at a hospital without one-on-one nursing care and want the additional help. Others just like having a helping hand, and others believe it will enhance the birthing experience. See Chapter 7 for some additional information on doulas.

Immersing yourself in a water birth

Water births refer to spending much of labor immersed in water, with the option of even delivering the baby in the water. Water births usually take place in a birthing center with the help of a midwife, although some hospitals may provide birthing pools or baths. The water temperature is kept about the same as the body temperature, and the woman's temperature should be monitored throughout labor. A recent review of randomized trials found a somewhat lower rate of anesthesia when water immersion was used in the first stage of labor. Interesting, prolonged immersion for more than two hours may actually slow down labor by decreasing the production of oxytocin. Although some professionals in the medical community feel that a water birth is a safe procedure, others have more serious concerns about its safety for both the patient and newborn. Water immersion during the second stage is not well studied. There have been a few cases reported of water aspiration and snapped umbilical cords, difficulty regulating body temperature, and infections in the newborn.

Chapter 9

Special Delivery: Bringing Your Baby into the World

*W*hen you're nearing the end of the second stage of labor, you're very close to the point of delivery. Now is the time you've been waiting and preparing yourself for. Keep in mind that you don't have to worry too much ahead of time. You *can* prepare yourself — by taking childbirth classes and by reading this book, for example. And remember that your practitioner and her assistants in the delivery room will guide you through the process. Accept and rely on their help. Trust in yourself, too, and let this natural process move along one step at a time.

Basically, babies are delivered in one of three ways: through the birth canal by your pushing, through the birth canal with a little assistance (that is, using forceps or a vacuum extractor), or by cesarean delivery. The method that's right for you depends on many different factors, including your medical history, the baby's condition, and your pelvis's size relative to your baby's size. Don't feel overwhelmed. This chapter gives you the lowdown on all three.

Having a Vaginal Delivery

Most expectant mothers spend a great deal of time during the 40 weeks of pregnancy thinking ahead to the actual delivery. If you're having a baby for the first time, it may seem pretty scary. Even if you've had a child before, worrying a bit until you see your beautiful baby is normal. A little knowledge goes a long way, though, and being informed and prepared for all possibilities is always helpful.

The most common method of delivery is, of course, a vaginal delivery. (Figure 9-1 gives you an overview of the process.) Most likely, you'll experience what doctors call a *spontaneous vaginal delivery,* which means that it occurs as a result of your pushing efforts and proceeds without a great deal of intervention. If you do need a little help, it may come in the form of forceps or a vacuum extractor. A delivery requiring the use of one of these tools to help pull the baby out is called an *operative vaginal delivery.* We cover both courses of events in this chapter.

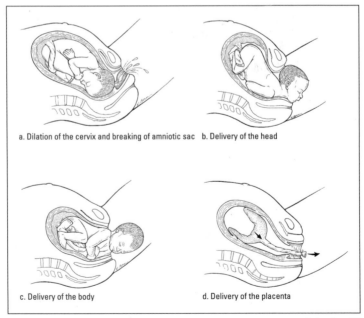

a. Dilation of the cervix and breaking of amniotic sac   b. Delivery of the head

c. Delivery of the body   d. Delivery of the placenta

Kathryn Born, MA

Figure 9-1: An overview of the delivery process.

During the first stage of labor, your cervix dilates and your membranes rupture. When your cervix is *fully dilated* (open to 10 centimeters), you reach the end of the first stage of labor and are ready to enter the second stage, in which you push your baby through the birth canal (vagina) and actually deliver the baby. At the end of the first stage, you may feel an overwhelming sensation of pressure on your rectum. You may feel as if you need to have a bowel movement. This sensation is likely to be greatest during contractions. Your baby's head descending in the birth canal and putting pressure on neighboring internal organs is causing this sensation.

If you have an *epidural* (a type of regional anesthesia used to take away the pain of labor — see Chapter 8), you may not feel this pressure, or the feeling may be less intense. If you do feel it, let your nurse or practitioner know because it's probably a sign that your cervix is getting close to being fully dilated and that it may be time for you to push. Your nurse or doctor performs an internal exam to confirm that your cervix is fully dilated. If it is, she tells you to start pushing.

 Whether your nurse, doctor, or midwife is actually coaching you during pushing varies from hospital to hospital and from practitioner to practitioner. The important factor is that someone is with you to help you through this stage of labor.

Occasionally, you may be fully dilated when the fetal head is still relatively high up in the pelvis. In this case, your practitioner may want you to wait until the contractions cause the head to descend more before you start to push.

Pushing the baby out

Pushing generally takes 30 to 90 minutes (though sometimes it takes as long as three hours), depending on the baby's position and size, whether you have an epidural, and whether you've had children before. (If this isn't your first delivery, your cervix may begin to dilate weeks before your due date, and, after you're fully dilated, you may push only once or twice to deliver!) Your nurse or practitioner gives you specific instructions on how to push. While you're pushing, your baby moves farther along its downward course. Women often begin pushing as soon as the baby's head has descended into the pelvis. How long you push depends on how far down the

head is when you start pushing, and how efficient you are at it. Sometimes it takes a while to get the hang of it. After you deliver the head, your doctor may tell you to stop pushing, so that she can suction some fluid out of the baby's mouth, and also feel to see if the umbilical cord is around the baby's neck. After that, you'll push one or two more times to deliver the rest of the baby.

You have several possible positions in which to push. Figure 9-2 points out three that can help:

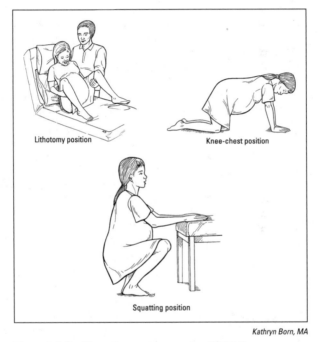

Lithotomy position

Knee-chest position

Squatting position

Kathryn Born, MA

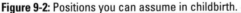

Figure 9-2: Positions you can assume in childbirth.

> ✔ **Lithotomy position:** In this position, which is the most common, you lean back and pull your flexed knees to your chest. At the same time, you bend your neck and try to touch your chin to your chest. The idea is to get your body to form a C. The position isn't the most flattering, but it does help to align the uterus and pelvis in a position that makes delivery relatively easy.

✔ **Squatting position:** An advantage of squatting is that you have gravity working with you. A disadvantage is that you may be too tired to hold the position for very long, and any monitoring equipment or an intravenous line you may have can be cumbersome.

✔ **Knee-chest position:** The knee-chest position is one in which you push while on all fours. This position is sometimes helpful if the baby's head is rotated in the birth canal in such a way that makes pushing the baby out in the lithotomy or squatting position difficult. The knee-chest position may be awkward for some women and difficult to stay in for very long.

TIP

Finding the one position that feels and works best for you may take a bit of experimentation. If you find that you're not making progress, try changing positions.

When you start to feel a contraction, your nurse or doctor usually tells you to take a deep, cleansing breath. After that, you inhale deeply again, hold in the air, and push like crazy. Focus the push toward your rectum and *perineum* (the area between the vagina and the rectum), trying not to tense up the muscles of your vagina or rectum. Push like you're having a bowel movement. Don't worry or be embarrassed if you pass stool while you're pushing. (If it happens, a nurse quickly cleans the perineum.) It's the rule rather than the exception, and all the people helping to take care of you have seen it many times before. In fact, passing stool is a sign that you're pushing correctly, so congratulate yourself. Trying to hold it in only impedes your efforts to push the baby out.

To watch or not to watch

Some partners want to see everything that's happening during childbirth; others feel uncomfortable even being in the delivery room. Likewise, some women want their partners to witness everything, and others prefer that their partners not see them in this situation.

However you feel about it, communicate your feelings to your partner so that you can make each other feel as comfortable as possible. The last thing you need is for you or your partner to be embarrassed during a time that should be one of joy and happiness.

Hold each push for about ten seconds. Many nurses count to ten or ask your coach to count to ten to help you judge the time. After the count of ten, quickly release the breath you have been holding, take in another deep breath, and push again for another ten seconds, exactly as before. You usually push about three times with each contraction, depending on the length of the contraction.

Between contractions, try your best to relax and rest so that you can get ready for the next one. If it's okay with your practitioner, your coach may give you some ice chips or pat your forehead with a damp, cool cloth.

After your baby gets far enough down the birth canal, the top of the head becomes visible during your pushing efforts. This first glimpse is called *crowning* because your practitioner can see the crown of the baby's head. Some labor rooms have mirrors so that you, too, can see the head crowning, but many women have no desire to look. (Don't feel bad or somehow inadequate if you don't want to — you're busy enough.) After the contraction, the baby's head may again disappear back up into the birth canal. This retraction is normal. With each push, the baby comes down a little farther and recedes a little less afterward.

Getting an episiotomy

Just before birth, the baby's head distends the *perineum* (the area between the vagina and the rectum) and stretches the skin around the vagina. As the baby's head comes through the vagina's opening, it may tear the tissues in the back, or *posterior,* part of the vaginal opening, sometimes even to the point that the tear extends into the rectum. To minimize tearing of the surrounding skin and perineal muscles, your practitioner may make an *episiotomy* — a cut in the posterior part of the vaginal opening large enough to allow the baby's head to come through with minimal tearing or to provide extra room for delivery. Although an episiotomy may decrease the likelihood of a severe tear, it doesn't guarantee that you won't get one (that is, the cut made for the episiotomy may tear open even further as the baby's head or shoulders are delivered).

Your practitioner doesn't know whether you need an episiotomy until the head is almost out. Some doctors routinely make an episiotomy, and others wait to see whether it's definitely

necessary. Episiotomies are more common in women having their first baby than in those who have delivered before because the perineum stretches more easily after a previous birth. Tell your practitioner if you have strong wishes regarding receiving an episiotomy. Keep in mind, though, that some natural tears can be worse than an episiotomy.

The type of episiotomy made depends on your body, on the position of the baby's head, or on your practitioner's judgment. Practitioners can choose from two main types of episiotomies:

- ✔ **Median:** Straight down from the vagina toward the anus
- ✔ **Mediolateral:** Angled away from the anus

A local anesthetic can numb the area if you haven't had an epidural.

Expectant mothers ask . . .

Q: "Do I really need an episiotomy?"

A: The answer to this question depends on many factors, including the point of view of your practitioner. It's an issue of frequent debate among people who deliver babies. And, as you may already know, it's also a big topic of discussion among pregnant women. Many practitioners believe that repairing a controlled cut in the perineum is easier than repairing any uncontrolled tear through the skin and perineal muscles that may occur without an episiotomy. The same people usually contend that episiotomies heal better, too. Although a doctor may see the layers of tissue in a cut better than in a tear, medical professionals aren't sure that makes any major difference. Compounding the issue is the fact that it's difficult to tell before labor whether the patient will need an episiotomy.

During delivery, the baby's head stretches the vagina's opening when the mother pushes. Sometimes the birth canal stretches enough that the baby's head doesn't need the extra room that an episiotomy provides. Then again, sometimes it doesn't. If you can "hold" the head at the perineum to let additional stretching occur, you may help matters. But holding the head there is easier said than done because of the incredible pressure that the baby's head exerts. One potential advantage of epidurals is that they allow for a slower delivery of the head and therefore reduce the chances that you'll need an episiotomy.

A median episiotomy may be less uncomfortable later on, and it may heal more easily. (See Chapter 11 for more coverage of the care and healing of an episiotomy.) However, a median episiotomy has a slightly greater chance of extending to the rectum. A mediolateral episiotomy, on the other hand, may be more uncomfortable later on and take longer to heal, but it has less chance of extending to the rectum when the baby's head passes through.

Most tears or lacerations that occur during delivery are in the perineum or are extensions of an episiotomy, which is also in that area. Occasionally, especially when the baby is exceptionally large or you have an operative vaginal delivery, lacerations can occur in other areas, such as the cervix, on the vagina's walls, the labia, or the tissue around the urethra. Your practitioner examines the birth canal carefully after delivery and sews up any lacerations that need to be repaired. These lacerations usually heal very quickly and almost never cause long-term problems. Don't worry about having the stitches removed — most doctors use the type of sutures that dissolve on their own.

Handling prolonged second-stage labor

If you're having your first child and you remain in the second stage of labor for more than two hours (or three hours if you have an epidural), the labor is considered prolonged. If you're having your second or subsequent child, a second stage nearing one hour (or two hours if you have an epidural) is also considered prolonged.

A prolonged second stage may be due to inadequate contractions or to *cephalopelvic disproportion,* which is a poor fit between the baby's head and the mother's birth canal (see Chapter 8). Sometimes, the baby's head is in a position that blocks further descent. Oxytocin (Pitocin) may help, or your practitioner may try to rotate the baby's head. You may also try changing your position to push more effectively. Sometimes forceps do the trick (see the "Assisting Nature: Operative Vaginal Delivery" section later in this chapter), if the baby's head is low enough in the birth canal. If all else fails, your doctor may recommend a cesarean delivery.

The big moment: Delivering your baby

When the baby's head remains visible between contractions, your nurse helps get you into position to deliver. If you're laboring in a birthing room, all she needs to do is to remove the platform at the foot of your bed and set up padded leg supports. If you need to be moved to a delivery room (more like an operating room), your nurse moves you and all your monitors to a stretcher. Whether you deliver in a birthing room or a delivery room depends both on the facility where you have your baby and on any risk factors you may have.

After you're in position to deliver, you still have to keep pushing with each of your contractions. Your doctor or nurse cleans your perineum, usually with an iodine solution, and places drapes over your legs to keep the area as clean as possible for the newborn. As you're pushing, your perineum is getting more and more stretched out. Whether you need an episiotomy is usually determined in these final moments.

With each push, the baby's head descends farther and farther until finally it comes out of the birth canal. After the baby's head delivers, your practitioner tells you to stop pushing so that she can suction secretions from the baby's mouth and nose before the rest of the body comes out.

 To stop pushing at this point can be difficult because of the intense pressure in your perineal area; panting may make it a little easier not to push. If you have an epidural, you may not feel this intense pressure.

Your practitioner also checks at this point to see whether the umbilical cord is wrapped around the baby's neck. A *nuchal cord,* as it's called, is actually quite common and very rarely a cause for worry. Your practitioner simply removes the loop from around the baby's neck before delivering the rest of the baby.

Finally, your practitioner instructs you to push again to deliver the baby's body. Because the head is typically the widest part, delivery of the body is usually easier. After your baby has made it fully into the world, her mouth and nose are suctioned again.

Normally, after the baby's head delivers, the shoulders and body follow easily. Occasionally, though, the baby's shoulders may be stuck behind the mother's pubic bone, which makes

delivery of the rest of the baby more difficult. This situation is known as *shoulder dystocia*. If you have this problem, your practitioner can perform various maneuvers designed to dislodge the shoulders and deliver the baby. These methods include

✔ Applying pressure directly above your pubic bone to push away the entrapped shoulder

✔ Flexing your knees back to allow more room for delivery

✔ Rotating the baby's shoulders manually

✔ Delivering the posterior arm of the baby first

Although shoulder dystocia can occur in women with no risk factors, certain characteristics make this condition more likely:

✔ Very large babies

✔ Gestational diabetes

✔ Prolonged labor

✔ A history of large babies or babies with shoulder dystocia

Delivering the placenta

After the baby is born, the third stage of delivery begins — the delivery of the placenta, also known as the *afterbirth* (refer to Figure 9-1). This stage lasts only about 5 to 15 minutes. You still have contractions, but they're much less intense. These contractions help separate the placenta from the uterus's wall. After this separation occurs and the placenta reaches the vagina's opening, your practitioner may ask you to give one more gentle push. Many women, exhilarated by and exhausted from the delivery, pay little attention to this part of the process and later on don't even remember it.

Repairing your perineum

After the placenta is out, your practitioner inspects your cervix, vagina, and perineum for tears or damage and then repairs (with stitches) the episiotomy or any tears. (If you didn't have an epidural and you have sensation in your perineum, your practitioner may use a local anesthetic to numb the area before repairing it.)

After the practitioner finishes with the repairs, a nurse cleans your perineal area, removes your legs from the leg supports, and gives you warm blankets. You may also continue to feel mild contractions; these contractions are normal and actually help to minimize bleeding.

Assisting Nature: Operative Vaginal Delivery

If the baby's head is low enough in the birth canal and your practitioner feels that the baby needs to be delivered immediately or that you can't deliver the baby vaginally without some added help, she may recommend the use of forceps or a vacuum extractor to assist. Using either of these instruments is called an *operative vaginal delivery*. Such a delivery may be appropriate to use when

- ✔ You've pushed for a long time, and you're too tired to continue pushing hard enough to deliver.

- ✔ You've pushed for some time, and your practitioner thinks you won't deliver vaginally unless you have this type of help.

- ✔ The baby's heart rate pattern indicates a need to deliver the baby quickly.

- ✔ The baby's position is making it very difficult for you to push it out on your own.

Figure 9-3 shows *forceps,* two smooth, curved, spatula-like instruments that are placed on the sides of the baby's head to help guide it through the outer part of the birth canal. The *vacuum extractor* is a suction cup that is placed on the top of the baby's head, to which suction is applied to allow your practitioner to gently pull the baby through the birth canal.

Both techniques are safe for you and the baby if the baby is far enough down in the birth canal and the instruments are used appropriately. In fact, these techniques can often help women avoid cesarean delivery (but not always — see the next section). The decision to use forceps or a vacuum extractor often depends on your practitioner's judgment and experience and the baby's position and station.

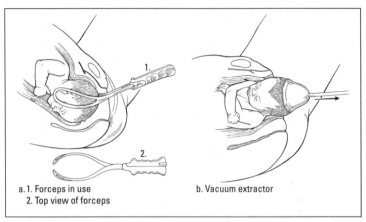

a. 1. Forceps in use
2. Top view of forceps

b. Vacuum extractor

Figure 9-3: Two ways to help the process of a vaginal delivery along: (a) using forceps or (b) using a vacuum extractor to help guide the baby through the birth canal.

If you haven't had an epidural, you may need extra local anesthesia for a forceps or vacuum delivery, and most practitioners perform an episiotomy to make extra room. After the forceps or vacuum is applied, the practitioner asks you to continue to push until the head emerges. The forceps or vacuum extractor is then removed, and the rest of the baby is delivered with your pushing.

If forceps are used, very often the baby is born with marks on her head where the forceps were applied. If this happens to your baby, remember that it's quite typical, and the marks disappear within a few days. A vacuum extractor may cause the baby to be born with a round, raised area on the top of the head where the extractor was applied. This mark, too, goes away in a few days.

Having a Cesarean Delivery

Many patients wonder whether they'll need a cesarean. Sometimes your doctor knows the answer before labor even begins — if you have placenta previa (see Chapter 14), for example, or if the baby is in a *breech or transverse lie* (that is, the baby is lying sideways within the uterus rather than

head-down). But most of the time, neither you nor your doctor can know whether you'll need a cesarean until you see how your labor progresses and how your baby tolerates labor.

Because a cesarean is a surgical procedure, a doctor performs a cesarean delivery in an operating room under sterile conditions. A nurse inserts an intravenous line in the patient's arm and a catheter in the bladder. After a nurse or nurse's assistant scrubs the patient's abdomen with antiseptic solution, a nurse places sterile sheets over the patient's belly. One of the sheets is elevated to create a screen so that the expectant parents don't have to watch the procedure. (Although childbirth is usually an experience shared by both parents, a cesarean delivery is still a surgical operation. Most doctors feel that the procedure isn't something that expectant parents should watch because it involves scalpels, bleeding, and exposure of internal body tissue that's normally not seen, which is disturbing to many people.)

Many hospitals allow the coach or partner to stay in the operating room during a cesarean delivery, but this decision depends on the nature of the delivery and on hospital policy. If the cesarean is an emergency, the doctors and nurses are moving quickly to ensure the safety of both the mother and the baby, which may make it necessary for the partner or coach to wait elsewhere.

The exact place on the woman's abdomen where the incision is made depends on the reason she's having the cesarean. Most often, it is low, just above the pubic bone, in a transverse direction (perpendicular to the torso). This cut is known as a *Pfannensteil incision* or, more commonly, a bikini cut. Less often, the incision is vertical, along the midline of the abdomen.

After the doctor makes the skin incision, she separates the abdominal muscles and opens the inner lining of the abdominal cavity, also called the *peritoneal cavity,* to expose the uterus. She then makes an incision in the uterus itself, through which the infant and placenta are delivered. The incision in the uterus can also be either transverse (most common) or vertical (sometimes called a *classical incision*), depending again on the reason for the cesarean and previous abdominal surgery. After delivery, the uterus and abdominal wall are closed with sutures, layer by layer. A cesarean delivery takes 30 to 90 minutes to perform.

Understanding anesthesia

The most common forms of anesthesia used for cesarean deliveries are epidural and spinal. (See Chapter 8 for more information on anesthesia.) Both kinds of anesthesia numb you from mid-chest to toes but also allow you to remain awake so that you can experience your child's birth. You may feel some tugging and pulling during the operation, but you don't feel pain. Sometimes the anesthesiologist injects a slow-release pain medication into the epidural or spinal catheter before removing it in order to prevent or greatly minimize pain *after* the operation.

If the baby has to be delivered in an emergency and there's no time to place an epidural or spinal, general anesthesia may be needed. In that case, you're asleep during the cesarean and totally unaware of the procedure. Also, general anesthesia may be needed in some cases because of complications in pregnancy that make it unwise to place epidurals or spinals.

Uncovering cesarean's roots

Cesarean delivery, in which the baby is born through an incision in the mother's abdomen, is hardly a new medical innovation. Cases have been documented since the beginning of recorded history. In fact, many famous works of medieval and Renaissance art depict abdominal deliveries.

The origin of the term *cesarean section* is a subject of some controversy. Julius Caesar, it turns out, probably wasn't delivered this way, according to *Cesarean Delivery,* a history written by physicians Steve Clark and Jeffrey Phelan (published by Chapman & Hall). In those days, it was rare for the mother to survive the procedure. Yet Caesar's mother survived her delivery and was depicted in Renaissance art that recounted the life of Caesar as an adult.

One theory is that the name comes from the *Lex Cesare,* the laws of the ancient Roman emperors. One of those laws mandated that any woman who died while she was pregnant be delivered by an abdominal incision so that the infant could be baptized. This rule later became canon law of the Catholic church. A third possible explanation for the term *cesarean* is its relationship to the Latin term *cadere,* which means *to cut.* The term *section* also implies surgical cutting, so if *cadere* is indeed the origin of *cesarean,* then *cesarean section* is redundant. In modern obstetrics, we prefer the phrase *cesarean delivery* or *cesarean birth.* Still, many people continue to call the operation a cesarean section or *c-section.*

Looking at reasons for cesarean delivery

Your doctor may perform a cesarean delivery for many reasons (see the list later in this section), but all are about delivering the infant in the safest, healthiest way possible while also maintaining the mother's well-being. A cesarean delivery can be either planned ahead of labor *(elective),* unplanned during labor (when the doctor determines that delivering the baby vaginally isn't safe), or done as an emergency (if the mother's or the baby's health is in immediate jeopardy).

 If your practitioner feels that you need a cesarean delivery, she will discuss with you why it is needed. If your cesarean is elective or proposed because your labor isn't progressing normally, you and your partner have time to ask questions. In cases in which the baby is in a breech position, you and your practitioner may consider together the pros and cons of having either an elective cesarean delivery or a vaginal breech delivery (see Chapter 14). Both carry some risks, and often your practitioner asks you which risks are most acceptable to you. If the decision to perform a cesarean is due to a last-minute emergency, the discussion between you and your doctor may happen quickly, while you're being wheeled to the operating room.

 If things seem hurried or rushed when you're on your way to the operating room for an emergency cesarean, don't panic. Doctors and nurses are trained to handle these kinds of emergencies.

Your practitioner may suggest that you have a cesarean delivery for one of many different reasons. This list describes the most common ones.

Reasons for elective, or planned, cesarean delivery:

✔ The baby is in an abnormal position (breech or transverse).

✔ You have placenta previa (see Chapter 14).

✔ You've had extensive prior surgery on the uterus, including previous cesarean deliveries or removal of uterine fibroids. (See Chapter 13 for more information on vaginal births after cesarean delivery.)

✔ You're delivering triplets or more.

Reasons for unplanned but nonemergency cesarean delivery:

✔ The baby is too large in relation to the woman's pelvis to be delivered safely through the vagina — a condition known as *cephalopelvic disproportion (CPD)* — or the position of the baby's head makes vaginal delivery unlikely.

✔ Signs indicate that the baby isn't tolerating labor.

✔ Maternal medical conditions preclude safe vaginal delivery, such as severe cardiac disease.

✔ Normal labor comes to a standstill.

Reasons for emergency cesarean delivery:

✔ Bleeding is excessive.

✔ The baby's umbilical cord pushes through the cervix when the membranes rupture.

✔ Prolonged slowing of the baby's heart rate.

Other than the fact that the baby and placenta are delivered through an incision in the uterus rather than through the vagina, for the baby, there's not much difference between cesarean and vaginal delivery. Babies delivered by a cesarean before labor usually don't have cone-shaped heads, but they may if you're in labor for a long time before having a cesarean. As the baby is trying to make its way through the vaginal canal, the head often molds, forming a cone-shape as it is squeezing through. Sometimes, the early formation of swelling or leading to a cone-head shape, occurring way before the pushing stage, may be a sign that the baby is not fitting through. (For more on cone-shaped heads, see Chapter 10.)

Women who have labored for a long time only to find they need a cesarean delivery are sometimes, understandably, disappointed. This reaction is natural. If it happens to you, keep in mind that what is ultimately most important is your safety and your baby's safety. Having a cesarean delivery doesn't mean that you are a failure in any way or that you didn't try hard enough. Roughly 20 to 30 percent of women need a cesarean delivery for a variety of reasons. Practitioners stick to basic guidelines when monitoring progress through labor, and those guidelines are all about giving you and your baby the best chance for a normal, healthy outcome.

All surgical procedures involve risks, and cesarean delivery is no exception. Fortunately, these problems aren't common. The main risks of cesarean delivery are

- ✓ Excessive bleeding, rarely to the point of needing a blood transfusion

- ✓ Development of an infection in the uterus, bladder, or skin incision

- ✓ Injury to the bladder, bowel, or adjacent organs

- ✓ Development of blood clots in the legs or pelvis after the operation

Recovering from a cesarean delivery

After the surgery is finished, you're taken to a recovery area, where you stay for a few hours until the hospital staff can make sure that your condition is stable. Often, you can see and hold your baby during this time.

The recovery time from a cesarean delivery is usually longer than from a vaginal delivery because the procedure is a surgical one. Typically, you stay in the hospital for two to four days — sometimes longer, if complications arise. Check out Chapter 11 for details about recovering from a cesarean delivery.

Debunking cesarean rates

Some women choose their practitioner or the hospital where they're going to deliver based on the number of cesarean deliveries (as a percentage of total deliveries) that the practitioner, group, or hospital has done. However, that number is meaningless, unless you also know the demographics of the practice or hospital. For example, a maternal-fetal medicine specialist who predominantly cares for older women, women with many medical problems, or women carrying twins or more is expected to have a higher cesarean rate than a doctor or midwife who takes care of young, healthy women. The important issue isn't the cesarean delivery rate, but whether the cesareans were done for appropriate reasons.

Congratulations! You Did It!

Women may experience any and every kind of emotion after their babies are born. The spectrum of feelings is truly infinite. Most of the time, you're completely overcome with joy when your long-awaited baby finally is born. You may be incredibly relieved to see that your baby appears healthy and obviously okay. If your baby requires extra medical attention for some reason and you can't hold her right away, you may be upset or, at the very least, disappointed. Just remember that very soon you'll have her to hold and enjoy for the rest of your life. Some women feel too scared or overwhelmed to care for their baby right away. Don't feel guilty about any such feelings — they, and most others, are completely normal. Just take one moment at a time. You've come through a phenomenal event.

Shaking after delivery

Almost immediately after delivery, most women start to shake uncontrollably. Your partner may think that you're cold and offer you a blanket. Blankets do help some women, but you aren't shivering because you're cold. The cause of this phenomenon is unclear, but it's nearly universal — even among women who have cesarean deliveries. Some women feel nervous about holding their babies because they're shaking so much. If you feel this way, let your partner or your nurse hold your baby until you feel up to it.

Don't be concerned at all about this shaking. It usually goes away within a few hours after delivery.

Understanding postpartum bleeding

After delivery — either vaginal or cesarean — your uterus begins to contract in order to squeeze the blood vessels closed and thus slow down bleeding. If the uterus doesn't contract normally, excessive bleeding may occur. This condition is known as *uterine atony*. It can happen when you have multiple babies (twins or more), if you have some infection in the uterus, or if some placental tissue remains inside the uterus after the placenta is delivered. Then again, in some

cases, excessive bleeding happens for no apparent cause. If it happens to you, your doctor or nurse may first massage your uterus to get it to contract. If massage doesn't solve the problem, you may be given one of several medications that promote contracting, like oxytocin, methergine, or hemabate.

If you have some placental material remaining in your uterus, it may need to be removed by reaching inside the uterus or by a *D&C (dilation and curettage)*, which involves scraping the uterus's lining with an instrument. The vast majority of the time, the bleeding stops without a problem. However, if it doesn't stop with these medications and procedures, your doctor will discuss other forms of treatment with you.

Hearing your baby's first cry

Shortly after delivery, your baby takes her first breath and begins to cry. This crying is what expands your baby's lungs and helps clear deeper secretions. In contrast to the stereotype, most practitioners don't spank a baby after she's born, but instead use some other method to stimulate crying and breathing — rubbing the baby's back vigorously, for example, or tapping the bottom of the feet. Don't be surprised if your baby doesn't cry the very second after she's born. Often, several seconds, if not minutes, pass before the baby starts making that lovely sound!

Checking your baby's condition

All babies are evaluated by the Apgar score, named for Dr. Virginia Apgar, who devised it in 1952. This score is a useful way of quickly assessing the baby's initial condition to see whether she needs special medical attention. Five factors are measured: heart rate, respiratory effort, muscle tone, presence of reflexes, and color, each of which is given a score of 0, 1, or 2 for each parameter with 2 being the highest score. The Apgar scores are calculated at both one and five minutes following birth and each parameter is added up. The lowest is a 0 (very rare) and the highest a 10. An Apgar score of 6 or above is perfectly fine. Because some of the characteristics are partially dependent on the infant's gestational age, premature babies frequently get lower scores. Factors such as maternal sedation also can affect a baby's score.

Many new parents anxiously await the results of their child's Apgar score. In fact, an Apgar score taken one minute after the baby is born indicates whether the baby needs some resuscitative measures but is not useful in predicting long-term health. An Apgar score taken five minutes later can indicate whether resuscitative measures have been effective. Occasionally, a very low five-minute Apgar score may reflect decreased oxygenation to the baby, but it correlates poorly with future health. The purpose of the Apgar score is merely to help your doctor or pediatrician identify babies who may need a little extra attention in the very early newborn period. It certainly is no indication of whether your baby will get into Harvard or Yale.

Cutting the cord

After the baby is actually delivered, the next step is to clamp and cut the umbilical cord. Some practitioners may offer your labor coach the opportunity to cut the cord — but your partner is under no obligation to do so. If having the opportunity to cut the cord is something you feel strongly about, let your practitioner know ahead of time.

At the time of this writing, there has been a lot of discussion about the risks and benefits of delayed cord clamping. The idea is that by delaying the clamping of the cord by 2 or 3 minutes, you can give your baby more blood that is stored within the cord and placenta. Recent data based on an analysis of about 15 different studies showed a significant benefit in premature infants. For these preemies, delayed cord clamping showed lower rates of transfusion for anemia, lower rates of a complication called necrotizing enterocolitis, and lower rates of intraventricular hemorrhage (known as IVH, a potentially serious complication in very preterm babies). While the levels of bilirubin (a breakdown product of hemoglobin, which in high levels can cause problems) were higher, there was no greater need to treat these babies with phototherapy (a way of breaking down bilirubin). In contrast, in full-term babies, the studies did show that while hemoglobin levels were higher in the immediate newborn period, and there was less iron deficiency at 3 and 6 months, there was a 40 percent increase in the need for phototherapy for high bilirubin levels and jaundice. Therefore, the decision to perform delayed cord clamping should be individualized. There doesn't seem to be large proven benefits in term infants and there are some significant risks, so at this time it is not routinely performed. However, in premature infants, the decrease in the risk of IVH is compelling and should be considered.

After cutting the cord, your practitioner either lays your baby on your abdomen or gives the baby to your labor nurse to put under an infant warmer. The choice depends on your baby's condition, your doctor's or nurse's standard practice, and the institutional policy where you're delivering. (See more on newborn care in Chapter 10.)

Banking cord blood and tissue

Cord blood is blood that is left in the umbilical cord and placenta after birth. Recently, couples have the option of collecting this blood either through a private or public bank. The rationale for collecting the cord blood is that it contains certain types of stem cells that may be used to treat some specific diseases. These blood-forming stem cells that may be used to treat some disorders of the blood or immune system, and even for complications associated with certain cancer treatments. There are some important things to know about cord blood cells. If a baby is born with a genetic disorder, the practitioner can't use the baby's own stem cells for treatment because the baby has the same genes that caused the disorder in the first place. Also, if a child gets leukemia, you can't use that child's own stem cells for treatment. However, stem cells from a healthy child can be used to treat another child's leukemia. Very recently there has also been the capability to store umbilical cord tissue, which contains stem cells that may be used for the treatment of other conditions.

- ✔ **Public cord banks** store umbilical cord blood that is available for anyone who needs it. There is no charge for the collection and storage of the blood. You don't, however, have control over your child's own cord blood, but it is available for use by anyone who needs it. Public cord banking is not available in all, or even many, institutions.

- ✔ **Private cord banks** store your blood specifically for your own use. The blood may be used to treat your child or other relatives. There is an annual fee for storage of the blood, and often a charge for collecting the blood.

Many couples ask whether it is worth paying the money to bank their child's cord blood. The chance that the cord blood will actually be needed to treat your child or a relative is low, about 1 in 2,700. However, that number may change as research to treat various conditions advances. The cord stem cells are not miracle cells, and they can't treat all conditions. It is also

not currently known how long the cells will last. If you do decide to store the umbilical cord blood privately, you should find out the specific fees, and also ask what would happen if the company goes out of business.

Finding out about new uses for your placenta

The placenta is an amazing organ that provides nutrients and oxygen to your baby, and provides for elimination of waste from your fetus. It is known to be rich in hormones and protein. Occasionally we have couples ask us if they can take their placenta home for other uses. You would need to discuss with your doctor or find out from the hospital if you can take your placenta with you. Some potential uses (not necessarily scientifically proven) are as follows: Some cultures advocate eating the placenta, for nutritional as well as cultural significance. Others believe that eating the placenta can ward off postpartum depression. Many companies sell skin treatments containing extracts of animal placenta, especially sheep placenta. Don't be surprised at ads for anti-aging properties and elimination of dark spots! Placentas have also been found in hair products and claims to strengthen hair. Many come from cow or sheep placentas. Believe it or not, horse placenta is thought to heal sport injuries. We are not advocating the placenta for these causes, but thought you might find it interesting. Of course, if you have had any complications, such as preeclampsia, or a baby measuring small, or you delivered prematurely, your placenta should be sent to pathology for scientific evaluation.

Chapter 10

Hello, World! Meet Your Newborn

- -

In This Chapter

▶ Examining your newborn's appearance

▶ Viewing the hospital's role in the first days of life

▶ Knowing what the pediatrician looks for

- -

*F*or almost 40 weeks, you and your baby have been in one body, and if you're like most women, you've focused on staying healthy to help your baby grow — and on preparing to deliver your baby safely. Now suddenly, your baby is out in the world, and you finally get to take your first real look at him. You may find that in some ways, your baby's appearance surprises you. Newborns typically look a little funny. Remember that many superficial aspects of your baby's appearance — the cone-shaped head, the blotches, and especially the white, pasty goo — will soon disappear.

In this chapter, we give you an idea of what to expect when you first meet your little darling. We also explain the role of the hospital and the pediatrician who visits your baby in the first hours or days.

Looking at Your Bundle of Joy

Immediately after delivery, your practitioner puts your baby on your belly or hands him over to a nurse for some judicious cleansing and toweling off before putting the baby in your arms.

In the first moments after your baby is born, you may be overwhelmed by feelings of love. The shock and relief of it all may

daze you. Most likely, you also think that your baby is the most beautiful thing you've ever seen. Then again, maybe you don't. Contrary to the fairy tales you see on TV soap operas, *I Love Lucy* reruns, and cartoons, babies don't always come out clean and smelling like a spring shower. Your baby is far more likely to be covered with some of your blood, amniotic fluid, and white goo known as *vernix*. His skin may be blotchy, and he may even have a few bruises from delivery. So you may need to keep an open mind when assessing his appearance right off the bat.

Feeling a little hesitant at first or overwhelmed at the sight of your new baby actually isn't uncommon. Often it takes a few days before you establish a true connection or bond with your baby. If you're feeling a little detached, don't worry. As reality sets in and you get to know your baby, you feel much better.

You notice many other features about your new baby's appearance — from his little stump of an umbilical cord to the amazingly long fingernails and toenails. And you observe his first behaviors — from the initial cry to the way he startles at loud noises. In this section, we go over many of your newborn's characteristics.

Varnished in vernix

A thick, white, waxy substance typically covers a newborn baby from head to toe. The formal name for this substance is *vernix caseosa,* a phrase with Latin roots meaning "cheesy varnish." Vernix is a mixture of cells that have sloughed off from the outer layer of the baby's skin and of debris from the amniotic fluid.

Experts have several theories about this substance. Some doctors believe that vernix acts as an emollient to protect the tender fetal skin from the dryness that may result from living within a bag of amniotic fluid. Others believe that the vernix acts as a lubricant to help the baby slide through the birth canal. Some babies have more vernix than others; some have none at all. The amount isn't significant. If your baby passed meconium while inside the uterus (see Chapter 7), the vernix may look a little greenish.

Regardless of what it looks like, most of the vernix usually comes off when the nurses dry off your baby. There's no reason

to leave the vernix on the baby's skin. Any vernix that doesn't come off in the drying process is usually absorbed within the first 24 hours.

The shape of the head

Caput succedaneum — more commonly called *caput* — refers to a circular area of swelling on the baby's head, located at the spot that pushed against the cervix's opening during delivery. The exact location of the swelling varies, depending on the position that the baby's head was in. The swollen area can range in size from only a few millimeters in diameter to several centimeters (a few inches). Caput generally goes kaput within 24 to 48 hours after birth.

Babies who are born headfirst *(vertex)* often go through a process known as *molding*. This molding occurs because throughout labor, as the baby descends gradually through the birth canal, he "fits" his way along (see Figure 10-1). In fact, sometimes your practitioner may tell you that he can feel the baby's head molding to the canal even before the baby is born. Molding doesn't cause any harm. The bones and soft tissues in the baby's head are designed to allow this molding to happen. The result is often a baby with a cone-shaped head (see Figure 10-2). By 24 hours after delivery, the molding usually disappears, and the baby's head appears round and smooth.

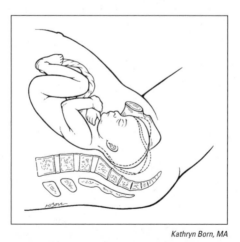

Kathryn Born, MA

Figure 10-1: A baby's head is often molded as it descends through the birth canal.

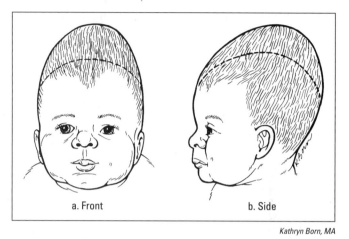

a. Front   b. Side

Kathryn Born, MA

Figure 10-2: The cone shape usually goes away after about 24 hours.

Some women, particularly those who have had children before or who had rapid labor, have babies with no molding. Also, babies born in the breech presentation or by cesarean may not have molding.

Sometimes, during the passage through the birth canal, a baby's ears can also fold down into strange positions. The same thing can happen with the baby's nose, so that at first, it may appear *asymmetric,* or pushed to one side, but these features are no reason to rush your baby to a plastic surgeon. These minor oddities are temporary and disappear during the first few days.

Black-and-blue marks

Quite often, babies are born with black-and-blue marks on their heads from the labor and delivery process. These marks usually happen because the forces of labor put so much pressure on the baby's scalp, or as a result of a forceps or vacuum delivery. A bruise doesn't indicate that anything harmful has occurred; it's merely a reflection of how vigorous the labor process can be. Most black-and-blue marks go away within the first few days of life.

Blotches, patches, and more

Most people think of newborn skin as blemish-free — the very definition of perfection — but newborns have all kinds of spots

and markings. Most disappear within a matter of days or weeks. Some of the most common newborn skin conditions include

✔ **Dry skin:** Some babies, particularly those who are born late, have an outer layer of skin that looks shriveled like a raisin and peels off easily shortly after birth. You can use lotion or baby oil, if needed, as a moisturizer.

✔ **Hemangiomas:** A type of reddish spot, known as a *hemangioma,* may not appear until a week or so after delivery. It can be almost any size, large or small, and can occur anywhere on the infant's body. Although the majority of these spots go away in early childhood, some persist. You can treat the spots that become bothersome (because of their appearance). Discuss treatment options, if needed, with your pediatrician.

✔ **Mongolian spots:** Bluish-gray patches of skin on the lower back, buttocks, and thighs are especially common in Asian, Southern European, and African-American infants. These patches are sometimes called *mongolian spots.* They often disappear in early childhood.

✔ **Neonatal acne:** Some babies are born with tiny white or red pimples around the nose, lips, and cheeks, and some develop them weeks or months later. These bumps are completely normal and are sometimes called *neonatal acne* or *milia.* No need to rush to the dermatologist, though. The little bumps disappear in time.

✔ **Red spots:** Reddish discoloration on the skin, whether very deep and dark or light and hardly noticeable, is very common in newborns. Most of these discolorations go away or fade, but some may persist as birthmarks. One type of discoloration in particular, *erythema taxicum,* can be extensive. It looks like bad hives, and it comes and goes over the baby's first few days of life.

✔ **Stork bites:** You may notice small ruptured blood vessels around your baby's nose and eyes or on the back of the neck. These marks are commonly known as *stork bites* or *angel kisses.* They're common in newborns, and they also disappear after a while, although it sometimes takes weeks or months.

Baby hair

Some babies enter the world totally bald, whereas others come out looking like they need a haircut. The amount of hair

present at birth doesn't necessarily predict what the baby's hair will look like later on. Most often, newborn hair thins out and is replaced by new hair. Different babies grow hair at different rates; some have relatively little hair even at a year of age, whereas others already need a trip to the beauty salon.

Often, a soft, fine layer of dark hair, which can be especially prominent on the forehead, shoulders, and back, covers babies' bodies. This hair is called *lanugo,* and like so many aspects of a newborn's appearance, is quite normal. Lanugo is most common in preterm babies and in infants of mothers who have diabetes. It falls out within several weeks of life.

Extremities

Newborn babies often assume a position similar to the one that they became familiar with inside the uterus, the so-called *fetal position.* You may notice that your baby likes to be curled up a bit, with his arms and legs bent and fingers balled into a fist.

Watch out for those nails, though! Newborn fingernails and toenails may be surprisingly long and sharp. Many hospitals dress newborn babies in little shirts with mitten-like attachments to cover the hands so that the babies can't scratch themselves. To minimize this risk, keep the nails relatively short. Pick up a pair of baby nail scissors or clippers from your local drugstore.

A good time to trim fingernails and toenails is when your baby is fast asleep and oblivious to what you're doing.

Eyes and ears

At birth, a baby's vision is quite limited. Newborns can see only objects that are close-up and see things best at a distance of about 7 to 8 inches away. They also respond to light and appear to be interested in bright objects.

All newborn babies have dark blue or brown eyes, regardless of what color eyes the parents have. By the age of 4 months, baby eye color changes to the permanent hue. Right after birth, the whites of your baby's eyes may have a bluish tint. This tint is normal and disappears in time.

Often, a newborn's eyes may appear a little swollen or puffy. The whole delivery process causes this puffiness; it's perfectly

normal, and it quickly subsides. Some puffiness may also be due to an antibiotic ointment put in the eyes after birth (see the "Caring for your baby's eyes" section later in this chapter).

Babies are fully able to hear from the moment they're born, which is why you may notice that your baby reacts with a startled motion to loud or sudden noises. Newborns also can distinguish various tastes and smells.

Genitalia and breasts

Babies are often born with a swollen or puffy scrotum or labia. The breasts also may appear slightly enlarged. Maternal hormones that cross the placenta cause this swelling. Sometimes, high maternal hormone levels can even cause the baby to secrete whitish or pinkish discharge from the breasts (known as witch's milk) or from the vagina (like a period) in female babies. Like so many newborn characteristics, these secretions are both normal and transient; they go away within a few weeks after birth.

Umbilical cord

The stump of your baby's umbilical cord probably has a little piece of plastic attached to it. After delivery, your practitioner closes the cord with a small plastic clamp and then cuts it. Usually, your practitioner removes this clamp before you take the baby home. Then the umbilical cord stump quickly dries up and shrivels so that it looks like a hard, dark cord. Within one to three weeks, the stump usually falls off. Don't try to pull it off.

To keep the stump clean, you can dip a cotton swab in water, alcohol, or peroxide and clean around the base. However, some pediatricians think this cleaning is unnecessary — unless a lot of goopy stuff is around the base.

Newborn size

In general, newborn babies weigh anywhere from about 6 to 8 pounds (about 2,700 to 3,600 grams) and measure 18 to 22 inches (46 to 56 centimeters) long. The exact size depends on the baby's gestational age (the number of weeks the pregnancy lasted), genetics, and many other factors, such as

whether the mother had diabetes, whether she smoked, and how healthy her diet was during pregnancy.

You may notice that your baby's head seems disproportionately large compared to his body. This feature is true of all newborns. Your baby can't hold up his head and needs time to develop muscles strong enough to hold it up without assistance. You also may notice soft spots on the back and top of your baby's head. These are *fontanelles,* areas where the baby's skull bones meet. Fontanelles allow for the rapid growth of the baby's brain. The back spot (posterior fontanelle) usually closes within a few months, but the anterior or top fontanelle (the one most typically called the soft spot) usually remains until the baby is 10 months to 1 year old.

Seeing how your baby breathes

Often, the baby starts to cry spontaneously shortly after delivery, but not every baby cries right away. A full-throated cry is music to the ears of the hospital staff because they know that the cry triggers the baby's first breathing efforts. Healthy breathing can begin without a loud cry, however, and some babies give only a little whimper. Some babies have normal respiration even if they don't wail at high decibels.

If your baby is slow to start breathing spontaneously, you may notice the doctor, nurse, or midwife stimulating your baby by rubbing his back, drying him off, or tapping his feet. Contrary to the stereotype portrayed in old movies, your practitioner is unlikely to turn your baby upside down and give him a little spank on the behind to elicit that first cry.

During pregnancy, a fetus receives oxygen through the placenta. After delivery, the baby takes over respiratory function by using his own lungs. While in the womb, a special fluid bathes your baby's lungs, and this fluid is often pushed out during delivery. Sometimes, however, a baby needs extra time and help — in the form of suctioning or stimuli — to expel all the fluid in the lungs.

You may notice that your baby breathes differently than you do. Most babies breathe 30 to 40 times a minute. A newborn's respiratory rate also can increase with physical activity. Newborns breathe through their noses rather than their mouths. This great natural adaptation enables them to breathe while nursing or bottle-feeding.

You may also think that your baby's belly looks unusually large and protuberant, but it's just a normal new baby's belly. The fact that the belly rises up and down quite noticeably during breathing and gets somewhat distended as the baby starts to swallow some air only enhances the effect. This movement is also normal because babies use their diaphragms to breathe, not their chest muscles, as older children and adults usually do.

Knowing What to Expect in the Hospital

After your nurse and practitioner are assured that your baby is fine (usually determined by an Apgar test — see Chapter 9 for details), the hospital staff starts cleaning the baby and helping him make a comfortable transition to life outside the womb. Like butterflies emerging from their cocoons, newborns must adjust to a new state of being in various ways. Suddenly, and for the first time, they can breathe on their own and see the wide world around them. This section points out what happens in the hospital after your baby is born to ensure that he is warm, safe, and healthy.

Bracelets are for security, not a fashion statement

At the hospital, your baby wears an identification bracelet to identify him as yours. All hospitals also require that the mother wear a bracelet with the baby's ID number on it. (Many hospitals now also require every new partner to wear an ID band to identify the proud partner.) Each time the staff brings the baby to the mother, the staff member reads off the numbers to ensure that the right baby is given to the right mother. Most hospitals also take additional security measures to prevent any mix-ups and to prevent unauthorized individuals from gaining access to the nursery. Many nurseries are locked and all are closely supervised.

Preparing baby for life outside the womb

A lot happens in the few hours immediately after your baby is born. He has made a pretty significant change and has a lot to adjust to. The medical staff takes immediate action to give him the best start in life.

Keeping your baby warm and dry

Because body temperature drops rapidly after birth, keeping your new baby warm and dry is important. If newborns become cold, their oxygen requirements increase. For this reason, a nurse dries the baby off, places him in a warmer or warmed bassinet, and then watches his temperature closely. Often the nurse wraps or swaddles him in a blanket and puts a little hat on him to reduce the loss of heat from the head — the site of most heat loss (just as your mother told you). When the baby gets to the nursery, a nurse usually dresses him in a little shirt and then wraps him again in a blanket.

Caring for your baby's eyes

Most hospital staffs routinely place an antibiotic ointment into a newborn's eyes to lower the chance that he may develop an infection from passage through the vagina of a mother who has chlamydia or gonorrhea. The ointment doesn't appear to be bothersome to babies and is completely absorbed within a few hours.

Some parents worry that the ointment may blur the baby's vision and thus hinder parent-child bonding. You don't have any reason to be concerned about possible blurring, however. Babies don't see clearly in any case (see the "Eyes and ears" section earlier in this chapter).

Boosting vitamin K

Most hospitals give newborns an injection of vitamin K to decrease the risk of serious bleeding. Vitamin K is important in the body's production of substances that help the blood clot. This nutrient doesn't pass through the placenta to a baby very easily, however, and newborn livers, because they're immature, produce very little of it. So babies are typically low in this nutrient. Giving the baby vitamin K is an important preventive measure.

Making tracks: Baby's footprints

Most likely, a nurse takes your baby's footprints shortly after he is born to make a permanent record of identity. (The unique ridges that form on a baby's feet are actually present several months before birth.) Some hospitals give you a copy of your baby's footprints for your scrapbook. Although most hospitals still use this technique of identification, not all do.

Vaccinating for hepatitis B

Many hospitals now routinely start the vaccination process against hepatitis B for newborn babies, whereas others prefer that a pediatrician administer the first of the three shots after the baby is discharged from the hospital. (The last two are given over the course of the next six months.) Wherever your baby receives the vaccine, this shot is an important tool to reduce his chance of contracting hepatitis B later in life.

Understanding baby's developing digestive system

Most babies wet their diapers six to ten times a day by the time they're one week old. The frequency of bowel movements depends on whether you bottle- or breast-feed. Typically, a breast-fed baby has two or more bowel movements per day, whereas a formula-fed baby has only one or two per day.

Don't be surprised if your baby's first stool looks like thick, sticky, black tar — that's normal. It's called *meconium*. Ninety percent of newborns pass their first stool within the first 24 hours, and almost all the rest do so by 36 hours. Later on, the color of the stools lightens, and the texture becomes more normal. A formula-fed baby typically has semi-formed, yellow-green stools, whereas a breast-fed baby has looser, more granular, yellowish stools.

Most newborns urinate within the first few hours after birth, but some don't urinate until the second day. The passage of meconium and urine is an important sign that your baby's gastrointestinal and urinary tracts are functioning well.

Considering circumcision

Circumcision is the surgical removal of a male infant's penis foreskin. Parents of boy babies must decide whether they want their son to have this procedure performed. The decision to have a circumcision may involve cultural and religious considerations, as well as personal preferences. More than half of newborn boys in the United States are circumcised, but in many other countries, circumcision is rarely performed. The frequency of circumcision in the United States is on the decline, as new information is emerging that challenges the medical arguments for performing the procedure.

Doctors once thought that circumcision helped reduce the incidence of penile cancer, that it prevented infections, and that it reduced the incidence of changes in the appearance of a penis related to a tight foreskin. However, these advantages haven't proved to be true. In fact, the American Academy of Pediatrics has issued a formal statement that existing evidence is not sufficient to recommend routine circumcision. That said, there is some data that shows that circumcision may decrease the risk of a male infant contracting a urinary tract infection, or a male contracting HIV from an infected female partner. Some possible complications associated with circumcision include bleeding, infection, and scarring. Circumcision based on cultural or religious views is still relatively common. The decision, of course, is one that both parents should be comfortable with.

Some people feel that circumcision is beneficial for hygienic reasons. For example, some uncircumcised males build up a thick white discharge called *smegma* under the foreskin, which may lead to a bad odor or infection. However, boys can be taught to wash their penis and prevent this from happening.

If you decide to circumcise your son, your obstetrician or pediatrician performs the procedure within a day or two after your son is born — as long as he is healthy, full-term, or nearly full-term, and without any congenital abnormalities that would cause your doctor not to do the procedure. For some Jewish and Muslim families, male circumcision is part of their religious practice. For Jewish families, they often have a ceremonial circumcision after the baby is discharged from the hospital, performed by a *mohel.*

Many hospitals offer injectable anesthetics or an anesthetic cream that doctors apply to the baby's penis prior to the procedure. The emphasis on pain medication is a humane and

important medical advance, prompted by studies that show that newborns do indeed react to the pain and stress associ-ated with circumcision. Just doing comforting things like swad-dling the baby, giving sugary fluid by mouth and Tylenol are not enough to decrease the pain associated with circumcision, although they can help reduce the stress level. Good options for real pain management, or *analgesia,* include a topical anes-thetic cream (EMLA cream), a nerve block called a *dorsal nerve block,* which reduces pain sensation to the area, or a *subcuta-neous ring block,* again acting as a block to pain sensation.

After circumcision, the doctor wraps the baby's penis in petro-leum jelly-soaked gauze. When this gauze falls off after about four hours, the top of the penis may look reddish and slightly swollen.

If the gauze doesn't fall off, don't pull at it. Squeeze warm water over the gauze to help it loosen. In the first few days, clean the area with warm water and keep it dry. After each diaper change, apply an antibacterial ointment or petroleum jelly until the penis heals.

The penis is usually completely healed within one week. During this time, you may notice a crusty substance at the tip; this substance is normal and goes away with time. But if the penis looks unusually swollen and discolored or if your baby has a fever, call your pediatrician.

Spending time in the neonatal intensive care unit

During the hospital stay after delivery, most newborns room with their mothers or stay at least part of the time in the regular hospital nursery — sometimes called the *well-baby nursery.* But sometimes newborns need the kind of extra attention they can get only in a *neonatal intensive care unit* — sometimes called a *special care nursery.* Within such a nursery, you may find a special area for critical care, where one-on-one nursing, sophis-ticated monitors, breathing machines, and so on are available. You may also find the so-called *step-down area,* for babies who aren't yet ready to go to the well-baby nursery but don't need critical, one-on-one care.

If your pediatrician thinks that your baby needs care in the neonatal intensive care unit, it doesn't automatically mean

that something is wrong. Often, doctors place babies in special care nurseries for a short while just for observation — for any number of reasons. These are some of the most common (this list is far from inclusive):

✔ The baby was born prematurely.

✔ The baby does not weigh quite enough to make the birth weight cutoff established by your particular hospital.

✔ The baby may need antibiotics — for example, because the mother had a fever during labor or because she had a prolonged rupture of membranes prior to delivery.

✔ The baby's breathing seems somewhat labored. This reason is a relatively common one for putting a baby under observation for a short period of time.

✔ The baby has a fever or a seizure.

✔ The baby is anemic.

✔ The baby is born with certain congenital abnormalities.

✔ The baby requires surgery.

Checking In: Baby's First Doctor Visit

Before or after delivery, someone from the hospital asks for your pediatrician's name. Your pediatrician should be someone who is authorized to work at the hospital where you have delivered but may or may not be the same pediatrician you plan to use after you leave the hospital. If you live some distance from the hospital and have selected a pediatrician close to your home who doesn't have privileges at the hospital where you deliver, you still need another pediatrician to care for your baby during the hospital stay. Depending on the time you deliver, the pediatrician may see the baby on the same day, or he may see the baby the next day.

When the pediatrician examines your baby, he checks the baby's general appearance, listens for heart murmurs, feels the *fontanelles* (the openings in the baby's skull where the various bones come together), looks at the extremities, checks the hips, and generally makes sure that the baby is in good condition. The pediatrician orders a variety of standard blood

tests and newborn screening tests. The specific screens that are required vary from state to state but often include tests for thyroid disease, *PKU* (a condition in which a person has trouble metabolizing some amino acids), and other inherited metabolic disorders. The results of these screening tests usually don't come back until after you take your baby home. The pediatrician gives you the results at your baby's first office visit. If any of the tests come back positive, the state also notifies you by mail. Be sure to ask the pediatrician upon discharge when your baby should be seen again.

Considering heart rate and circulatory changes

Remember how your practitioner checked the fetal heart rate during prenatal visits? You may have noticed then how fast the beat was. In utero, the baby's heart rate is, on average, 120 to 160 beats per minute, and this heart rate pattern continues during the newborn period. Your baby's heart rate also can increase with physical activity and slow down when he sleeps.

After your baby is born, important changes in circulation occur. In utero, because a fetus doesn't use the lungs to breathe, a structure called the *ductus arteriosus* shunts away much of the blood from the lungs. Normally, this shunt closes on the first day of life. Sometimes, a murmur is heard in the first days after the baby is born, which indicates changes in blood flow. This murmur, which is called a PDA for *patent ductus arteriosus,* is usually normal and nothing to worry about. However, some heart murmurs may require further investigation — specifically, by having a special sonogram, or *echocardiogram,* of the baby's heart. Even when a cardiologist finds murmurs due to small structural problems (like a small hole in the heart's septum), many murmurs go away on their own. If your baby is diagnosed with a murmur, discuss it thoroughly with the baby's pediatrician or a pediatric cardiologist who specializes in these conditions.

Looking at weight changes

Most newborns lose weight during their first few days of life — usually about 10 percent of their body weight — which, of course, if you weigh only 7 or 8 pounds (3,200 or 3,600 grams),

amounts to less than a pound (454 grams). This phenomenon is completely normal and is usually caused by fluid loss from urine, feces, and sweat. During the first few days of life, the typical infant takes in very little food or water to replace this weight loss. Preterm babies lose more weight than full-term babies, and it may take them longer to regain their weight. In contrast, babies who are small for their gestational age may gain weight more rapidly. Generally, most newborns regain their birth weight by the tenth day of life. By the age of 5 months, they're likely to double their birth weight. By the end of the first year, they triple it.

For Partners: Home at Last — with the New Family

In the hospital, the primary focus is on the patient — in the case of childbirth, the mother and her baby. But the hospital stay is usually short, and as soon as Mom and baby come home, the partner is expected to join them on center stage. In fact, you're likely to find yourself in a starring role.

If pregnancy, labor, and delivery weren't enough to jolt you into the realization that your life is changing forever, getting home from the hospital with your new family certainly does. You and your partner now have a new set of responsibilities. For dads, long gone are the days when it was normal for men to assume that the mother would take on those responsibilities all by herself. Men can help change diapers (they even have changing tables in men's restrooms these days), feed the baby, shop, and do household chores. Even if your partner is breast-feeding, you can sometimes feed the baby breast milk she has pumped and put into a bottle. In fact, parents may want to pre-pare bottles this way regularly because feeding the baby is an important and highly satisfying way to bond.

Your partner is going to need at least six weeks to get back to her pre-pregnancy shape, and probably longer. During the first couple of months, she may be exhausted. She's recovering from labor and delivery, after all. And chances are good that both you and she are somewhat sleep-deprived. Conditions like these make it easy for anyone to lose patience from time to time or to lose her temper more often than usual. Simply

being aware of the fact that you're operating under special circumstances for a while is helpful. See that your partner has time for rest — and try to take naps yourself.

In a somewhat stressful (even if very joyful) situation such as having a new baby, sex may not be a huge priority. Give yourself and your partner the time you both need to adjust your sex drives. Even after your partner's practitioner gives her the go-ahead to resume sex (usually about six weeks after delivery) and you're both ready, take things slow and easy at first. The tissue around your partner's vagina and *perineum* (the area between her vagina and rectum) may still be a little sore. And the fact that it has been some number of weeks or months since the two of you have had intercourse may add to the discomfort. Many couples find it useful to use a water-based lubricant for the first few times; some new mothers need to wait longer than six weeks after delivery before they're comfortable enough for sex.

Finally, don't be surprised if you feel unprepared for parenthood, lacking not only skills, but also an understanding of what it takes to do a good job. Unlike cats, dogs, or jungle animals, humans aren't born with surefire instincts about how to be perfect parents. Both you and your partner need time to develop the skills it takes to handle babies — and children, and teenagers. Along the way, you often work by trial and error. Just realize and accept this situation. Talk about it with each other — often. And fasten your seat belts. You're in for an incredible adventure.

Chapter 11

Taking Care of Yourself after Delivery

*A*ccording to the old adage, it takes nine months for a woman to make a baby and nine months for her body to return to normal afterward. In reality, the time it takes to recover from childbirth varies widely from woman to woman. But most of the changes that your body goes through during pregnancy revert to normal during the postpartum period — sometimes called the *puerperium* — which begins immediately after delivery of the placenta and lasts for six to eight weeks.

As you go through this period of change, you're likely to have many questions about what you can do to make the postpartum transition as easy as possible. In this chapter, we tell you what life may be like as your body gets back into its old shape, as you begin to have sex again, and as you deal with all the physical and psychological challenges of new motherhood.

Recuperating from Delivery

The average hospital stay after an uncomplicated vaginal delivery is 24 to 48 hours. After a cesarean, you may stay in the hospital for two to four days. In some hospitals, you spend this recovery period in the same room in which you delivered.

In others, you move to a separate postpartum unit. The nurses continue to monitor your vital signs (blood pressure, pulse, temperature, and breathing) and check your uterus to make sure that it's firm and well-contracted. Nurses (often the same ones taking care of you) also monitor your baby's vital signs. Your nurses can provide you with pain medication that your practitioner has prescribed, if you need it, and help you care for your tear or episiotomy if you have either one.

The following sections outline the different ways your body begins to recuperate after a delivery and what you can expect.

Looking and feeling like a new mom

Only in movies and on TV do women throw on a sassy pre-pregnancy outfit and leave the hospital looking like they did before they even considered having a baby. Delivery takes a toll, and although most of the changes are fleeting, you'll notice that you look and feel different.

After delivery, your face may be swollen, very red, and possibly splotchy. Some women even have black marks under the eyes or broken blood vessels around their eyes and, all in all, look as though they've just been in a prize fight. All these characteristics are to be expected; pushing causes the rupture of tiny blood vessels in your face. Don't be alarmed. You'll look like your old self again in a few days.

You'll also feel like yourself before long, but you're likely to experience *afterpains,* or contractions that persist sporadically after delivery. These pains are similar to the contractions you experienced during labor and delivery, and they gradually fade away within a few days. You may find the afterpains are more noticeable while you're breast-feeding.

Understanding postpartum bleeding

Experiencing vaginal bleeding after delivery is completely normal, even if you had a cesarean delivery. Average blood loss after a vaginal delivery is about 500 cc, or one pint. After a cesarean, the average blood loss is twice that — about a liter,

or a quart. In order to minimize excessive blood loss, many practitioners give oxytocin (Pitocin) through the mother's intravenous (IV) line or methylergonovine malleate (Methergine) as an intramuscular injection. These medications help keep the uterus contracted. When the uterus contracts, it squeezes shut the blood vessels from the placental bed to reduce bleeding. If your uterus doesn't seem to be contracting well, your doctor or nurse may massage your uterus, through your abdomen, to promote contractions.

The blood coming from your vagina, called *lochia,* may initially appear bright red and contain clots. Over time, it takes on a pinkish and later a brownish color. It gradually diminishes in volume, but the flow may persist for three to four weeks after delivery. You may notice that the amount of bleeding increases each time you breast-feed. This increase happens because the hormones that help produce breast milk also cause your uterus to contract, and this contraction squeezes out any blood or lochia in the uterus. Many patients tell us that the bleeding is heavier when they stand up after being in bed for a while. This extra bleeding happens simply because the blood pools in the uterus and vagina while you're lying down, and when you stand up, gravity draws it out. It's perfectly normal.

If you have very heavy bleeding with clots that lasts for several weeks after your delivery, let your practitioner know.

The best way to deal with postpartum bleeding is to use sanitary napkins. Pads are available in varying thicknesses to accommodate whatever amount of bleeding you have. Don't use tampons, because they may promote infection during the time that your uterus is still recovering. Although the bleeding usually subsides after two weeks, some women experience bleeding for six to eight weeks. Occasionally, fragments of placental tissue stay within the uterus, and this condition can lead to extensive bleeding.

Traditionally, doctors told women not to take deep tub baths after delivery if they were still bleeding. Today, many practitioners say that tub baths are okay, and most feel that shallow baths — called *sitz baths* — are perfectly acceptable. If your practitioner says to avoid tub baths until your bleeding has subsided, she may be concerned that full baths may increase the chance of developing some infection inside your uterus. The trouble is that doctors really have no data on this topic — no studies demonstrate a risk from taking full baths. Ask your practitioner what she thinks you should do.

If your lochia takes on a foul odor, which may be a sign of infection, let your nurse or practitioner know.

Dealing with perineal pain

The amount of pain or soreness you feel in your *perineum* (the area between the vagina and the rectum) depends largely on how difficult your delivery was. If your baby came out easily after only a couple of pushes and you have no episiotomy or lacerations, you probably feel little pain. If, on the other hand, you pushed for three hours and delivered a ten-pound budding linebacker, you're more likely to have perineal discomfort.

The pain you feel has several causes: The progression of the baby through the birth canal causes stretching and swelling of the surrounding tissues. Also, an episiotomy or tears in the perineum naturally hurt, just as an injury to any other part of your body would. The pain is worse during the first two days after delivery. After that, it rapidly improves and is usually nearly gone within a week.

Your perineum may be swollen, and if you had an episiotomy, you have stitches closing it up. Sometimes these stitches are visible on the outside, and sometimes they're buried underneath the skin.

Many women are concerned about the stitches used to sew up their episiotomy or lacerations. These sutures aren't meant to be removed. They gradually dissolve over the next one to two weeks. They're strong enough to handle most activities, so don't worry that a sneeze, a difficult bowel movement, or lifting your ten-pound baby will cause the stitches to tear open.

It's important to keep the perineal area clean to prevent an infection from developing. Such an infection is a rare complication, but call your doctor if you notice a foul-smelling discharge or increasing pain and tenderness in the area, especially if you have a fever higher than 100.4 degrees Fahrenheit.

Here are the best ways to care for your perineum as it recovers from your delivery:

✔ Keep the perineal area clean. You may want to use a squirt bottle filled with warm water to help clean places that are difficult to reach. Sometimes your nurse at the hospital can give you one to take home with you.

✔ Some women get relief from pain by taking a sitz bath. A sitz bath consists of soaking your bottom in a small amount of warm water. In the hospital, the nurses provide you with special basins for taking sitz baths. At home, you can sit in a few inches of warm water in the bathtub. If you have a lot of swelling in the area, putting Epsom salts in the water may give you added relief.

✔ You can buy various kinds of anesthetic sprays and pads that you can apply to the perineum to help ease the pain. Or you can soak gauze pads in witch hazel and apply them to the area. Some women find that chilling the witch hazel increases its effectiveness. (You can also buy little gauze pads that are presoaked in witch hazel — Tucks, for example.) Other women find that ointment or petroleum jelly is soothing, too. It keeps the skin moist and soft and prevents it from sticking to sanitary pads.

✔ An ice pack applied to the perineum during the first 24 hours after delivery helps minimize swelling and discomfort.

✔ Over-the-counter pain relievers — such as acetaminophen (Tylenol is a well-known example) or ibuprofen (such as Motrin or Advil) — or some prescribed pain medications further ease the pain. Taking these medications isn't a problem if you're breast-feeding.

✔ Avoid standing for long periods of time, which can make the pain worse.

✔ After a bowel movement, try not to contaminate the area with the toilet tissue you use to wipe yourself. Clean the area around the anus with a separate toilet tissue, and don't wipe from back to front. If the areas around the anus or the perineum are tender, try to just pat the area dry, instead of wiping. You may find that using baby wipes is really helpful, because they clean the area very well, don't shred, and are gentle on healing tissues.

✔ Don't insert anything into your vagina (such as a tampon) for six weeks and don't douche.

✔ Avoid intercourse for 6 weeks after delivery. Your doctor will see you for a routine postpartum checkup at the six-week mark. As long as you are well healed, sex should be okay at that time!!

You can relieve the gravitational pressure on your perineum from time to time by getting off your feet and lying down for a short while. Finding the time may be hard given that you're incredibly busy caring for a new baby, but make it a priority. And take heart — usually in a week and certainly by two weeks, most of your discomfort is gone.

If you're extremely uncomfortable, you may want to ask your doctor to prescribe pain medications. If you notice that your perineal area is very red or purple and tender, if you run a fever, or if you notice a foul-smelling discharge, let your practitioner know.

If you had any lacerations that extended near your rectum, you may want to take a stool softener (such as Colace), *not* a laxative, so that bowel movements aren't too terribly painful. At least make sure that you drink extra fluids and consume extra fiber in your diet so that your stool is soft. When you anticipate having a bowel movement, you may want to take a pain reliever ahead of time — acetaminophen (Tylenol), perhaps, or some other nonsteroidal anti-inflammatory agent, such as ibuprofen (Motrin or Advil).

Surviving swelling

Immediately after delivery, especially after a vaginal delivery, you may discover that your entire body looks swollen. Don't freak out — this is normal. Many women develop swelling during the last few weeks of pregnancy, and this swelling often persists for a few days to a few weeks into the postpartum period. The intense pushing efforts required to deliver the baby may further cause your face and neck to swell, but this also goes away a few days after delivery. In general, it can take up to two weeks for the swelling to completely disappear.

Don't step on the scale the day after you deliver. You may find that you have actually gained weight from all the water you retain during delivery.

Many patients ask, "Isn't there something you can give me to help relieve the swelling, like a diuretic or something?" Prescribing medication usually isn't necessary because the swelling goes away on its own in a few days, when you're back up and around. Just be patient. You *will* have ankles again.

Coping with your bladder

When you were pregnant, you probably felt like all you did was pee, right? Now, after you've given birth, you may actually find urinating difficult immediately after delivery, or you may feel discomfort when you do urinate. This discomfort is a result of the way the bladder and urethra are compressed when the baby's head and body come through the vagina. The tissues around the opening to the urethra are often swollen after delivery, and this swelling can add to the discomfort.

Some women may need to be *catheterized* (a thin, flexible plastic tube is inserted through the urethra into the bladder) after delivery to help empty the bladder. The problem is sometimes worse if you have an epidural because the anesthesia can hang around in your system for several hours and temporarily make the bladder more difficult to empty. But your bladder regains its normal tone a few hours after delivery, so urinary discomfort is usually a short-lived problem.

 If you feel a burning sensation primarily during urination, let your doctor or nurse know because it may be a sign that you're developing a urinary tract infection.

Some women experience the opposite problem: They find that they don't have good control over their bladder function — that they leak a little urine when they stand up or laugh, or that they have to run like a cheetah to make it to the john in time. If this incontinence happens to you, don't worry too much because time usually solves the problem. In some cases, it may take a number of weeks to get things under control.

 Kegel exercises (see the "Doing Kegel exercises" section later in this chapter) may be useful if the problem persists. Another good strategy is to make a conscious effort to go to the bathroom at regular intervals to empty your bladder before it becomes an emergency!

Battling the hemorrhoid blues

Most of your pushing efforts during delivery are focused toward the rectum, a fact that causes many women to develop *hemorrhoids* — dilated veins that pop out from the rectum. Unfortunately, having no problems with hemorrhoids before

you go into labor is no guarantee that they won't appear after delivery. If you develop hemorrhoids during the last part of your pregnancy, they may get worse after delivery. At times, hemorrhoids can be more uncomfortable than an episiotomy, and they last a little longer. Turn to Chapter 7 for tips on dealing with hemorrhoids.

The good news is that the problem is usually temporary. Postpartum hemorrhoids typically go away within a few weeks. Sometimes they don't go away completely, but for the most part they aren't bothersome. They may not trouble you at all for a few months, and then they may be uncomfortable again for a few days, and then get better again.

Consider taking a stool softener (such as Colace), as we mention earlier, and make sure you consume plenty of fluids and fiber. This way, bowel movements won't hurt so much and you won't have to push too hard (which makes hemorrhoids worse). Your hemorrhoids are likely to go away within one to two weeks.

Understanding postpartum bowel function

Many women find that they don't have a bowel movement for a few days after delivery. This lack of bowel function may be because you haven't eaten much or because epidurals and some other pain medications sometimes slow down the bowels a little. Your system may take a few days to return to normal.

Many women are afraid of bearing down because they don't want to tear the stitches used to repair their episiotomy, so they try avoid having a bowel movement altogether. But avoiding a bowel movement isn't a great idea. You have no reason to be afraid of tearing the stitches. Your episiotomy is repaired in several layers with strong sutures. Tearing the sutures is extremely difficult, especially by having a bowel movement.

Here are a few ways to make having a bowel movement easier:

- ✔ Walk around the postpartum ward as much as you can. Walking improves circulation to the bowels and can help to eliminate any residual effects of the epidural.
- ✔ Try taking a stool softener, such as Colace.
- ✔ Try not to think about it too much. Things happen in time.

If you have hemorrhoids or a laceration that reaches back to the rectal area (see Chapter 7), a bowel movement may be painful. You can reduce the discomfort by using a local anesthetic cream and by using a stool softener. Also, you may want to take a pain reliever shortly before you anticipate having a bowel movement.

Continuing to recover at home

By the time you're discharged from the hospital after a vaginal delivery, most of the acute pain is gone. After you get home, however, you can still expect some soreness. The main area of discomfort is around your perineum. No matter how easy your delivery may have been, this part of your body has undergone some real trauma, and it simply needs time to heal.

Try not to let the lingering discomfort associated with having just given birth frustrate you. Keep in mind what an amazing miracle your body has just been through. In addition to dealing with the soreness from delivery, you need to adjust to a new lifestyle — getting up at all hours of the night, changing diapers, and feeding your new baby.

Recovering from a Cesarean Delivery

The hospital stay after a cesarean delivery is generally a few days longer than after a vaginal delivery — usually three to four days in total. If you have a cesarean delivery, you're put on a stretcher immediately afterward and transported to the recovery room. You may even feel up to holding your baby during the trip. Just like any surgery, the first few days can be uncomfortable. Don't worry, though, because after the initial few days, most people recover quite easily.

Going to the recovery room

When you're in the recovery room, your nurse and anesthesiologist monitor your vital signs. The nurse periodically checks your abdomen to make sure that the uterus is firm and that the dressing over the incision is dry. Your nurse also checks for signs of excessive bleeding from the uterus. More than likely, you have a catheter in your bladder, and

it stays in place for the first night so that you don't have to worry about getting up to go to the bathroom. You also have an intravenous (IV) line in place to receive fluids and any medications your doctor prescribes. If you had an epidural or spinal anesthetic, your legs may still seem a little numb or heavy. This feeling wears off in a few hours. If you had general anesthesia (that is, if you were "put to sleep"), you may feel a little groggy when you get to the recovery room. Just as with a vaginal delivery, you may experience some shaking (see Chapter 9). If you're up to it and if you want to, you can breast-feed your baby while you're in the recovery room.

Most likely, you received pain medication in the operating room, and you may not need any more while you're in the recovery room. In some hospitals, if you have an epidural or spinal, your anesthesiologist injects a long-lasting medication into the catheter that keeps you almost pain-free for about 24 hours. If, however, your pain medication doesn't seem to be working, by all means let your nurse know.

Taking it one step at a time

When your nurse and anesthesiologist are confident that your vital signs are stable and that you're recovering normally from the anesthesia, you're discharged from the recovery room — generally about one to three hours after delivery. You're transported on a stretcher to a hospital room, where you spend the rest of your recovery time.

The day of delivery

On the day of your cesarean, you should plan on just staying in bed. Thanks to your catheter, you don't need to worry about getting up to go to the bathroom. If you had your surgery early in the morning, you may feel like getting up later in the evening, if only to sit in a chair. Just be sure to check with your nurse first to see whether getting up is okay. When you get up the first time, make sure someone is there to help you.

Although some doctors still prefer that patients not have any food immediately after a cesarean, many doctors now allow women to eat and drink shortly after the surgery. Often, we find that the patient is the best judge of what she should and shouldn't do: If you feel queasy and nauseous, you're better off

not eating. But if you feel hungry, drinking liquids and having small amounts of solid food is probably fine.

Like women who have had a vaginal delivery, expect some vaginal bleeding (lochia) after a cesarean. The bleeding may be quite heavy during the first few days after your surgery (see the "Understanding postpartum bleeding" section earlier in this chapter).

As far as care for the incision, many practitioners will remove the dressing on the first or second day after the cesarean. Once the dressing is removed, you are usually able to shower. Our advice is that during the shower, don't rub the incision, just let the water run over it and pat it dry immediately after the shower. Some women's incisions are closed by sutures which will reabsorb over time with no need for removal, while others may be closed by staples, which do need to be removed.

Most women who have a cesarean delivery and have staples in their skin worry that removing the staples will hurt. But don't worry. Staple removal is a quick and painless procedure.

The day after

The first day after your surgery, your doctor is likely to encourage you to get out of bed and start to walk around. The first couple of times you get up to walk may be pretty uncomfortable — you may feel pain around the incision in your abdomen — so you may want to ask for a so-called *top-up* dose of pain medication 20 minutes or so before getting up.

Make sure someone is with you the first few times you get up to make sure you don't fall.

Depending on your fluid needs, your doctor may also discontinue your IV line. Most of the time, you're able to drink liquids on the first day, and many doctors also let you eat solid food.

Most likely, you have a bandage over your abdominal incision. Sometimes this bandage comes off on day one, but other times doctors prefer to leave it on longer.

Many women ask about *rooming in* — that is, having the baby stay in the room with them — after a cesarean delivery, especially after they've had a day or so to recover a bit from the

procedure. Having the baby in the room with you is certainly fine if you feel up to it. But by no means should you feel that you have to. Keep in mind that you just had abdominal surgery, and you may not be physically able to attend to every single one of your baby's needs during the first few days afterward. The hospital nurses are there to help, so during this time devote as much energy as possible to your own recovery. You'll be that much better able to care for your baby after you get home.

Understanding post-cesarean pain

You may feel a kind of burning pain at the site of your abdominal skin incision. This pain is worse when you get out of bed or change positions. Eventually, the burning diminishes to a sort of tingling sensation and is much improved within a week or two after surgery.

You may also feel pain from post-delivery uterine contractions — just as women who deliver vaginally do. Your doctor is likely to give you oxytocin (Pitocin) for the first few hours after your surgery to encourage contractions and thus minimize blood loss. Pain from contractions diminishes by the second day, although it may recur when you breast-feed because breast-feeding can trigger more contractions.

You may feel pain in tissues deep beneath your skin. A cesarean isn't a simple slit through the surface of a woman's belly. The physician must cut through several layers of tissue in order to reach the uterus. Each layer must then be repaired. And every one of the repaired incisions can generate pain, which is why you may feel pain deep in your abdomen after a cesarean. This pain usually takes one to two weeks to fade away. Many women tell us that they feel more pain on one side or the other, possibly because the stitches are a little tighter on one side. Whatever the reason, uneven pain is very common and nothing to worry about.

Many women say the worst pain of all is gas pain. The intestines accumulate a large amount of gas after a cesarean delivery, in part because of the way the intestines are manipulated during the surgery but also as a result of the medications — the anesthetics used during the operation and the painkillers given afterward. Gas pains typically begin on the second or third day

after delivery and improve when you start to pass gas. Get up and walk around as much as possible, because doing so gets the gastrointestinal tract moving again.

If you have a cesarean delivery after going through labor for hours, you may have perineal pain — from pushing and from any number of internal exams — on top of everything else. This pain disappears soon after delivery.

Dealing with post-op pain

The amount of pain or discomfort experienced after a cesarean delivery varies from woman to woman, depending on the circumstances of her delivery and on her tolerance for pain. Your practitioner can prescribe pain medication, but she probably will specify that the medication shouldn't be given unless you ask for it. (Sometimes this is hospital policy.) So if you want the pain relief, ask for it — before your pain becomes excruciating. Ask for the medication when you anticipate getting out of bed or just before your next dose of medication is due (usually after three or four hours), so that you give your nurse enough time to get it for you.

Some hospitals offer a PCA *(patient-controlled analgesia)* pump, which is attached to your IV line. When you feel your pain increasing, you simply press a button on the pump to release a small amount of pain medication into your IV line. Because you receive the medication intravenously, you can feel its effects quickly, and by using the medication only when you feel you need it, you can often get by with much less medication in total. Don't worry about overdosing, though, because the pump has special settings that prevent you from getting too much medication.

Getting ready to go home

After surgery, you find that each day is noticeably easier and more comfortable than the one before. Over the course of three days, you gradually find it easier to get out of bed and walk around. You start to eat normally again. You're also able to shower — and many women find that first shower a truly big relief. But please keep in mind that you have just been through not only major surgery but also nine months of pregnancy! And you must recover from both. Some women

really do recover quickly and feel like going home after only a couple of days. But many women need more time to feel strong enough to leave the hospital.

The length of your stay may be determined to some extent by what your insurance plan allows and what individual state laws mandate. And occasionally, a post-operative infection or some other complication necessitates a longer-than-usual hospital stay. But typically, you're ready to go home after about three days.

Here are some indications that you may be ready to go home:

✓ You tolerate food and liquids without any problem.

✓ You urinate normally and without difficulty.

✓ Your bowels are on their way to recovering normal function.

✓ You have no signs of infection.

Continuing to recover at home

When you're discharged from the hospital after a cesarean delivery, you're well on your way down the road to recovery. However, getting back on your feet after a cesarean delivery takes longer than after a vaginal delivery, so take it easy for the first week or two after you return home. Keep the following pointers in mind as you recover.

Taking good care of yourself

Get the help you need from family and friends, if possible. If you can afford it, consider hiring a baby nurse for the first few weeks. (A baby nurse can be quite helpful for women who've had vaginal births, too.) Make sure, however, that any caregivers you recruit to help you have all of their vaccinations up to date. Specifically, make sure that they have had a TDap vaccine booster within the past ten years (see Chapter 1). When you are on your own, try to keep the household chores you do to a minimum. Avoid running up and down stairs a lot. Devote your energy to taking care of your new baby and taking care of yourself. Pay attention, and your body will clearly let you know how much activity you can handle.

Some doctors recommend that you not drive a car for the first week or two. This restriction isn't because of the anesthesia you may have had — the anesthesia really doesn't affect your reflexes for more than a day or two after delivery. The problem is simply that any leftover pain you may be experiencing after delivery may make it difficult for you to quickly move your foot from the gas pedal to the brake if you need to stop suddenly. When your pain is gone, you can safely resume driving.

Most doctors also advise you to postpone any abdominal exercises until after your six-week checkup, so that the incisions in all the layers of your abdomen have time to heal completely.

Most women feel pretty much back to normal by the six-week point. But some need as long as three months to fully recover.

By the time you're home from the hospital, you should be able to eat normally. If you lost a great deal of blood during your surgery, however, you may want to ask your doctor whether you should take extra iron supplements.

Noticing changes in your scar

At first, the scar from your cesarean delivery looks reddish or pinkish. In time, it may turn a darker shade of purple or brown, depending to some extent on your skin color. Over the course of a year, the scar will fade and, eventually, assume a very pale color. If you have dark skin, it may be brownish. Most of the time, a cesarean scar is pencil-thin or even thinner. A scar from a cesarean delivery may look prominent immediately after the procedure, when the staples are still in place, but after they're removed and the scar has had several weeks to heal, you'll observe how it begins to fade into something far less obvious.

Many factors can affect the healing process and thus determine what the scar ultimately looks like. Some women are naturally prone to forming a thick type of scar, called a *keloid*. In these cases, doctors really can't do much to change the situation. Some over-the-counter products claim to help wounds heal, but none have been proven to be beneficial.

You may notice that the area around your incision becomes numb. This numbness occurs because in making the incision, your doctor cut through some of the nerves that transmit sensation in that area. The nerves do grow back, however, and in time the numbness turns into a mild tingling sensation and then returns to normal.

Some women notice a blood-tinged fluid discharge coming from the center or side of their incision. This drainage sometimes happens when blood and other fluids accumulate under the incision and then seep out. If only a small amount oozes out and the drainage then stops, it's okay. Applying a little pressure to this area with a clean bandage is a good idea.

If you notice persistent blood-tinged or yellowish discharge from your incision, let your doctor know. Occasionally, the incision may open at the point where the drainage occurs. If so, your doctor may want you to take special measures to keep the opening clean so that it heals on its own.

Recognizing causes for concern

Most women who have cesarean deliveries recover without any problems. In some cases, however, you may not heal quickly and smoothly. Call your doctor if you notice any of the following:

- ✔ If pain from your incision or from your abdomen increases, rather than decreases

- ✔ If large amounts of blood or blood-tinged fluid drain from your incision

- ✔ If you have a fever higher than 100.4 degrees Fahrenheit

- ✔ If your incision begins to open up

- ✔ If you notice any odor associated with the discharge that may occur from your incision

Going through More Postpartum Changes

Many aspects of postpartum life are the same whether you had a vaginal or a cesarean delivery. Now that you're no longer pregnant, your body begins shifting back to its pre-pregnancy state, and you're in for a number of changes. This section overviews many of the common changes you may experience.

Sweating like a . . . new mom

If you're managing to get any sleep at night despite having a new baby in the house, you may find that you wake up drenched in sweat. Even during the daytime, you may notice that you perspire significantly more than usual. This sweating is very common and is thought to have something to do with fluctuations in hormone levels that occur as your body returns to a nonpregnant state. It's very similar to the night sweats and hot flashes that menopausal women get, due to a drop in estrogen levels. As long as the sweating isn't associated with any fever, it's not a problem. It goes away over the course of the next month or so.

Dealing with breast engorgement

A woman's breasts typically begin to *engorge*, or fill with milk, three to five days after she delivers her baby. You may be amazed to see how huge your breasts can really be! If you're breast-feeding, your baby lessens the problem for you as she gets the hang of nursing, figures out how to take in more milk, and establishes a pattern of feeding. (See Chapter 12 for more information about breast-feeding.)

If you're not breast-feeding, you may find that your breasts stay engorged for 24 to 48 hours (which can be quite painful), and then you begin to feel better. Wearing a tight-fitting supportive bra may make the process a little less uncomfortable. Applying ice packs or bags of frozen peas to your breasts helps the milk to "dry up," as does taking cold showers. Cold temperature causes the blood vessels in the breasts to constrict, lessening milk production, whereas warmth causes the blood vessels to dilate, promoting milk production. (Doctors no longer prescribe a medication to help a woman's milk dry up, because the drug they once used has been associated with some significant complications.)

Understanding hair loss

One of the stranger aspects of the postpartum return to normalcy is hair loss. A few weeks or months after delivery, most women notice that they're shedding like crazy. This shedding is normal. It is one of the effects that estrogen has on your

body during pregnancy. This common problem doesn't last long. Your hair is usually back to normal by nine months after delivery.

All hair follicles go through three phases of development: a *resting* phase, a so-called *transitional* phase, and a *shedding* phase. The elevated levels of estrogen that are present during pregnancy essentially freeze your hair in the resting phase. Within a few months after delivery, all that hair proceeds on to the shedding phase. Suddenly, you notice large amounts of hair sticking in your brush or washing down the drain.

Chasing away the baby blues

Studies show that the vast majority of women — as many as 80 percent — suffers a bout of the blues during the first days and weeks after they deliver. Typically, you begin to feel a little down a few days after the birth, and you may continue to feel vague sadness, uncertainty, disappointment, and emotional discontent for a few weeks. Many women are surprised at the feeling; after all, they've looked forward to motherhood, and they feel sure that they're really thrilled about it.

No one knows for sure *why* women get the blues postpartum, but a few explanations are plausible. First, the shift in hormone levels that comes after delivery can affect mood. Also, when pregnancy ends, a mother must change her whole focus. After focusing on the birth for so many months, she suddenly finds that the big event is over, and she may feel almost a sense of loss. And face it — parenthood brings tremendous anxiety, especially for a first-time mother. Feeling overwhelmed by all the responsibility and all she needs to figure out about caring for a baby isn't unusual for a woman. Add in the physical discomfort — episiotomy repair, breast tenderness, hemorrhoids, fatigue, and the rest — and you begin to wonder how any new mother can avoid feeling a little blue.

Fortunately, postpartum blues tend to fade away rather quickly, usually by about two to four weeks after the birth. Keep in mind that what you're feeling is extremely common and that it doesn't mean you don't love your child or that you won't be a fabulous parent. Be open about it; let your partner, family members, and friends know how you feel, because you need love and support at this time.

If you find yourself suffering from the baby blues, remember that you're not the first woman to feel this way. The feeling is as normal as pregnancy itself. And take heart: Those who have already grappled with the problem have found a number of ways to ease the blues. Consider this list of some of the best strategies:

✔ Lack of sleep compounds the problem of the baby blues. Everything is worse when you're physically fatigued. The amount of stress that you can handle when you've had your rest is much greater than if you haven't slept enough. So try to get more sleep. If the baby is napping, try to lie down and snooze.

✔ Accept other people's offers of help. In most cases, you don't have to take care of your baby entirely by yourself. You're a great mom, even if you do let Aunt Suzie or Grandma Melba change a diaper or burp the baby.

✔ Talk about how you feel with other mothers, close family members, and friends. You're likely to find that they felt exactly as you do now. They can empathize with you and offer suggestions for how to cope.

✔ If possible, try to get some time to yourself. Often, new parents are overwhelmed by the realization that their time is no longer their own. Get out of the house, if you can. Take a walk, read, watch a movie, or get some exercise. Have dinner with your partner or with a friend.

✔ Pamper yourself with a manicure or pedicure, a trip to the hair salon, or a massage. Often the blues are exacerbated by the fact that your body still isn't back to what it used to be, and doing something that makes you feel beautiful may help.

If you don't begin to feel better in three or four weeks, let your practitioner know. Some women go beyond the blues into full-blown postpartum depression. Check out the next section for more information.

Recognizing postpartum depression

True *postpartum depression* isn't nearly as common as the blues, but it does affect more women than you may imagine. Between

10 and 15 percent of women develop depression within six months after they deliver. Symptoms include

✔ Severe unhappiness

✔ Inability to enjoy being with the baby (or to enjoy life in general)

✔ Lack of interest in caring for the baby

✔ Insomnia

✔ Weak appetite

✔ Inability to function from day to day

✔ Extreme anxiety or panic attacks

✔ Thoughts of harming the baby or yourself

Although postpartum blues are usually mild and transient, full-blown depression can be severe and lasting. Despite the severity of the symptoms, postpartum depression often goes unrecognized, or the mother may attribute the problem to something else.

No one knows exactly why postpartum depression occurs, but certain characteristics put a woman at higher than normal risk. These risk factors include

✔ History of postpartum depression

✔ History of depression in general

✔ Experience of anxiety before the birth

✔ Life stress

✔ Lack of a good support system

✔ Marital dissatisfaction

✔ An unplanned pregnancy

✔ Unhappiness about the labor and delivery process

If you have postpartum blues and it doesn't go away after three or four weeks, if the feeling seems to be getting worse, or if you develop the blues more than two months after your delivery, discuss the situation with your doctor. Your blues may have blossomed into full-fledged postpartum depression.

Treatment for postpartum depression includes counseling (group or individual psychotherapy), antidepressant medications, and, rarely, hospitalization. Recent studies have suggested that in some cases, taking small doses of estrogen under the tongue can help. Of course, only follow this treatment under your doctor's supervision. Your doctor may want to check to see whether you have postpartum thyroid disease, which can mask itself as depression or make your depression worse. Discuss all these with your doctor.

To get further information about how to handle postpartum depression, you may want to get in touch with one of the following resources:

- ✔ **Postpartum Support International:** www.postpartum. net or call 1-800-944-4PPD.

- ✔ **PPDMOMS.ORG:** www.1800ppdmoms.org or call 1-800-PPD-MOMS.

- ✔ **March of Dimes:** Go to www.marchofdimes.com. Enter "postpartum depression" in the search field on its home page (it's really prominent and in the middle of the top of the page). There are numerous links to help you find the information that applies to your particular situation.

Checking your progress: The first postpartum doctor visit

Most practitioners ask their patients to come in for a checkup about six weeks after delivery if both the pregnancy and the birth were uncomplicated. If you had a cesarean or some complication, you may be asked to come in earlier.

During a postpartum checkup, your practitioner performs a complete exam (including a breast and vaginal exam) and obtains a PAP smear, if needed. In most cases, the six-week checkup suffices for your annual gynecological exam. Your practitioner probably also talks with you about your birth control options. Discuss the "spacing" of future children (see Chapter 13) and other precautions before conceiving again — such as taking folic acid a few months beforehand and, if this pregnancy had complications, getting whatever special blood tests your practitioner may advise.

Returning to "Normal" Life

Your body typically needs six to eight weeks for the changes that you experience during pregnancy to disappear. After delivery, your body needs some time to get back in shape for your day-to-day activities, let alone for vigorous exercise or sex. This section focuses on what you can do to help make the transition easier.

Getting fit all over again

Making exercise a priority after delivery is important for every new mom. Fitness has many benefits for both your physical and emotional well-being. It can help your body recover from the stress of pregnancy, and it helps you feel more even-tempered and better about yourself.

Resume your sports and workouts gradually. Naturally, the amount of exercise you can handle depends on what kind of shape you were in before and during your pregnancy.

After pregnancy, restoring strength to your abdominal muscles is especially important. In some women, pregnancy causes the abdominal or *rectus* muscles to separate a little, as shown in Figure 11-1. The medical term for this separation is *diastasis*. Doing abdominal exercises to restore their strength and draw them together is important.

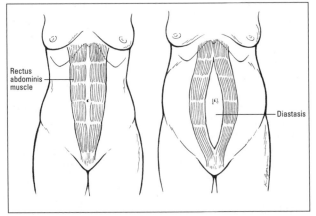

Rectus
abdominis
muscle

Diastasis

Kathryn Born, MA

Figure 11-1: After pregnancy, your abdominal muscles may be separated a bit, one side from the other.

Over the course of two weeks, depending on how you feel, you can gradually increase your exercising until you're fully active again. Finding the time may be a problem, of course. But fitting exercise into your schedule is worth every effort. Taking care of a newborn can make you feel as though you've just run a marathon, but real exercise is what your body needs. In fact, by improving your overall sense of well-being, exercise can make the whole challenge of caring for a new baby much easier.

 Walking is great exercise for just about everyone. During the first two weeks after delivery, take it slow. But after that, you may find that long or brisk walks are enjoyable for both you and your baby — and a great form of exercise.

Losing the weight

You may feel like jumping onto a scale right after delivery to see how much weight you've lost. But take caution. Some women do lose a lot of weight quickly after delivery, but some actually gain weight from all the fluid retention. Rest assured that you'll soon weigh less than you did before you delivered — probably about 15 pounds less — but the loss may not register until a week or two after delivery.

Refer to Table 11-1 to see what accounts for the initial weight loss.

Table 11-1	Losing Weight after Birth
Baby	*6 to 9 pounds*
Placenta	1 to 2 pounds
Amniotic fluid	1 to 2 pounds
Maternal fluids	4 to 8 pounds
Shrinking uterus	1 pound

Your uterus continues shrinking for several weeks. Immediately after you deliver, it still extends up to about the level of your navel — about the same point as when you were 20 weeks pregnant. However, because of the excess skin you now have, you probably still look pregnant when you stand up. Don't let your appearance get you down! Your uterus keeps contracting and your skin regains much of its tone until, about two months after delivery, your belly is down to its pre-pregnancy size.

Most women need two to three months to get back to their normal weight, but, of course, the time varies according to how much weight you gain during pregnancy. If you gain 50 pounds (and have just one baby), don't expect to look fabulous in a bikini six weeks after you deliver. Sometimes a woman needs an entire year to get back into shape. A healthy diet and regular exercise help the weight come off.

Try to get as close to your pre-pregnancy weight — or your ideal body weight (see Chapter 4) — as soon as is reasonably possible. You don't have to let a pregnancy turn into a permanent weight gain. If you let each successive pregnancy cause a little more accumulation, your health may suffer in the long run.

Pondering your postpartum diet

Any woman who's just had a baby needs to once again examine her diet. If you're breast-feeding, you want to ensure, as you did when you were pregnant, that you're eating a healthy combination of foods that provide both you and your baby with good nutrition and that you're also getting enough fluid. (For more information about how to follow a balanced, nutritious diet, see Chapter 4.)

The best approach to weight loss involves exercise plus a well-balanced diet that's low in fat and includes a mix of protein, carbs, fruits, and vegetables. You may find that a program such as Weight Watchers, which has been around for years and provides a sensible, well-balanced way to lose weight, may offer the motivation and support you need to get your diet on track. Weight Watchers isn't based on rapid initial weight loss and is designed to change your way of eating so that you discover how to eat healthily, yet still lose weight. You can check out the Web site at www.weightwatchers.com. You may also want to check out other commercial diet programs, such as Jenny Craig and LA Weight Loss.

Taking your vitamins

Regardless of whether you breast-feed, continue taking your prenatal vitamins for at least six to eight weeks after you deliver. If you do breast-feed, keep taking vitamins until you stop breast-feeding. Taking care of a new baby may make it hard for you to eat properly, and the childbirth experience may have left you

anemic. If you lost a particularly large amount of blood during your delivery, your practitioner may suggest that you take iron supplements to help restore your blood count. Calcium is also very important for any woman, especially one who's breast-feeding, in order to maintain strong bones. A calcium supplement or extra calcium in your diet is a good idea.

Doing Kegel exercises

Kegel exercises are squeezing motions aimed at strengthening the muscles of the pelvic floor that surround the vagina and rectum. These muscles give support to the bladder, rectum, uterus, and vagina. Keeping them strong is key to reducing the adverse effects that pregnancy and delivery can have on this part of the body. If the pelvic floor muscles are very weak, the chances are greater of developing *urinary stress incontinence* — a leakage of urine when you cough, sneeze, laugh, or jump — or *prolapse* or *protrusion* of the rectum, vagina, and uterus — in which these organs begin to sag below the pelvic floor.

Pregnancy places extra weight on the pelvic floor muscles, and vaginal delivery stretches and puts added pressure on them. The net result is a general weakening. Some women seem to naturally maintain excellent muscle tone in the pelvic floor after delivery. But others notice symptoms of weakness: a little urinary incontinence, the feeling that their vagina is loose, or pressure on their pelvic floor from a sagging uterus, vagina, or rectum. The way to strengthen the pelvic floor muscles — to avoid or diminish these symptoms — is to perform Kegel exercises.

To perform these exercises, you tighten the muscles around your vagina and rectum. Here's a simple way to find out what it feels like to do the exercises correctly: Sometime when you're urinating, try to stop the flow of urine midstream. Or insert a finger in your vagina and try to tighten the muscles around your finger. If you're doing Kegels correctly, your finger feels the squeeze. (Both of these techniques are simply ways of figuring out how to squeeze the muscles, not the way you normally practice the exercise.)

When you're first doing Kegels, squeeze the muscles for as long as ten seconds and then release. Squeeze five to ten times per session, and try to do three to four sessions a day. Ultimately, you can build up to the point where you hold each squeeze for

ten seconds and do 25 squeezes per session. Continue to do the Kegels four times a day. You can do them while you're sitting, standing, or lying down, and you can do them while you're also doing something else — bathing, cooking, talking on the phone, watching television, driving your car, or standing in line at the grocery store.

Having sex again

If you're like most postpartum women, sex is the last thing on your mind. Many women find that their interest in sex declines considerably during the first weeks and months after pregnancy. But at some point, the fatigue and emotional stress of childbirth ease up, and your thoughts are likely to be more amorous again. For some women (and their lucky partners), the rebound occurs fairly quickly. For others, it may take 6 to 12 months.

The drastic hormonal shifts that occur after delivery directly affect your sex organs. The precipitous drop in estrogen leads to a loss of lubrication for your vagina, and less engorgement of blood vessels as well. (Increased blood flow to the vagina is a key aspect of sexual arousal and orgasm.) For these reasons, intercourse after childbirth can be painful and sometimes not all that satisfying. With time, as hormone levels return to their pre-pregnancy norm, the problem tends to correct itself. In the meantime, using a lubricant sold specifically for this purpose helps.

The exhaustion and stress of caring for an infant further reduces the desire for sex in some women. Your attention, and your partner's, too, is likely to be focused more on the baby than on the relationship between the parents. Set aside some time for the two of you to be alone together. This time together need not even include sex — just holding, hugging, and expressing feelings for each other.

Most doctors recommend that women refrain from intercourse for four to six weeks after the baby is born in order to give the vagina, uterus, and perineum time to heal and for the bleeding to subside. At your six-week follow-up doctor visit, you can ask your practitioner about resuming sex.

Choosing contraception

Many people believe that breast-feeding prevents a woman from becoming pregnant. Although breast-feeding *usually* delays the return of ovulation (and, thus, periods), some women who are nursing do ovulate — and do conceive again (see Chapter 12). You may not ovulate the entire time that you breast-feed, or you may start again as early as two months after delivery. And if you don't breast-feed, ovulation begins, on the average, ten weeks after delivery, although it has been reported to occur as early as four weeks. If you breast-feed for less than 28 days, your ovulation returns at the same time as it does for non-nursing women.

It's important to consider your options for birth control before you have sex again. Most women have a wide range of birth-control options regardless of whether they're breast-feeding. But some women have medical conditions that prevent them from using certain methods. Discuss your options with your practitioner at a postpartum visit.

Chapter 12

Feeding Your Baby

●●●

In This Chapter

▶ Breast or bottle — making the decision that's right for you

▶ Getting into the breast-feeding routine

▶ The basics of formula feeding

●●●

*O*ne of the first big decisions any new parents make is whether to breast-feed their infant or use formula and bottles. Although the majority of parents these days choose to breast-feed, the decision is by no means an easy one. If you find the decision difficult, take comfort in the fact that both choices are sound and legitimate. In this chapter, we lay out the basic first steps you need, no matter which way you go.

Deciding between Breast and Bottle

Ask almost anyone — your obstetrician, your pediatrician, your friends, total strangers — and they will advise you to breast-feed. In fact, the American Academy of Pediatrics, the World Health Organization, and the Institute of Medicine all recommend exclusive breast-feeding for six months, followed by a combination of breast milk and complementary foods for up to at least 12 months of age. "Exclusive" breast-feeding means no food or drink other than breast milk — including water — unless medically indicated. Back in the 1950s, bottle-feeding became all the rage when scientists developed techniques to pasteurize and store cow's milk in formulas appropriate for infant nutrition. Breast-feeding has regained popularity largely because people and scientific studies have recognized its many medical benefits.

However, the decision whether to breast-feed isn't simply a medical one. It also involves issues of convenience, aesthetics, body image, maternal bonding, and even conditions surrounding delivery. The decision about how to feed your baby is a personal one that every mother must decide for herself. Figuring out how to breast-feed takes an incredible commitment, so don't feel pressured to do it if your heart isn't in it or if the thought of doing it makes you feel stressed or uncomfortable. If you decide that bottle-feeding is the best decision for you and your baby, don't feel guilty about it.

You may hear that breast-feeding offers the best opportunity for a mother to bond with her baby, but bottle-feeding can also be a very warm and loving way to interact with your baby — not only for the mother, but also for her partner and whoever else may be helping care for the baby. And although breast-feeding offers certain undeniable benefits, the vast majority of bottle-fed babies is — and remains — perfectly healthy.

This section looks at these two options a bit closer and helps you make a decision that's right for you. Whatever your decision, make it before you deliver, so that you have adequate time to prepare for the moment when your baby starts feeding. Some women elect to try out breast-feeding for a little while to see how they like it. Some decide from the beginning to use a combination of both breast and bottle (filling the bottle with either formula or breast milk that has been pumped and refrigerated).

Sizing up the advantages of breast-feeding

Breast-feeding gives your baby a tailor-made formula for good nutrition and a whole lot more.

The following are some advantages to breast-feeding for the baby:

- ✔ Human breast milk can strengthen the baby's immune system and help reduce the risk of allergies, asthma, and sudden infant death syndrome (SIDS). It can also decrease the chances of pneumonia in the baby's first year of life.

- ✔ Babies who are exclusively breast-fed for six months have a decreased number of ear infections (otitis media), fewer

gastrointestinal infections, and a lower chance of developing necrotizing enterocolitis (NEC), a serious illness more commonly seen in premature babies, but also occasionally seen in term infants.

✔ When breast-fed babies grow up, they have lower chances of developing inflammatory bowel disease (Crohn's disease or ulcerative colitis), celiac disease (a problem with digesting gluten), diabetes, childhood leukemia, and lymphoma. They also have a lower risk of adolescent and adult obesity.

✔ Breast-fed babies, when they enter school, have higher intelligence scores and higher ratings by their teachers.

✔ Mother's milk contains nutrients that are ideally suited to a baby's digestive system. The most commonly used formulas contain proteins from cow's milk which aren't as easily digested, and your baby can't readily use the nutrients it contains.

✔ Human milk also contains substances that help protect a baby from infections until his own immune system matures. These substances are especially plentiful in the *colostrum* that mothers' breasts secrete during the first few days after the baby is born.

✔ Babies are more likely to have an allergic reaction to formula than to mother's milk.

Following are some advantages to breast-feeding for the mom:

✔ Moms who breast-feed have less postpartum blood loss and an increased rate of involution (the uterus getting back to its normal, pre-pregnancy size). They also have lower rates of postpartum depression and are less prone to child abuse and neglect.

✔ If you breast-feed your baby, you have lower risks of adult-onset diabetes, rheumatoid arthritis, hypertension (high blood pressure), hyperlipidemia (high cholesterol), cardiovascular disease, breast cancer, and ovarian cancer later in life.

✔ Breast-feeding is emotionally rewarding. Many women feel that they develop a special bond with their baby when they breast-feed, and they enjoy the closeness surrounding the whole experience.

✔ Breast-feeding is convenient. You can't leave home without it. You never have to carry bottles or formula with you.

✔ Mother's milk is cheaper than formula and bottles.

✔ You don't have to warm up breast milk; it's always the perfect temperature.

✔ Breast-feeding provides some degree of birth control (although it's not totally reliable — see the "Looking at birth control options" section later in this chapter).

✔ *Lactation (milk production)* causes you to burn extra calories, which may help you lose some of the weight you gained during pregnancy.

✔ A breast-fed baby's bowel movements don't have as strong an odor as those of babies who are formula-fed.

✔ Breast milk is pretty much organic — no additives, no preservatives.

✔ Some studies suggest that women who breast-feed may reduce their lifetime risk of breast cancer.

There are a few situations where breast-feeding is not recommended:

✔ If the infant has a rare genetic disorder called classical galactosemia

✔ If the mother is HIV-positive (see the next section)

✔ If the mother has untreated tuberculosis or brucellosis

✔ If the mother is taking certain medications, like amphetamines, chemotherapeutic agents, ergotamines, or statins. Patients often ask if they can breast-feed if they are taking medications for psychiatric problems (psychotropic drugs — some antidepressants fall in this category). The jury is still out on this issue, but most providers feel that medications commonly used today for depression and anxiety are relatively safe and that NOT treating the problem could cause more danger to the baby than any small risk these medications may pose. Ask your doctor about medications you take on a regular basis.

Checking out why some moms may choose bottle-feeding

You may decide to choose the option of bottle-feeding for any of the following reasons:

✔ You don't want to breast-feed. If your heart isn't in it, it ain't gonna happen. Too much trial and error is involved in making breast-feeding work for someone who's not truly committed to succeeding.

✔ You've tried breast-feeding, and your breasts don't produce enough milk to feed your baby (or babies!).

✔ Bottle-feeding better fits your lifestyle. Although many working mothers breast-feed, others feel that juggling the requirements of their job with those of breast-feeding is just too difficult.

✔ Some women find the whole concept of feeding their baby a "bodily secretion" unpleasant.

✔ Bottle-feeding enables others to feed the baby.

✔ If you have a chronic infection — HIV, for example — bottle-feeding helps ensure that you don't pass the infection to the baby via breast milk. (Women who carry the hepatitis B virus can breast-feed as long as the baby has received the hepatitis B vaccine.)

✔ If you or your baby is very sick after delivery, bottle-feeding may be your only option. A mother or baby who's in the intensive care unit (ICU) because of a complicated delivery often can't initiate breast-feeding. The mother can use a mechanical pump to empty the milk from her breasts and freeze the milk to feed to the baby up to six months later. Even if the baby can't use the pumped milk at this time, pumping at least keeps the supply of milk flowing. Occasionally, a mother can restart the flow of milk later on, when she or the baby recovers, but this option isn't always possible and often requires the assistance of a lactation specialist.

✔ If you've had previous surgery on your breasts, bottle-feeding may be your best bet (you may not be able to lactate). No medical evidence indicates that lactation has any effect on the progression of breast cancer after it has already been diagnosed, but some women who have had

surgery or other treatment for breast cancer are unable to lactate. Also, some evidence suggests that women who have had breast implants produce less milk. However, many of these women produce some milk and can still breast-feed.

Latching onto Breast-Feeding

Pregnancy goes a long way toward preparing your body for breast-feeding. The key pregnancy hormones cause the breasts to enlarge and prepare the glands inside the breasts to lactate. But you can prepare yourself for day-to-day nursing. You can, for example, toughen your nipples a bit — and thus minimize soreness later on — in a few different ways:

✔ Wear a nursing bra with the flaps down (allowing your clothing to rub against your nipples).

✔ Roll your nipples between your thumb and forefinger for a minute or so each day.

✔ Rub your nipples briskly with a terry washcloth after bathing or showering.

Be aware, however, that stimulating your nipples late in your pregnancy can elicit uterine contractions. When you are near the end of your pregnancy, ask your practitioner before doing this kind of stimulation. One way to get around this problem is to avoid the nipple itself and just rub petroleum jelly, an antibacterial ointment, or baby oil over the areola.

Some women have inverted nipples and worry during pregnancy that their nipples will make breast-feeding difficult. Usually, the problem corrects itself before the baby is born, but a few techniques can help things along:

✔ Use the thumb and forefinger on one hand to push back the skin around the areola. If this doesn't bring out the nipple, gently grasp it with your other thumb and forefinger, pull it outward, and hold it for a few minutes, as shown in Figure 12-1. Do this exercise several times a day.

✔ You can also try wearing special plastic breast cups (available at most drugstores) designed to help draw out the nipple over time.

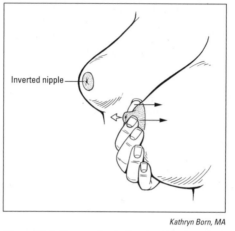

Kathryn Born, MA

Figure 12-1: One method of correcting inverted nipples.

Start one of these preparation techniques for short sessions during the second trimester and then gradually increase the amount of time you work your nipples or wear the cups until your nipples stay out on their own.

Looking at the mechanics of lactation

The flood of estrogen and progesterone that your body experiences during pregnancy causes your breasts to grow — sometimes to an astonishing size. This growth starts early, within three to four weeks of conception, which is why the first sign of pregnancy for many women is breast tenderness. As pregnancy progresses, small amounts of serum-like fluid can leak from the nipples. But serious milk production doesn't start until after the baby is born.

During the first days after delivery, the breasts secrete only a yellowish fluid known as colostrum, which doesn't contain much milk but is rich in antibodies and protective cells from the mother's bloodstream. These substances help the newborn fight off infections until his own immune system matures and can take over. Colostrum is gradually replaced by milk.

Don't be alarmed if your baby doesn't seem to get much milk during the first few days. The colostrum is very beneficial on its own. Your baby probably doesn't even have much of an appetite until he is 3 to 4 days old. And he is likely to need the first few days to practice sucking movements.

When your baby starts sucking on your breasts, it signals your brain to have the breasts produce milk. About three or four days after delivery, milk production sets in. When milk enters the ducts, the breasts become engorged with milk (see Figure 12-2). The engorgement can be so great that your breasts feel rock-hard and sometimes very tender. Don't worry, though. When your baby starts feeding regularly and your milk starts flowing, the engorgement is no longer so intense. The *letdown reflex* (milk entering the ducts) occurs each time your baby feeds. After you have been nursing for a while, you may find that the mere sound of your baby crying or the feel of your baby cuddling next to you can trigger the reflex.

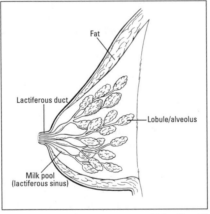

Kathryn Born, MA

Figure 12-2: Your breasts contain a network of milk ducts, which start delivering colostrum during the first days after delivery.

Lactating women typically produce about 600 milliliters (10 ounces) of milk per day by the end of the first postpartum week. This increases to about 800 milliliters (14 ounces) by the end of the third week and peaks at 1½ to 2 liters (25 to 35 ounces).

Checking out breast-feeding positions

You can breast-feed in one of three basic positions, as shown in Figure 12-3. Use whichever position works and is comfortable for you and your baby. Most women alternate among the positions.

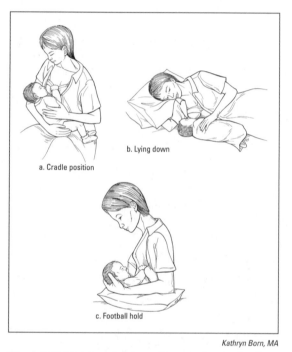

b. Lying down

a. Cradle position

c. Football hold

Kathryn Born, MA

Figure 12-3: The three basic positions for breast-feeding.

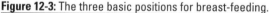

- ✔ **Cradling:** Cradle your baby in your arms with his head next to the bend in your elbow and tilted a bit toward your breast. (See Figure 12-3a.)

- ✔ **Lying down:** Lie on your side in bed with the baby next to you. Support the baby with your lower arm or pillows so that his mouth is next to your lower breast, and use your other arm to guide your baby's mouth to the nipple. This position is best for late-night feedings or after a cesarean delivery when sitting up is still uncomfortable. (See Figure 12-3b.) One concern about breast-feeding while in bed is that you may fall asleep and unknowingly

roll over your baby. You may decide to keep a cradle or crib next to your bed so you can put your baby back to sleep right after you finish feeding, without disrupting your night's sleep too much.

✔ **Football hold:** Cradle your baby's head in the palm of your hand and support the body with your forearm. For extra support, you can place a pillow underneath your arm. Use your free hand to hold your breast close to the baby's mouth. (See Figure 12-3c.)

Getting the baby to latch on

If you choose to breast-feed, you can get started immediately after delivery, wherever you happen to be — the birthing room, the delivery room, or the recovery room. Begin as soon as the nurses have checked your baby's health and your baby has settled down a bit from the delivery. Expect to feel a little awkward at first, and try not to get too frustrated. Many babies don't want to breast-feed immediately. Have patience — you and your baby will eventually get the hang of it.

Babies are born with a suckling reflex, but many of them don't follow it enthusiastically right off the bat. Sometimes babies need some coaxing to latch onto the breast:

1. **Arrange yourself and your baby in one of the basic breast-feeding positions (see the preceding section).**

2. **Gently stroke the baby's lips or cheek with your nipple.**

   This action usually causes the baby to open his mouth. If your baby doesn't seem to want to open his mouth, try expressing (gently pressing out) a little milk — colostrum, really — and rubbing some on the baby's lips.

3. **When the baby's mouth is wide open, bring his head to your breast and gently place his mouth over your entire nipple.**

   This prodding usually causes the baby to start sucking. Make sure that the entire areola is inside the baby's mouth, because if it isn't, he doesn't get enough milk and you get sore nipples. However, don't stuff your breast into your baby's mouth. Rather, bring the mouth to your nipple, and let the infant take in the breast.

The tip of the baby's nose should be barely touching the skin around your breast. The only way the baby can breathe while feeding is through his nose, so be careful not to completely cover the baby's nose with your breast. If your breast obstructs the baby's nose, use your free hand to depress your breast in front of his nose to let some air in.

Orchestrating feedings

After your baby latches on, you know that he is sucking when you see regular, rhythmic movements of the cheeks and chin. Several minutes of sucking may go by before your milk letdown occurs. In the beginning, let your baby feed for about five minutes on each breast per nursing session. Over the course of the first three or four days, increase the amount of time on each breast to 10 to 15 minutes. Don't get too hung up about timing the feedings, though; your baby lets you know when he has had enough by not sucking and letting your nipple slip away.

If your baby stops sucking without letting go of your nipple, insert your finger into the corner of his mouth to break the suction. (If you just pull your breast straight out, you'll end up with sore nipples.)

When switching from one breast to the other, stop to burp your baby by laying him either over your shoulder or your lap and gently patting his back. Figure 12-4 shows you some of the various burping positions. Burp him again when the feeding is finished.

Typically, mothers initially breast-feed about 8 to 12 times a day (averaging 10). This pattern enables your body to produce an optimal amount of milk, and it allows your baby to get the proper amount of nutrition for healthy growth and development. Try to space the feedings fairly evenly throughout the day; of course, your baby has some influence on the schedule. You don't have to wake your baby for a feeding unless your pediatrician specifically advises you to do so. You especially don't have to wake your baby at night; if the baby's willing to sleep through, just count yourself lucky. Nor do you have any reason to withhold a feeding if your baby is hungry — even if only an hour or so has passed since the last feeding. (Also keep in mind that the number of feedings in a day may be less than average if you supplement breast-feeding with some formula feedings.)

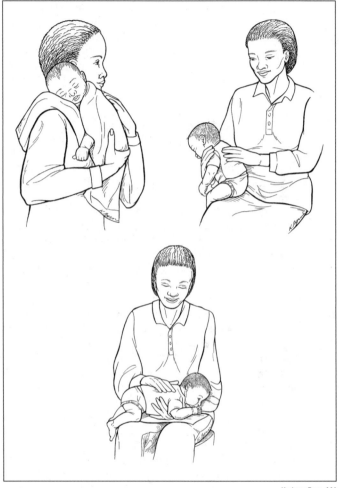

Kathryn Born, MA

Figure 12-4: There's more than one way to burp a baby. Here are a few of the tried-and-true positions.

You can tell that your baby is getting enough milk if your baby

- ✓ Nurses ten times a day on average
- ✓ Gains weight
- ✓ Has six to eight wet diapers a day
- ✓ Has two to three bowel movements a day
- ✓ Produces urine that's pale yellow (not dark and concentrated)

If your baby isn't meeting these criteria or if you have any concern that your baby isn't getting enough milk, call your pediatrician. Some women, no matter how diligent they are, need to supplement breast milk with formula because they just can't produce enough breast milk to totally meet their baby's needs.

Maintaining your diet

During breast-feeding, as during pregnancy, your nutrition is largely a matter of educated common sense. Your breast milk's quality isn't significantly affected by your diet unless your eating habits are truly inadequate. However, if you don't take in enough calories or water, your body has a difficult time producing adequate milk. You may also find that your baby reacts a different way to certain foods. For example, he may be extra gassy if you've eaten particular foods. If you pay attention to how your baby responds to different foods, you can figure out what foods to avoid.

Breast-feeding women should take in 400 to 600 calories a day more than they would normally eat. The exact amount varies according to how much you weigh and how much fat you gained during pregnancy. Because lactating does burn fat, breast-feeding helps get rid of some of the extra fat stores you may have. But avoid losing weight too fast, or your milk production will suffer. Also, avoid gaining weight while you're breast-feeding. If you find that you're putting on more pounds, you're most likely taking in too many calories or not exercising enough.

You also need extra vitamins and minerals — especially vitamin D, calcium, and iron. Keep taking your prenatal vitamins or some other balanced supplement while you're nursing. Also, consume extra calcium — either a supplement or extra servings of milk, yogurt, and other dairy products. Omega-3 fatty acids are also important for your developing baby — you should consume about 200 to 300 mg of these every day.

Breast milk is mainly water (87 percent). To produce plenty of breast milk, you must take in at least 72 ounces of fluid per day, which is about nine glasses of milk, juice, or water. Don't go overboard, however, because if you drink too many fluids, your milk production may actually decrease. You also don't want to markedly increase your calorie intake with high-sugar, high-carbohydrate, or high-calorie fluids. A good way to tell

whether you're getting the right amount of fluid is to monitor your urine output. If you urinate infrequently or if the color is a deep yellow, you probably aren't getting enough. If you constantly run to the bathroom, you may be drinking too much.

If you find that your baby is fussy and has a hard time sleeping, you may be consuming too much caffeine. Try cutting back on the coffee or cola until you find the level your baby tolerates.

Looking at birth control options

Although breast-feeding decreases the likelihood of ovulation, it by no means guarantees that you won't become pregnant. For a woman who chooses not to breast-feed, it takes an average of 10 weeks after the birth to resume ovulation — that is, to become fertile again. About 10 percent of women who do breast-feed also begin ovulating again after 10 weeks, and about 50 percent start up again by 25 weeks — about six months — after their babies are born. Clearly, breast-feeding isn't a great form of birth control.

Before you resume intercourse, consider using some effective form of birth control, because chances are you don't want to become pregnant again right away. You can use birth control pills (some are okay with breast-feeding), barrier methods (condoms, a diaphragm, and so on), or long-acting progesterone shots (such as Depo-Provera). One of the newer forms of birth control (Nexplanon) is a tiny reservoir which contains a progesterone-like substance and is placed below the surface of the skin on the inner part of your arm. The reservoir slowly releases the medication and can prevent you from getting pregnant for up to three years. They can even be implanted while you are in the hospital recovering from your delivery and do not interfere significantly with breast feeding. Discuss your options with your practitioner before discharge from the hospital or at your six-week checkup.

Determining which medications are safe

Just about any medication you take gets into your breast milk, but usually only in tiny amounts. If you need to take a medication while breast-feeding, try taking the lowest dose possible

and, as a rule, take it just after you finish a breast-feeding session. That way, your body breaks down most of the medication by the time you need to breast-feed again. In general, don't deprive yourself of medications that you really need just because you're afraid that some of it may get to the baby and cause harm. Check with your doctor about medications to be sure that they're fine to take while breast-feeding.

The following medications are okay to take while breast-feeding:

- ✔ Acetaminophen (such as Tylenol)

- ✔ Antacids

- ✔ Most antibiotics

- ✔ Most commonly used antidepressants (see the "Sizing up the advantages of breast-feeding" section earlier in this chapter)

- ✔ Antihistamines

- ✔ Aspirin

- ✔ Most asthma medications

- ✔ Decongestants

- ✔ Most high blood pressure medications

- ✔ Ibuprofen (such as Advil or Motrin)

- ✔ Insulin

- ✔ Most seizure medications

- ✔ Most thyroid medications

Expectant mothers ask . . .

Q: "Can I breast-feed while I'm on the Pill?"

A: It's fine, although it may affect the amount of milk you produce. Pills that contain estrogen decrease the amount of milk that you produce, and if you take them too soon after giving birth, they may make it difficult for your body to start milk production. However, after breast-feeding is well established, they're fine. Some women find that the newer progestin-only pills are a better alternative — they have less effect on milk production — but they're slightly less effective.

Handling common problems

One of the greatest misconceptions about breast-feeding is that it comes easily and naturally to everyone. Breast-feeding takes practice. Problems can range from a little nipple soreness to, in rare cases, infections in the milk ducts.

Sore nipples

Many women experience some temporary nipple soreness during the first few days that they breast-feed. For most women, the pain is mild, and it goes away on its own. For some, however, the soreness gets progressively worse and can lead to chapped or cracked nipples and moderate to severe pain. If your breasts are heading in this direction, take action before your suffering gets out of hand. The following list outlines some remedies:

- ✔ Review your technique to make sure that your baby is positioned correctly. If the baby isn't getting the entire nipple and areola in his mouth, the soreness is likely to continue. Try changing the baby's position slightly with each feeding.

- ✔ Increase the number of feedings and feed for less time at each feeding. This way, your baby won't be as hungry and may not suck as hard.

- ✔ Definitely continue to feed on the sore breast, even if only for a few minutes, to keep the nipple conditioned to nursing. If you let it heal completely, the soreness will only start all over again when you feed from that nipple again. We suggest that you feed on the least sore breast first, because that's when your baby's sucking is most vigorous.

- ✔ Express a little breast milk manually before you put the baby to the breast. This action helps initiate the letdown reflex so that the baby doesn't have to suck as long and hard to achieve letdown.

- ✔ Don't use any irritating chemicals or soaps on your nipples.

- ✔ After your baby finishes feeding, don't wipe off your nipples. Let them air-dry for as long as possible. Wiping them with a cloth may cause needless irritation.

- ✔ Exposing the nipples to air helps to toughen the skin, so try to walk around the house with your nipples exposed as much as possible. If you wear a nursing bra, leave the

flaps open while you're at home. Your nipples toughen from the fabric of your clothes rubbing against them.

✔ If you're using pads to soak up leakage from your breasts, change them as soon as they get moist, or they may chafe your nipples.

✔ Try massaging vitamin E oil or ointment, olive oil, or lanolin into sore nipples and then letting them air dry. Udder Cream and Bag Balm, products developed to treat chapped teats on milk cows (yes, cows), have found new popularity among breast-feeding women. Many drugstores and cosmetics stores now sell these creams.

✔ Apply dry (not moist) and warm (not hot) heat to the nipples several times a day. You can use a hot water bottle filled with warm water.

Pain from breast engorgement

As we mention earlier, when the breasts become engorged with milk, they can hurt. One way to avoid painful engorgement is to begin breast-feeding right after the baby is born. Other strategies that help include wearing a firm, but not tight, bra and massaging the breasts before feeding. Massaging facilitates letdown and relieves some of the engorgement. You can also try placing warm compresses on your breasts. (Some women feel that ice packs work better — try both and see which works best for you.)

Clogged ducts

Sometimes, some of the milk ducts in the breast become clogged with debris. If this happens, a small, firm, red lump may form inside the breast. The lump may be tender, but it's usually not associated with a fever or excruciating pain. The best way to treat a clogged breast duct is to try to completely empty that breast after each feeding. Start the baby out on that breast when he is most hungry. If the baby doesn't completely empty the breast, use a breast pump on that side until all the milk is drained. Applying heat to the lump and massaging it manually is helpful. You can also try letting the spray from a warm shower fall on your breast to promote milk release. Most important, keep feeding.

If the lump persists for more than a few days, becomes very painful or is associated with a fever, call your doctor to make sure that you're not developing an abscess.

Mastitis (breast infection)

Breast infections (mastitis) occur in about 2 percent of all breast-feeding women. Bacteria from the baby's mouth usually cause the infections, which are most likely to happen two to four weeks after delivery (but can occur earlier or later than that). Infections are more common in women who are breast-feeding for the first time, who have chapped nipples with cracks or fissures, and who don't empty their breasts completely at feedings.

The symptoms of mastitis include a warm, hard, red breast; high fever (usually over 101 degrees Fahrenheit); and malaise (like when you have the flu and your whole body feels achy). The infection in the breast may be diffused, or it may be localized to a particular segment of the breast (known as a lobule). If the infection is localized, the redness may appear as a wedge-shaped area over the infected portion of the breast (see Figure 12-5). If these symptoms develop, call your doctor immediately. More than likely, he will prescribe an antibiotic and may even want you to come into the office for an examination.

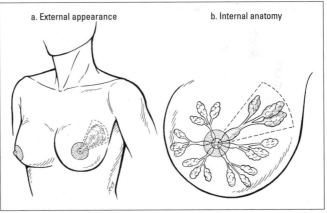

a. External appearance   b. Internal anatomy

Kathryn Born, MA

Figure 12-5: An outer view and an inner view of a wedge-shaped mastitis.

Continue to breast-feed your baby while you have the infection. It's not harmful to the baby; after all, the bacteria probably came from the baby's mouth. If you stop breast-feeding, the breast becomes engorged, making your discomfort even worse. Acetaminophen (such as Tylenol), ibuprofen, or warm compresses may help relieve the pain from mastitis while the antibiotics take effect (usually in about two days). Drink plenty

of fluids, and get as much rest as you can to allow your body's natural healing powers to work. Take your medication for the fully prescribed amount of time to help make sure that the infection doesn't recur.

Breast abscess

If mastitis isn't treated aggressively or if a milk duct remains clogged, a breast abscess can develop. In fact, breast abscesses form in as many as 10 percent of all cases of mastitis. Symptoms of a breast abscess are extreme pain, heat and swelling over the area of the abscess, and high fevers (over 101 degrees Fahrenheit). Sometimes doctors can treat abscesses with antibiotics, but often the abscess needs to be drained surgically.

Breast-feeding resources

If you have special problems or if you want more in-depth information about breast-feeding, contact one of the following organizations:

✔ La Leche League International or La Leche League USA, 1400 N. Meacham Rd., Schaumburg, IL 60173; phone 1-877-4 LA LECHE; Web site www.llli.org or www.lllusa.org

✔ American College of Obstetricians and Gynecologists, 409 Twelfth St. SW, Washington, D.C. 20024; phone 800-673-8444; Web site www.acog.org

✔ American Academy of Pediatrics, 141 Northwest Point Rd., Elk Grove Village, IL 60007; phone 800-433-9016; Web site www.aap.org

✔ International Board of Lactation Consultant Examiners; phone 703-560-7330; Web site www.iblce.org

✔ International Lactation Consultant Association; phone 919-861-5577; Web site www.ilca.org

✔ American College of Nurse-Midwives, 818 Connecticut Ave. NW, Ste. 900, Washington, D.C. 20006; phone 240-485-1800; Web site www.midwife.org

Other methods for getting information and assistance with breast-feeding include

✔ Calling the hospital where you intend to deliver or hospitals in the area where you live and asking to speak with a lactation consultant or lactation specialist

✔ Asking your practitioner for breast-feeding information

✔ Talking to friends and family members who have breast-fed their babies

If you develop a breast abscess, you can continue to breast-feed on the other side, but you should stop feeding on the side of the abscess until the problem subsides. Check with your doctor before resuming feedings on that side.

Breast-feeding multiples

It may seem daunting, but some women with multiples successfully breast-feed. Your body can make enough milk for two or more babies at once, especially if you're persistent and work up your milk production to a high level. Even so, arriving at a system that works for you takes some experimentation. You may breast-feed two babies at once or each one separately. The advantage to the first alternative is that you don't spend all your time breast-feeding, but the second method is easier. You don't have to deal with one baby finishing first and needing to be burped while the other one is still sucking. (Holding one baby over your shoulder and keeping another one at your breast can be very tricky, no matter how many pillows and props you use.) You may breast-feed one baby, bottle-feed the other, and then alternate at the next feeding. You may breast-feed each baby a little at each feeding and then supplement with the bottle. Or you may breast-feed the babies for most of the day and then supplement with a bottle before bedtime when your milk supply is low.

Women who breast-feed twins need to take in even more extra calories and fluids. You need about 400 to 600 extra calories per day for each baby you are breast-feeding. (Imagine how much you'd have to consume to breast-feed triplets! About 1,200 to 1,800 extra calories per day!) Also, you need to increase your fluid intake from 8 to 10 glasses per day to about 10 to 12 glasses per day.

If you do decide to try breast-feeding multiples, count on needing help from other family members and friends. Don't be afraid to ask for it.

Bottle-Feeding for Beginners

Suppose you've decided to forego breast-feeding in favor of formula. Or you've been breast-feeding for a while, and you want to switch. In this section, we go over what you need to know to get your baby started on bottles.

Stopping milk production

If you decide to formula-feed, you need to stop the process of milk production in your breasts. Milk production is triggered by warmth and breast stimulation. To stop the production of milk, create the opposite environment. Here are some suggestions:

- Wear a tight-fitting bra.

- Apply ice packs to your breasts when they become engorged (usually around the third or fourth day after your baby is born).

- Keep ice packs inside your bra, or use small packages of frozen vegetables, like peas or corn, which you can easily fold to fit within a bra. (We don't recommend going out in public this way, though.)

- Place cold cabbage leaves inside your bra. Cabbage works chemically to reduce the production of milk.

- Let cold water run over your breasts during a shower.

 If you're going to breast-feed for a short period of time (6 to 12 weeks), consider giving your baby one bottle of formula per day while nursing to help make the transition easier.

Engorged breasts can be very uncomfortable. If you're in a great deal of discomfort, you may want to ask your doctor about pain medication. Fortunately, the engorgement usually lasts only 36 to 48 hours and seldom requires medical help.

Choosing the best bottles and nipples

 You won't have any trouble finding a wide choice of bottles and nipples. Some babies definitely demonstrate a preference for one type of bottle or nipple over another. You may have to experiment to discover what tools work best for you and your baby. Four-ounce bottles are good for the first few weeks or months. Later, when your baby drinks more, you can switch to the larger eight-ounce bottles.

Here is some information on bottles:

✔ Some bottles are actually plastic holders in which you insert little transparent plastic bags that hold the milk or formula. The advantage of this type is that you can throw away the empty milk bag, and you don't have to worry about sterilizing the plastic container. Also, because the plastic bag is designed to collapse, less air gets into the bag and into the baby's stomach.

✔ Some bottles are angled, which also helps to allow less air to be taken in by the baby, leading to less gas.

✔ Nipples come in a wide variety. Newborn nipples have a smaller hole, and the size of the hole increases with the age of the baby (nipples generally come in newborn, 3- and 6-month sizes, and then larger ones for older babies). Orthodontic nipples are designed for a more natural fit. Some nipples are made out of latex, and others of silicone. Silicone nipples are clear, have less of an odor, and are firmer. Your baby may demonstrate a strong preference for one type over another or may not notice much of a difference.

Feeding your baby from a bottle

Your mother, grandmother, or any number of well-intentioned friends may tell you to sterilize bottles by boiling them in water. But we — and most pediatricians — think that this step is unnecessary. After all, a mother who breast-feeds doesn't have to boil her nipples!

Many parents choose to warm their baby's bottle, but heating it isn't necessary. If you choose to, though, you can warm a bottle in different ways. You can place it in a container filled with hot water or use a bottle warmer.

If you use the microwave to heat your baby's bottle, be careful. The breast milk or formula may heat unevenly, and some parts of it may be too hot for the baby. However, if you shake the bottle after warming it, it may be okay. Just make sure you squirt some onto your wrist to check the temperature first. Some formula manufacturers don't recommend microwaving their product, so make sure to read the information on the side of the packaging.

Saving leftover formula or breast milk generally isn't a good idea. However, some pediatricians say that reusing a bottle once is okay, so talk it over with your baby's doctor. In any case, don't leave a bottle filled with milk sitting outside the refrigerator for very long, because warmth encourages the growth of bacteria that can upset your baby's stomach.

Your choice of formula is one you should make with your pediatrician. Call his office prior to delivery and find out what he suggests you use. Many formulas come premixed, but some come in either a powder or concentrated liquid form, both of which require you to add water. The powder and concentrated liquid forms cost less, but they may not be available in as wide a variety of formulas.

All kinds of formulas are available, including organic formulas. The jury is still out as to whether there are clear medical benefits to organic formulas. They may be more costly, and some have extra sugar, so check with your pediatrician about whether organic is the way to go.

Some babies develop an allergic reaction to their formula; they may have an upset stomach or develop a skin rash. If your baby becomes allergic, talk with your pediatrician. He may want to switch your baby to a soy-based formula or some other hypoallergenic formula.

Pediatricians generally caution against propping up a baby's bottle by laying it on a pillow next to the baby's mouth, because propping implies that the baby is being left unattended. Also, laying a baby flat on his back with the bottle propped creates more potential for choking. Propping a bottle may also promote tooth decay.

The most common position for bottle-feeding your baby is to hold the baby cradled in one arm, close to your body. Put a pillow on your lap, which eases the strain on your arms and neck. Most parents find it easier to always hold the baby in the same arm and in the same direction. For example, if you're right-handed, you may want to hold your baby in your left arm and the bottle in the right. When the baby is a little older and has better control of his head and neck muscles, you may want to lay him in front of you along your legs for a change of pace. This way, you and your baby can make eye contact.

Here are some other tips for moms who are bottle-feeding (whether with formula or breast milk):

✔ Don't swaddle the baby too much or keep him too warm during feeding. The baby may get so comfortable that he falls asleep instead of feeding.

✔ Change the baby's diaper in the middle of a feeding. This may help to wake him up, so that he can finish the rest of the bottle.

✔ If your baby has trouble finding the nipple to put in his mouth, stroke his cheek, and he will turn in that direction.

✔ To check to see whether your baby is hungry, put the tip of your finger (a clean finger) into his mouth to see whether he starts to suck.

✔ Keep the bottle tilted in such a way as to completely fill the nipple with the formula, thereby minimizing the amount of air your baby gets.

Burp your baby at least once midway through a feeding and again at the end of a feeding. (Refer to Figure 12-4 for various burping positions.) Babies often take in air along with the milk or formula they drink, and burping helps them get rid of it. It also makes them more comfortable and able to eat more.

Dealing with Baby's Developing Digestive System

Your baby has a brand-new digestive system, and one that requires considerable breaking-in. Long story short: Babies spit up. A lot. Whether they're breast-fed or bottle-fed, newborn babies are likely to vomit as often as two times per day. Try these suggestions for dealing with spitting up:

✔ Keep a cloth over your shoulder when burping or holding your baby so that you don't have to constantly change, or ruin, your clothes.

✔ Keep a small bib on your baby during and after feeding so that you don't have to constantly change, or ruin, all the baby's clothes.

✔ Burp your baby after each feeding. Refer to Figure 12-4 to see some of the most common positions.

✔ If you're bottle-feeding, stop partway through the bottle to burp the baby, rather than allowing the baby to drink the entire bottle in one shot.

✔ Don't play with the baby too much after feeding. Jiggling the baby or moving the baby around a lot can lead to more spitting up.

✔ If your baby seems to be spitting up large quantities or if the spitting up is very forceful, let your pediatrician know.

Sometimes, spitting up or vomiting several times a day can be a sign of something as simple as overfeeding, or it may indicate a condition known as *gastroesophageal reflux disease,* or GERD, which is a digestive disorder caused by gastric acid from the stomach flowing into the esophagus. It is common in babies, although it can occur at any age. If your newborn is showing symptoms such as pain when spitting up, irritability, inconsolable crying, gagging, choking, or refusal to eat, you should definitely speak to your pediatrician.

Your pediatrician diagnoses GERD by conducting a medical history, physical exam, and certain diagnostic tests. These tests may include an upper gastrointestinal series, *endoscopy* (placement of a flexible tube with a light and camera lens into the organs of the upper digestive system), pH testing, and gastric emptying studies.

The need for treatment for reflux depends on your baby's age, overall health and medical history, the extent of the problem, and your baby's tolerance for specific medications, procedures, and treatments. Sometimes reflux can be improved through feeding changes. Try these suggestions:

✔ After feeding, place your baby on his stomach with his upper body elevated at least 30 degrees, or hold him in a sitting position for about 30 minutes.

✔ If bottle-feeding, keep the nipple filled with milk or formula, so that your baby doesn't swallow too much air.

✔ Adding a feed thickener, such as rice cereal, may be beneficial for some babies who are about 6 months or older. Check with your pediatrician.

✔ Burp your baby frequently during feedings.

Part IV
Dealing with Special Concerns

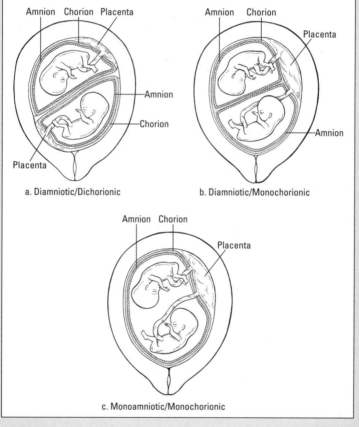

Amnion Chorion Placenta

Amnion

Chorion

Placenta

a. Diamniotic/Dichorionic

Amnion Chorion

Placenta

Amnion

Amnion

b. Diamniotic/Monochorionic

Amnion Chorion

Placenta

c. Monoamniotic/Monochorionic

Kathryn Born, MA

Discover more about placenta previa in a bonus article at www.dummies.com/extras/pregnancy.

In this part . . .

✔ Focus on the unique circumstances that go along with pregnancy. From the mother's age to having multiples to preparing siblings for the new arrival, we cover all that you need to know about special considerations.

✔ In pregnancy, problems can occur. Get a grasp on some of the things that can go wrong and how to deal with them.

✔ Discover what to do if you get sick while pregnant and how to handle preexisting conditions.

✔ Find ways to handle anything unexpected that may come during pregnancy. Know where to turn for support should a miscarriage occur and understand what to do if your baby has an abnormaility.

Chapter 13

Pregnancies with Special Considerations

*N*o two pregnancies are exactly alike. If you're like most women, you figure out pretty early in the game that your experience is different in some way from every friend and relative you talk to. You're not as nauseous as your sister was during the first three months — or your morning sickness is 20 times worse than your best friend's. You feel comfortable exercising throughout your pregnancy, although your Cousin Millie was put on bed rest. Plenty of variation occurs within the boundaries of what is considered to be a "normal" pregnancy. But some special kinds of pregnancies come with their own particular characteristics and challenges. This chapter focuses on them.

Figuring Out How Age Matters

Whether you're a prospective father or mother, age can make a difference — as many baby boomers are now finding out. Special problems and issues arise for men and women in their late 30s and older who are preparing to have children. Teen moms also face unique challenges. This section covers these challenges.

Over-30-something moms

Long gone are the days when almost all pregnant women were in their early 20s — and many were in their teens. Now, a greater number of women postpone having families until they've not only finished their education, but also have had time to become established in their careers. These days, too, divorce is more common, and many women find themselves having children with a second husband — often when they're well into their 30s or 40s (and sometimes 50s).

How old is too old? The answer used to be when you reach menopause — or even some years earlier — when your body no longer produces healthy eggs that can be fertilized to become embryos. But today, because of advances in assisted reproductive technologies like in vitro fertilization (IVF), which may use eggs donated by another woman, even women who are past the age of menopause can become pregnant. Also, over the last few years, there have been incredible advances in *egg freezing,* so that even if you are not ready to have children, eggs can be frozen and stored until the time is right.

Today, a more useful question is "At what age do you need to watch out for special problems?" And here, the answer is more specific. Any woman who is at least 35 years old during her pregnancy falls into the medical category of advanced maternal age, or AMA. (An impersonal term, to be sure, but perhaps less insulting than the alternatives that are also used: older gravida, mature gravida, and the particularly unfortunate elderly gravida.) The reason for singling out older mothers with any special term at all is that the incidence of certain chromosomal abnormalities increases with advancing maternal age. At age 35, the risks begin to increase significantly, as shown in Figure 13-1.

Doctors formerly concluded that at age 35, the risk of the fetus carrying some chromosomal abnormality was great enough to equal the risk of pregnancy loss after undergoing amniocentesis (about 0.5 percent at that time, although now the risks are thought to be much lower, 1/300 to 1/500, or even lower). Genetic testing — either amniocentesis or chorionic villus sampling — was routinely offered for pregnant women older than 35 in the United States. Some practitioners still adhere to the traditional age 35 dictum, but the American College of Obstetricians and Gynecologists now recommends women of all ages be offered the option of screening for Down syndrome — either by nuchal translucency screening, chorionic villus sampling, or amniocentesis (see Chapters 5 and 6).

Maternal Age and Chromosomal Abnormalities (Live Births)		
MATERNAL AGE	RISK FOR DOWN SYNDROME	TOTAL RISK FOR CHROMOSOME ABNORMALITIES*
20	1/1667	1/526*
21	1/1667	1/526*
22	1/1429	1/500*
23	1/1429	1/500*
24	1/1250	1/476*
25	1/1250	1/476*
26	1/1176	1/476*
27	1/1111	1/455*
28	1/1053	1/435*
29	1/1000	1/417*
30	1/952	1/384*
31	1/909	1/384*
32	1/769	1/322*
33	1/602	1/286
34	1/485	1/238
35	1/378	1/192
36	1/289	1/156
37	1/224	1/127
38	1/173	1/102
39	1/136	1/83
40	1/106	1/66
41	1/82	1/53
42	1/63	1/42
43	1/49	1/33
44	1/38	1/26
45	1/30	1/21
46	1/23	1/16
47	1/18	1/13
48	1/14	1/10
49	1/11	1/8

©John Wiley & Sons, Inc.

*Data of Hook (1981) and Hook et al. (1983). Because sample size for some intervals is relatively small, confidence limits are sometimes relatively large. Nonetheless, these figures are suitable for genetic counseling. *Excluded for ages 20–32 (data not available).*

Figure 13-1: As maternal age rises, so do the risks of chromosomal abnormalities.

Recently, non-invasive prenatal screening (NIPS, or non-invasive prenatal testing, NIPT) has become available for women 35 and older. This actually identifies fetal DNA in mom's blood and has a high detection rate for Down syndrome and disorders involving an extra chromosome 13 or 18. This can also tell the sex of the baby. It's important to remember that it is still a screening test

and not a definitive test. Currently the test is not available to women carrying multiple gestations, although research over the next few years may determine its utility in these situations.

The good news is that except for this increase in certain chromosomal abnormalities, babies born to women older than 35, or even older than 40, are as likely as any other babies to be healthy. The moms themselves do stand a higher-than-average risk of developing preeclampsia or gestational diabetes (see Chapters 14 and 15), and they stand an increased risk of delivering early or needing a cesarean delivery. Additionally, and for reasons we don't quite understand, women over age 35, and especially over age 40, are at a higher risk for stillbirth. Some doctors recommend closer surveillance in the last month of pregnancy, and even earlier delivery at about 39 weeks. Still, remember these risks aren't terribly high. Naturally, an older woman's experience with pregnancy depends to a large extent on her underlying health. If a woman is 48 years old or even 50, but she is in excellent health, she is likely to do extremely well.

A word about alternative conceptions

Thanks to assisted-reproductive technologies, more and more women older than 40 are becoming pregnant, some even with twins or triplets. Although many of these women conceive with their own eggs, many others conceive with someone else's. These women have unique issues to deal with, including what to tell their future children, friends, and family. Some, when they're pregnant, experience internal conflicts about the baby's genetic identity; they worry about the fact that their baby is biologically related to someone else and what that may mean. But often, these concerns disappear when the woman begins to feel her baby moving around inside her, and if not then, as soon as the baby is born.

Parents — even parents of children conceived the old-fashioned way — often discover after they meet their new baby in person that each child's identity is unique, and that the exact genetic ancestry doesn't matter nearly as much as they may have thought it would. So it makes sense that women who have had children conceived with donor eggs typically find that, after only a few days of caring for the new baby, they feel every bit as maternal as any biological mother would. The same is true of fathers of children who have been conceived with donor sperm. As the number of people having children with donated eggs or sperm grows, the whole experience is likely to become more comfortable for everyone involved.

Not-so-young dads

As we mention earlier, pregnancies in older women call for some special scrutiny because of the increased risk of genetic complications. To some extent, pregnancies involving older dads should likewise be singled out for observation. There is no absolute age cutoff for "advanced paternal age," but many people use 45 or 50 (although some argue it should be 35, just as it is for women).

Whereas for women the main genetic risk is having a fetus with a chromosomal abnormality (most commonly an extra chromosome), for men the risk is spontaneous gene mutations in the sperm, which can lead to a child with an autosomal dominant disorder, such as *achondroplasia* (a type of dwarfism) or neurofibromatosis. Only one copy of an abnormal gene can cause this kind of problem. (In so-called recessive genetic disorders — cystic fibrosis and sickle-cell anemia, for example — two copies of the abnormal gene are required for the problem to occur.) Autosomal dominant disorders are very rare, however, and many are impossible to test for, which is why no routine testing exists for advanced paternal age. Also, some studies suggest a slightly higher risk of autism with older dads, but again, the exact age at which this risk increases is not quite clear, and it still is an unusual cause of this disorder.

Very young moms

Pregnancy in teenage women raises a different set of concerns. Although this age group doesn't sustain any increase in chromosomal abnormalities, these women may experience a higher incidence of some birth defects. Because teenage moms tend to have less-than-optimal nutritional habits, they also experience a higher incidence of low-birth-weight babies. Teenage moms are also at a higher risk of developing preeclampsia, are more likely to deliver by cesarean delivery, and are less likely to breast-feed. Due to their unique situation, young moms need special guidance and counseling. If you're a teenage mom, we encourage you to receive adequate prenatal care, to follow a healthy diet, and to consider the benefits of breast-feeding (see Chapter 12).

Having Twins or More

Having twins may seem simple — to someone who's never faced the reality of it. It's either "double the pleasure" or a living nightmare (twice the work and only half the sleep). Twins are complicated, as any mother of twins can tell you — for hours and hours, if you're willing to listen. A sizable part of having twins, triplets, or more is the experience of pregnancy.

If you're having triplets or more, what applies to twins generally applies to triplets (and more), only to a much greater extent.

Although the vast majority of twin pregnancies proceed smoothly and result in the birth of two beautiful, healthy babies, some risks are involved for both the fetuses and the mom. As a result, most practitioners want women who are pregnant with twins to have checkups more frequently than other moms, and they may schedule plenty of extra ultrasound exams.

Ethnic background and family history can increase your chance of having twins; certain women are constitutionally more likely to ovulate more than one egg in a cycle. If twins occur in your family, let your practitioner know.

The odds (and oddities) of having twins, triplets, or more

The number of twins conceived is much larger than the number of twins that are actually born. Many pregnancies that begin as twin pregnancies end as single births because one of the fetuses never develops. In many cases, one of the fetuses disappears before the pregnancy is even diagnosed (the so-called *vanishing twin*). The incidence of twin births is usually estimated to be close to 3 percent of all births. However, the incidence is rising, mainly due to the increasing use of fertility techniques.

The incidence of spontaneous triplets is much rarer — about 1 in 7,000. Spontaneous quadruplets or more are exceedingly rare. However, with the increasing use of infertility treatments, the incidence of triplets has increased tenfold over the past few decades. Fortunately, though, the rate of increase is slowing because of refinements in infertility treatments.

This section takes a closer look at several questions and issues you may have if you're pregnant with twins.

Looking at types of multiples

Twins can be either identical or fraternal. These old-fashioned terms don't completely describe how twins occur. *Identical* twins look very much alike and are always the same sex. They come from a single embryo, meaning they're a product of the union of one egg and one sperm. (In other words, they are *monozygotic* — they come from the same zygote.) They have exactly the same genes as each other, which explains their resemblance. In the United States, roughly one-third of all twins are identical. An egg can split into three, leading to identical triplets, but it's very unusual.

A woman conceives *fraternal* twins when she ovulates more than one egg, two different sperm fertilize two eggs, and the resulting zygotes implant in her uterus at the same time. These *dizygotic* twins — who arise from two zygotes — don't share an identical set of genes. Instead, their genetic makeup is as similar as that of any pair of children born of the same parents. They're just born at the same time. They can be the same sex, or they can be of opposite sexes. Roughly two-thirds of all twins conceived spontaneously in the United States are dizygotic. If three eggs are fertilized, the result is fraternal triplets. A triplet pregnancy can also consist of two fetuses that are monozygotic and one from a second fertilized egg — leading to two babies that are identical and one that is fraternal.

 The chance that a woman will have identical twins increases after she reaches the age of 35. The chance a woman will have fraternal twins (because she ovulates more than one egg in any given month), on the other hand, rises until about the age of 35 and then drops off. Some families have more than their statistical share of fraternal twins. Some women are predisposed to ovulating more than one egg at a time, and that can lead to fraternal twins. If a woman has a history of twinning on her mother's side, she may stand a higher chance of twinning. Fraternal twinning also becomes more likely when a woman takes fertility drugs, because these medications boost her chances of ovulating more than one egg. Of course, a woman who takes fertility drugs can still produce an egg that gets fertilized and then splits in two to form identical twins.

Determining whether multiples are identical or fraternal

Many women who are pregnant with twins ask their doctor or sonographer during an ultrasound exam whether she can tell if her twins are fraternal or identical. In some cases, the technician or your doctor can tell: If the babies are two different sexes, they're fraternal. If they're the same sex, they may be either fraternal or identical. If they're the same sex or if the festuses' sexes aren't yet visible, other findings on ultrasound can suggest whether the twins are identical:

✔ An egg that splits very early after fertilization, within the first two or three days, results in two embryos that have separate placentas and separate amniotic sacs. This situation is called *diamniotic/dichorionic* (see Figure 13-2a). On ultrasound, they look no different than fraternal twins that come from two separately fertilized eggs. So with twins who have separate placentas and are of the same sex, it's impossible to tell on ultrasound if they're identical or fraternal.

✔ If an egg splits between the third and eighth day after fertilization, the resulting twins are in two separate amniotic sacs but share a single placenta (see Figure 13-2b). Your doctor may use the term *diamniotic/monochorionic* to describe this situation. If, on ultrasound, your doctor or sonographer can see that a set of twins shares a single placenta, chances are they're identical. (Keep in mind, though, that sometimes determining whether there is one placenta or two that are very close together is difficult on ultrasound.) The thickness of the membrane separating the sacs gives another clue — with two separate placentas, a thick membrane separates the two sacs, whereas with one placenta, the membrane is very thin.

✔ An egg that splits sometime between 8 and 13 days after fertilization results in twins that not only share a placenta but also are in a single amniotic sac (see Figure 13-2c). Twins like these are called *monoamniotic/monochorionic*. If your doctor does an ultrasound examination and sees twins sharing the same amniotic sac, she can be sure that they're identical. This is pretty rare (1 percent of all twins, or 1 in 60,000 pregnancies).

✔ An egg that splits after the 13th day of gestation results in conjoined or "Siamese" twins, which are exceedingly rare.

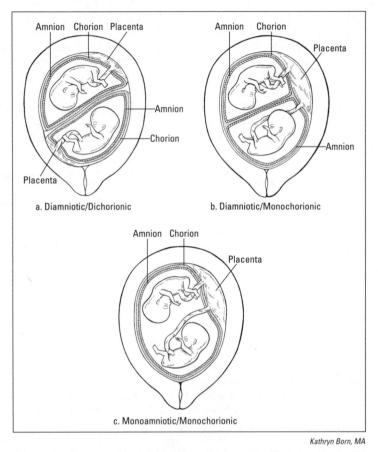

Amnion Chorion Placenta

Amnion

Chorion

Placenta

a. Diamniotic/Dichorionic

Amnion Chorion

Placenta

Amnion

b. Diamniotic/Monochorionic

Amnion Chorion

Placenta

c. Monoamniotic/Monochorionic

Kathryn Born, MA

Figure 13-2: Your practitioner can often tell what type of twins you're having by viewing the placenta(s) and amniotic sac(s) during an ultrasound exam.

An expert sonographer can use subtle signs to help differentiate the various types of twins, although sometimes it still may be hard to be absolutely certain. The sonographer establishes whether the twins have two separate placentas and, of less importance, whether they're actually fraternal or identical. Establishing the type of placentation (monochorionic or dichorionic) is easier in the first trimester than in the second or third trimester.

Because different types of twins are associated with different problems and risks, trying to figure out what type of twinning is present is important. If the ultrasound signs are ambiguous and the medical situation suggests that determining the type of twinning is especially important, special tests can be performed to answer this question. These tests are called *zygosity* studies and require an invasive procedure, such as amniocentesis, chorionic villus sampling (CVS), or fetal blood sampling (see Chapter 6).

Screening for Down syndrome in pregnancies with twins or more

For many years, the most common way of screening pregnancies for Down syndrome was by measuring different markers in the mother's blood at 16 weeks of pregnancy (see Chapter 6). The accuracy of this test with twins is fair, but with triplets or more, it doesn't help at all. The newer method of Down syndrome screening in the first trimester (*nuchal translucency,* see Chapter 5) appears to work pretty well for moms with multiple gestations because the doctor can obtain a nuchal-translucency measurement for each fetus, thus determining each fetus's individual risk of having Down syndrome. Using the nuchal translucency and mom's blood markers, doctors can detect about 70 to 75 percent of all cases of Down syndrome in twins. This is a little lower than the detection rate in single fetuses, but still pretty good. With triplets or more, using the nuchal-translucency measurement alone tends to be the most helpful approach, because it's difficult to determine how to use the mother's blood markers in this situation.

Conducting genetic testing in pregnancies with twins or more

Chorionic villus sampling and amniocentesis are a little trickier with twins or more. The two main challenges are to make sure each fetus is sampled separately and none of the tissue taken from one fetus contaminates the tissue taken from the other. In the case of identical twins, this issue isn't as critical, because the fetuses have the same genetic makeup. If you find a genetic abnormality (or lack of any genetic abnormalities) in one, the same is almost always true for the other. With fraternal twins, triplets, or more, testing each one separately is critical.

Our patients want to know . . .

Q: "Is doing an amniocentesis or CVS for twin or triplet pregnancies riskier than for singleton pregnancies?"

A: Although scientists have conducted little research on this question, it appears the chances of complications aren't substantially greater in multi-fetal pregnancies, if the person performing the procedure is experienced in doing it with mothers carrying twins or more.

Amniocentesis

Amniocentesis (see Chapter 6) is the most common way to do genetic testing in multi-fetal pregnancies. This method requires inserting a separate needle into the uterus for each fetus being tested. Of course, the amniocentesis is done under ultrasound guidance. After the doctor removes some fluid from the first fetus's amniotic sac, she may leave the needle in place to inject a harmless organic blue dye (called indigo carmine) into that fetus's amniotic sac. (Don't worry — you won't give birth to a Smurf. This blue dye is absorbed over time.) Then, if the fluid from the second needle comes out clear (not blue), the doctor knows that she has sampled the second sac. If you're carrying more than two fetuses, the doctor adds a few drops of blue dye to each consecutive sac after she taps it.

Chorionic villus sampling

Chorionic villus sampling, or CVS (see Chapter 5), can be somewhat complicated in multi-fetal pregnancies, but experienced doctors can usually handle the job. In some cases, the placentas are positioned in such a way that CVS is technically impossible. In these cases, the mother has the option of having an amniocentesis a little later in the pregnancy (at about 15 to 18 weeks, rather than 10 to 12 weeks for CVS).

Keeping track of which baby is which

Your doctor designates your babies before birth as Twin A and Twin B (or Triplets A, B, and C). These designations enable your doctor to communicate to you and others (nurses and other medical personnel) which baby is which and to follow

the progress of each baby separately and consistently through-out the pregnancy. By convention, the fetus closest to the cervix (the opening to the womb) is designated as Twin A (or Triplet A). This baby is usually born first. In a triplet pregnancy, the highest triplet (closest to your chest) is designated as Triplet C. (Some patients come up with their own clever names. We had one patient with twins who nicknamed her babies Gucci and Prada before birth so she could keep track of them.)

Living day-to-day during a multiple pregnancy

If you're pregnant with multiples, don't ignore everything else we've written in this book. In many ways, your pregnancy pro-ceeds like any other. The difference, as you may already know, is that your experience is more intense in various ways: You grow a larger belly quicker, your nausea may be worse, your amnio-centesis (if you have one) is a bit more complicated (as we describe earlier in this chapter), and the birth may take longer. With triplets or more, these physical changes and symptoms are even more exaggerated. In addition, certain complications are more frequent in multiples than in singletons. In the follow-ing list, we describe many of the ways your experience may be somewhat different:

- ✔ **Activity:** In the old days, doctors recommended women with twins be placed on bed rest beginning at 24 to 28 weeks. However, data shows women placed on bed rest appear to be no less likely than others to experience pre-term delivery or have babies of low birth weight. Whether you need to reduce your activity depends on your prior obstetrical history as well as how smoothly your preg-nancy goes from week to week. If you develop preterm labor or have problems with fetal growth, your doctor may recommend you take it easy. With triplets or more, the benefit is unclear, but many obstetricians routinely recom-mend bed rest starting in the second trimester.

- ✔ **Diet:** Many experts recommend women carrying twins con-sume an extra 300 calories a day above what is required for a singleton (in other words, an extra 600 calories per day above their pre-pregnancy intake). For triplets and more, no consensus exists, but obviously your food intake should be somewhat greater.

✔ **Iron and folic acid:** Women carrying twins, triplets, or more stand a greater chance of developing anemia, which is due to dilutional anemia (see Chapter 4) as well as greater demands for iron and folic acid. Doctors recommend supplemental iron and folic acid for women carrying two or more fetuses.

✔ **Nausea:** Most women carrying two or more fetuses definitely have more nausea and vomiting in early pregnancy than women with only one. This nausea may be related to higher levels of hCG (a pregnancy hormone) circulating through the bloodstream. The good news is that nausea and vomiting for mothers of multiples, as for mothers of single babies, usually goes away by the end of the first trimester.

✔ **Prenatal doctor visits:** Your practitioner is likely to follow pretty much the same routine she uses for mothers of single babies. That is, you have your blood pressure, weight, and urine checked at each visit.

But because you have more than one fetus, your practitioner may ask you to come in more frequently. Some practitioners perform routine pelvic exams to make sure your cervix isn't dilating prematurely; others may suggest your cervix be checked with an ultrasound exam. On the other hand, if you don't have any preterm labor symptoms, your doctor may decide you don't need these extra exams. (See the "Monitoring for preterm labor in twins" section later in this chapter for more details.)

✔ **Ultrasound examinations:** Most practitioners suggest that mothers of twins or more have ultrasound examinations every four to six weeks throughout their pregnancy in order to check fetal growth. If you have any problems, these exams may need to be more frequent.

With more than one fetus, your doctor can't use fundal height measurements to evaluate the growth. And because women with twins, triplets, or more are at a higher risk of having problems with fetal growth (see the "Intrauterine growth restriction" section later in this chapter), these periodic ultrasound exams are very important. Some doctors also may monitor the cervix every two weeks by transvaginal ultrasound during the second trimester to look for an increased risk of preterm birth. (For more on this, see the "Monitoring for preterm labor in twins" section later in this chapter.)

✔ **Weight gain:** The average weight gain for a twin pregnancy is 35 to 45 pounds (15 to 20 kg). But the exact amount you gain depends on your pre-pregnancy weight. The Institute of Medicine recommends that mothers with twin pregnancies gain about one pound per week during the second and third trimesters.

Recent studies show that you can achieve the optimal growth rates by taking into account your body mass index (see Chapter 4) prior to pregnancy, and that weight gain in the first two trimesters may be especially important. Doctors recommend weight gains of 45 to 50 pounds (20 to 23 kg) by 34 weeks for triplets and more than 50 pounds (23 kg) for quadruplets.

✔ **Delivery:** If you are carrying dichorionic twins and everything is going smoothly, many practitioners recommend delivery by 38 weeks 0 days to 38 weeks 6 days because this has the best outcome for your babies. If you are carrying uncomplicated monochorionic twins, doctors recommend delivery earlier, somewhere between 34 weeks 0 days to 37 weeks 6 days.

Going through labor and delivery

Although some studies have suggested that in very specific situations and with very strict criteria, vaginal delivery of a triplet pregnancy may be possible, almost all triplets are delivered by cesarean. The following section on birth positions and delivery is addressed to women carrying twins.

Often, pregnancy goes smoothly for mothers of twins, but labor and delivery can still be complex. For this reason, we recommend women carrying more than one fetus deliver in a hospital, where extra personnel are present to handle any complications that may arise.

Assuming the babies are full-term, your babies can be in different positions. Basically, their positions fall into one of three possibilities:

✔ Both fetuses can be head-down (vertex), as they are in about 45 percent of twin pregnancies (see Figure 13-3a). Vaginal delivery is successful 60 to 70 percent of the time when the babies are in this position.

✔ The first fetus can be head-down and the second not, as is the case about 35 percent of the time, making a cesarean delivery more likely unless your practitioner can turn the second baby to a head-down position. Whether trying to manipulate the baby in this way makes sense is a matter of some debate among practitioners. Your doctor's choice of trying to turn the baby around or delivering the baby breech depends on her training, experience, and professional bias.

✔ The first fetus can be breech or transverse (lying horizontally across the uterus), and the second can be breech, head-down, or transverse. This positioning occurs about 20 percent of the time (see Figures 13-3b and 13-3c).

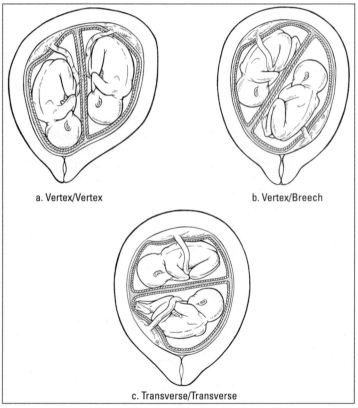

a. Vertex/Vertex   b. Vertex/Breech

c. Transverse/Transverse

Kathryn Born, MA

Figure 13-3: Three possible positions of twins before delivery.

With any of these combinations of positions, if the babies are preterm, the options may be different. In any case, discuss the possibilities with your doctor before the time of delivery.

Covering special issues for moms with multiples

If you're pregnant with twins or triplets (or more), your doctor puts you under closer surveillance, because the risk of certain complications is greater in multi-fetal pregnancies. The following topics are some of the things she is watching out for.

Don't let this list scare you. The important thing is to be aware of potential problems so that if they develop, you and your practitioner can recognize them early and manage them appropriately.

Preterm delivery

The biggest risk you face in carrying more than one baby is that you may have preterm labor and delivery. The average length of pregnancy for a singleton is 40 weeks, but for a twin pregnancy it's only about 36 weeks; for triplets, 33 to 34 weeks; and for quadruplets, about 31 weeks. A pregnancy is full-term if it lasts 37 weeks or more. Preterm delivery is technically between 24 and 37 weeks, but most babies born at 35 or 36 weeks are generally as healthy as babies delivered after 37 weeks.

Many women go into preterm labor without actually delivering their babies early. About 80 percent of mothers carrying triplets and 40 percent of those with twins experience preterm labor, but not all deliver early. (See details about preterm labor and delivery in Chapter 14.)

Chromosomal abnormalities

When you have more than one fetus and they aren't identical, the chance that either one of them has a genetic abnormality is somewhat higher. After all, each baby has its own individual risk of some abnormality, and the risks add up. Mothers of single babies are considered to be of advanced maternal age (AMA) at 35, as we describe earlier in the chapter, but in twin pregnancies derived from two separate eggs, AMA may be as early as 33, and for triplets, 31 or 32. This all becomes relevant for women considering the genetic testing we mention earlier.

Diabetes

Because the incidence of gestational diabetes is higher with twins or more, many practitioners recommend all women carrying more than one fetus be screened for this condition. (See Chapter 15.)

Hypertension and preeclampsia

Hypertension (high blood pressure) is more common in multifetal pregnancies. The risk is proportional to the number of fetuses present. Some women develop hypertension alone, without other symptoms or other physical signs. Others develop a condition unique to pregnancy called *preeclampsia*, which involves high blood pressure in association with spilling protein in the urine (proteinuria), or if proteinuria is absent, the presence of some other abnormalities (see the description of preeclampsia in Chapter 14). Forty percent of mothers carrying twins and 60 percent or more carrying triplets develop some form of hypertension during pregnancy. For this reason, your practitioner keeps a close eye on your blood pressure.

Intrauterine growth restriction

Problems with fetal growth occur in anywhere from 15 to 50 percent of all twins. The problem is even more common in triplets and in fetuses that share the same placenta. In the case of a single placenta, the blood may not be distributed equally, which may cause one twin to get more nutrients than the other. In multiples that have different placentas, growth restriction can result when one placenta is implanted in a more favorable position within the uterus and therefore provides better nourishment than the other. Your doctor is likely to schedule periodic ultrasound exams during your pregnancy to check that both (or all three) fetuses are growing properly.

Twin-twin transfusion syndrome

Twin-twin transfusion syndrome is specific to twins who share a single placenta. In some cases, the single placenta contains blood vessels that interconnect between the two fetuses. This connection enables the two fetuses to exchange blood — and allows the blood to become distributed unequally. The fetus that gets more blood grows bigger and produces extra amniotic fluid, whereas the one that gets less blood may suffer impaired growth and have significantly decreased amniotic fluid in its sac. This situation can be very serious, but fortunately, it affects only 10 to 15 percent of monochorionic twins.

Multi-fetal pregnancy reduction

Some doctors perform the multi-fetal pregnancy reduction procedure to decrease the number of fetuses a woman is carrying
in order to improve the chance that she delivers healthy babies.
Doctors more commonly use it in women who have at least
three viable fetuses resulting from fertility treatments because
of the high risk of preterm delivery if they try to carry all the
fetuses. Also, some women carrying twins want to reduce their
pregnancy to a singleton, and this is becoming increasingly
more common. Usually a maternal-fetal medicine specialist
performs a multi-fetal pregnancy reduction between 10 and
13 weeks in a special center. The risk involved is acceptably
low when an experienced physician specifically trained in this
procedure performs it. The important thing is to find out about
all possible options, so that you have as much information as
possible to make the best decision for you.

Selective termination

A selective termination procedure can be used in a multi-fetal
pregnancy to terminate one of the fetuses when that fetus has
a significant abnormality. A maternal-fetal medicine specialist
can perform this procedure if the fetuses have separate placentas, so that the medication used can't cross over and affect
the normal fetus. In the case of identical twins that share a
single amniotic sac, some other options are available (ask your
doctor). In the latter case, only a few centers in the United
States perform this procedure.

Monitoring for preterm labor in twins

Doctors aren't sure what exactly causes labor to start in any
pregnancy, but it has something to do with how distended the
uterus is. With twins, the uterus becomes larger much earlier
than it does with a single fetus, so the risk of going into labor
early — as well as delivering early — is increased. As we mention earlier, the average gestational age when a single fetus
delivers is 40 weeks. The average gestational age for the delivery of twins is 36 weeks.

Doctors have come up with ways to try to prevent premature
births in twin gestations. Some of the things that have been
tried are putting in a *cervical cerclage* (a stitch sewn into the

cervix to try to keep it closed — see Chapter 6) and using progesterone to keep the uterus from contracting. Unfortunately, neither of these two treatments has been shown to change the rate of premature delivery in twins.

Although no surefire treatments exist to prevent premature birth in twins, doctors have focused on trying to come up with strategies to predict which patients with twins are at the highest risk for delivering early. If your risk is high, your doctor may decide to admit you to the hospital for more intensive observation and to make sure you don't have preterm labor that is unrecognized. Your doctor may also give you steroid shots between weeks 24 and 34 to help your babies' lungs mature quicker in the event that you do deliver early.

Two factors that are indicators of early delivery can be examined via transvaginal ultrasound:

- ✔ **The length of the cervix:** The length of the cervix usually gets progressively shorter prior to delivery. Cervical length measurements are most helpful in twins between 16 and 24 weeks of pregnancy, but sometimes they are continued after that time if the situation warrants.

- ✔ **Whether or not the cervix is dilating:** Early dilation is sometimes called *funneling* because the cervix looks like a funnel on ultrasound.

The frequency of the measurements depends on your own individual situation, but they're typically taken about every two weeks. If your cervix is long and not dilated, your chances of a premature delivery are low. If it's short or showing signs of early dilation, your doctor will probably step up the frequency of your visits or even admit you to the hospital.

Another test to predict the likelihood of delivering early involves determining the level of *fetal fibronectin* (see Chapter 14). This substance is found in vaginal secretions obtained by using a special swab. Fetal fibronectin levels are higher in women with twins who are at an increased risk for early delivery. Even if your cervix is closed and you aren't in premature labor, if your fetal fibronectin test is positive, your doctor may decide to give you steroids.

Getting Pregnant Again

Doctors and parents haven't come to a consensus on the optimal time to get pregnant again. Probably the most important consideration is your overall health. If you can get back to your pre-pregnancy or ideal body weight quickly after you deliver, and if you can replenish any lost nutrients and vitamins (particularly folate, iron, and calcium) from your last pregnancy, you can probably consider getting pregnant again fairly soon — in about 12 to 18 months. A recent large study showed getting pregnant again in less than 18 months was associated with an increased risk of adverse pregnancy outcomes. If you've had a complicated pregnancy, a difficult delivery, or excessive loss of blood, wait until you're in better shape before trying again.

Also ask yourself what you consider to be the ideal age difference in your children. Some people feel having children close in age is better. That way, the older child doesn't have so many years to settle into the role of only child and, therefore, may not feel so jealous when the new baby comes. Others feel spacing the children further apart, so that the older child is mature enough to handle the introduction of a new sibling, is better. Most important is how you and your partner feel and how ready you are to take on another child. The decision may involve emotional and financial issues as well as physical ones. Ask yourself whether you can handle the pressure and the expense and can do the work that having another child takes.

Realizing how each pregnancy differs

Naturally, any mother compares her second pregnancy with her first, but every pregnancy is different. If your last pregnancy went smoothly, you may think any little thing out of the ordinary that happens in the next pregnancy is a signal that things aren't going well. By the same token, if your first pregnancy was difficult, you needn't assume the same complications are going to happen again. And no matter what anybody tells you, remember that different symptoms don't mean the second baby will be a different sex than your first child. See Chapter 2 for some myths about predicting your baby's sex.

These are some of the ways in which you may experience pregnancy differently the second (or third or fourth) time around:

- ✔ Many women feel that they're showing sooner or are at least more bloated and distended. This condition may be because their abdominal muscles have been stretched by their previous pregnancy and are now more lax.

- ✔ Many women find that nausea isn't as severe as it was the first time around, and others find that it's worse.

- ✔ You can usually identify fetal movement earlier.

- ✔ Labor is usually shorter, and delivery is easier.

- ✔ Many women find they feel Braxton-Hicks contractions earlier and more frequently than with their first child. (See Chapter 7 for more on Braxton-Hicks contractions.)

- ✔ Most women are less anxious the second time around.

One thing remains the same: As hard as it may be to believe, you will love your second child as much as your first.

In their third pregnancy, many women commonly experience a special kind of worry: They feel that because their first two pregnancies were healthy and problem-free, the third one's bound to have complications. Many feel that they were lucky twice in a row, and that going for a third time is pushing their luck. If you feel this way, believe us, you aren't alone. Keep in mind the chances of trouble aren't inherently greater in a third pregnancy, even if the first two went smoothly.

Giving birth after a prior cesarean delivery

If you've had a cesarean delivery and you get pregnant again, you may wonder whether you can deliver vaginally this time or need another cesarean. To some extent, the answer depends on which of the following kinds of cesarean you had:

- ✔ **Low transverse:** Most cesarean deliveries are done through a low-transverse incision (across the floor in the lower part of the uterus). (See Figure 13-4a.) Women who have this kind of incision usually can deliver vaginally in a subsequent pregnancy as long as they have no other complicating factors. The risk of uterine rupture is lowest with this kind of incision.

✔ **Classical:** If you have what's known as a classical cesarean, in which a vertical incision is made in the upper portion of the uterus (see Figure 13-4b), don't try to have a vaginal delivery in a subsequent pregnancy because this type of incision is more likely to rupture. Vertical incisions are sometimes performed in cases of very preterm birth or placenta previa (see Chapter 14), or when the mother's uterus is an abnormal shape or has large fibroids.

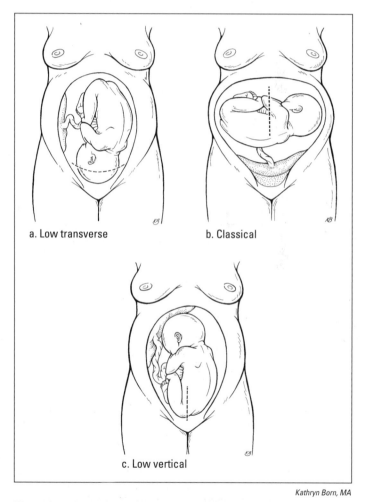

a. Low transverse   b. Classical

c. Low vertical

Kathryn Born, MA

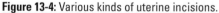

Figure 13-4: Various kinds of uterine incisions.

> ✔ **Low vertical:** A low-vertical incision (see Figure 13-4c) is performed less frequently than a low-transverse incision, but it does enable the mother to attempt labor and delivery in a subsequent pregnancy.

The incision made on your skin doesn't reflect the type of incision on your uterus. In other words, you may have a transverse incision on your skin (a bikini cut) but still have a vertical incision on your uterus.

Doctors used to think that after a woman had a cesarean delivery, all her babies would have to be delivered the same way and that trying a vaginal delivery risked the uterus rupturing through the old cesarean scar. But studies have demonstrated that the risk of such a rupture is actually quite low — less than 1 percent. Discuss the issues of uterine rupture with your doctor. Other recent studies show that 70 percent of the time, women can successfully deliver a baby vaginally after they've had a cesarean. Of course, the likelihood of success depends to some extent on why a cesarean was performed in the first place. If your doctor performed it because the baby was breech, the chance that the next baby can be delivered vaginally is nearly 90 percent. If the cesarean was performed because the baby was too large to fit through the mother's pelvis, the chance of a future vaginal delivery falls to 50 to 60 percent. Some smaller hospitals are unable to offer VBAC *(vaginal birth after cesarean)* to their patients because they don't have the capacity to meet the special requirements (like 24/7 availability of an anesthesiologist) needed to do so.

Why would you want to deliver your next baby vaginally? The main benefit is that if you're successful, your recovery is much shorter. Another potential benefit from a vaginal birth is that it's often associated with less postpartum pain. However, although most patients find the pain associated with vaginal birth to be less than that associated with cesarean delivery, some vaginal births have painful complications of their own. See Chapter 11 for more information.

Other benefits of a vaginal birth include the following:

> ✔ A lower risk of the kind of complications associated with abdominal surgery, including
>
>   • Anesthesia problems
>
>   • Inadvertent injury to adjacent organs

- Infection

- Possible blood clots from being immobile for a longer period of time

✔ For some women, a psychological benefit from experiencing a vaginal birth

✔ A shorter hospital stay

✔ The possibility, indicated by some studies, that the baby clears her secretions more efficiently if born vaginally

However, you do have some risk: If you try labor and then end up with another cesarean, studies show that the complication rate is higher than if you went straight to a repeat cesarean without labor. Additionally, your recovery may be longer than if you had elected to have a repeat cesarean.

If You're a Nontraditional Family

Single women and gay or lesbian couples bearing children are becoming more and more common. If you fall into one of these categories, discussing your situation with your practitioner is important. Don't worry that your doctor may judge or ridicule you. Practitioners are trained to be sensitive to all patients' needs, and you're no different. If your practitioner does seem to have a problem with your situation, move on to someone who's more understanding — the sooner, the better.

In many single-mother and lesbian pregnancies, the father of the baby isn't physically present. Still, try to have information about the father's family history and ethnicity so you and your practitioner can go over any genetic implications. (See Chapter 5.)

If the father isn't going to be around for the whole process, build your own support network. If you're a single mom, you may choose one or more people (family members or close friends) to share your pregnancy, labor, and delivery. If you're part of a lesbian couple, the nonpregnant partner can assume the primary support role. If the father is a gay male friend, include him as support. No matter the case, having your support people accompany you to any prenatal visits or prenatal classes and having them around for the labor and delivery process is completely appropriate.

Preparing Your Child (or Children) for a New Arrival

Many parents look forward to having a second child specifically because they want to provide a sibling for the first one. But your first child may not easily understand this reasoning. She may feel completely content about being the only child, and it may be months or years before the first one appreciates the second one. For those of you who are having your second child — or third or fourth (or more!) — the following sections offer a few ideas about how to help prepare the older one(s) for the new arrival. Many hospitals now offer sibling classes to help your child acclimate. Contact the hospital in which you plan to deliver for information.

Explaining pregnancy

The ease or difficulty you may have introducing a new baby sister or brother depends quite a bit on how old the elder sibling is. Explaining a new baby to a 15-year-old is easy; getting the concept across to a 15-month-old can be tricky. And the challenge begins at the time you tell the first child that you're pregnant. A 2-year-old has little concept of time and may not understand that Mom is pregnant for months before the baby comes. She may be frustrated the baby can't come immediately. So delay telling a very young child about your pregnancy until the second or third trimester, unless you don't mind being hounded every day about when the new baby is coming.

If your child is old enough — at least 2 or 3 years old — you may want to bring her along to prenatal doctor visits, ultrasound examinations, or when you're shopping for baby items. (While you're doing that shopping, consider getting a small present for your child so she doesn't feel neglected.) A child who is old enough may also like to join in discussions about what to name the new baby.

 If you anticipate moving your child to a new room or having her graduate from a crib to a bed, make the change before the baby is born. This change allows your older child to have a chance to acclimate so she doesn't associate the new situation directly with the new baby's arrival.

As you near the end of your pregnancy, don't be surprised if your child starts to act up or becomes unusually clingy and dependent. Many children get a sense that things are about to change when they see their mother getting physically bigger or when they overhear conversations about the impending arrival. During this time, be supportive and loving. Include your child in the preparations as much as possible. And remember that although having a new sibling affects almost all children in certain predictable ways, each child is unique, and how yours reacts depends in large part on her personality.

Making baby-sitting arrangements for your delivery

Obviously, you need to plan on having someone take care of your child when you and your partner go to deliver the new baby. If your delivery is scheduled (that is, you're having a planned cesarean or an elective induction), making arrangements is relatively easy. But most women don't know exactly when the big moment will arrive. And you still need to be ready beforehand.

If you go into labor spontaneously in the middle of the night, you want your child to be prepared in advance for what will happen and who will show up to take care of her while you're gone. Reassure your child you will be okay and that she can come to see you and the new baby in the hospital very soon. If possible, phone your child at home while you're in the hospital to tell her that you're doing well, especially if your labor is unusually long. Many hospitals now have special sibling visiting hours, and you may want to check out the details ahead of time.

Pack a couple of gifts to take with you to the hospital — one for your child to give to the new baby and one for the baby to give to the child.

Coming home

During the first few days that the new siblings live together, you may be amazed at how well-adjusted, happy, and excited your older child is. Part of this attitude is genuine enthusiasm. But keep in mind that part of it may also be your older child's

attempt to share the limelight with the new baby. Some children have a short period of difficulty coping; others do fine at first but develop longer-lasting sibling rivalry.

Don't be surprised if your child begins to regress in terms of some developmental milestones. A previously potty-trained child may resort to bed-wetting, for example. Or a child may resume thumb-sucking or have difficulty sleeping. You may notice your older child gets especially jealous while you're breast-feeding. During this period, understand your child may need extra reassurance that you still love her and the new baby hasn't replaced her in your heart at all.

Explain that your heart is big enough to love more than one child. If possible, allow your elder child to participate in helping to care for the baby. How much "help" your child is capable of providing depends on her age, but even small children can fetch a diaper if you need one or help give the baby a bath. Don't be surprised if at times your child expresses aggression toward you or the baby. Usually, these acts of aggression are harmless, but during this early stage of adjustment, don't leave your child alone with the baby unsupervised. She may not realize certain ways of handling the baby may be harmful.

Several months may pass before your older child feels secure, but eventually most children do deal with the change successfully. Quite often friends, neighbors, and family shower the new baby with gifts. Again, having a stash of inexpensive new toys for your older child to prevent excessive jealousy may be a good idea. It's also a good idea to occasionally spend some one-on-one time with the older child to maintain your special bond with one another. With extra love and understanding, you can help your child through what can be a difficult period.

Chapter 14

When Things Get Complicated

*T*he vast majority of pregnancies are smooth, uncompli-cated affairs — perfectly well managed by Mother Nature alone. Sometimes, though, your pregnancy can get a little complicated. Even when problems arise, ultimately both baby and mother are healthy in most cases. If you have no major medical problems going into your pregnancy and it remains uncomplicated, you may just as well skip this chapter. If, on the other hand, you're the type of person who wants to know about every possibility, and this kind of knowledge doesn't drive you nuts, you may find this chapter interesting. Just do yourself a favor: Don't take it too much to heart.

We have had many patients who, after reading other books about pregnancy, call us frantically, assuming they're experienc-ing every complication the books describe. This chapter's infor-mation is meant to either reassure you that your pregnancy is safe or — if you do have some particular problem — provide useful information to help you understand the situation better.

 We want to avoid writing yet another textbook in maternal-fetal medicine. To that end, we cover some conditions only briefly and omit some less common problems entirely. But our hope is that the following information gives you some famil-iarity with what can occur, so that if a problem develops, you know how to proceed.

Dealing with Preterm Labor

Normally, during the second half of pregnancy, the uterus contracts intermittently. As the end of your pregnancy approaches, these contractions grow more frequent. Finally, they become regular and cause the cervix to dilate. When contractions and dilation occur before 37 weeks of gestation, labor is considered *preterm*. Some women notice periods of regular contractions prior to 37 weeks. If the cervix doesn't dilate or efface, however, the condition isn't considered preterm labor.

Of course, the earlier preterm labor occurs, the more troublesome it can be. The problems that a premature baby has if he is born after about 34 weeks are usually much less worrisome than those he faces if born at only 24 weeks. Prior to about 32 weeks, the main problem is that the baby's lungs may still be immature, but other complications may exist as well. Nevertheless, the majority of babies born at 26 to 32 weeks are fine and healthy, especially if they have access to modern neonatal intensive care.

Premature babies stand a higher risk of contracting an infection, they may experience problems with the gastrointestinal tract (stomach and intestines), or they may experience an *intraventricular hemorrhage,* which is bleeding into an area within the brain.

The following can be signs and symptoms of preterm labor:

- ✔ Constant leakage of thin fluid from the vagina
- ✔ An increase in mucous-like vaginal discharge
- ✔ Intense and persistent pressure in the pelvis or vaginal area
- ✔ Menstrual-like cramps
- ✔ Persistent lower-back pain
- ✔ Regular contractions that don't stop with rest or decreased activity

Nobody knows for sure what causes premature labor, but clearly, some patients are at higher risk for developing it. If you fall into one of the high-risk categories, your practitioner

probably will want to follow you more closely than usual. The following are some factors that put you at risk for preterm delivery:

✔ An abnormally shaped uterus

✔ Bleeding during pregnancy, especially during the second half. (*Note:* This doesn't include occasional spotting during the first trimester.)

✔ A prior preterm delivery

✔ Some infections, like bacterial vaginosis, periodontal disease, or a kidney infection

✔ Smoking

✔ Abuse of certain illicit drugs

✔ Being African-American

✔ Poor nutrition and/or a low pre-pregnancy weight

✔ Being pregnant with twins or more

A lot of women ask whether certain working conditions can increase the risks of preterm birth. There does seem to be some association between premature birth and physically demanding work, prolonged standing, shift or night work, and significant fatigue. However, having a demanding job doesn't make preterm labor a certainty by any means.

The following suggestions can decrease your chances of preterm labor:

✔ **Stop (or decrease) smoking.** See Chapter 3 for more on how smoking affects your baby.

✔ **Avoid illicit drugs and alcohol.** To find out more about the risks posed by the use of these substances, turn to Chapter 3.

✔ **Reduce occupational fatigue.** Limit work to less than 42 hours per week, and minimize standing to less than 6 hours per day.

✔ **Make sure you are getting adequate nutrition and hydration.** Check out Chapter 4 for the details of a healthy diet.

✔ **Try 17-hydroxyprogesterone caproate.** If you have a history of spontaneous preterm delivery in a prior pregnancy, talk to your doctor about starting a medication called 17 hydroxyprogesterone caproate. See the "Preventing preterm labor" section later in this chapter for more information on this medication.

Some interventions that haven't been shown to be helpful in lowering your chances of preterm labor are

✔ Bed rest and hospitalization

✔ Avoiding intercourse

✔ Taking medications that are typically used to stop premature labor once it has set in (called tocolytics as a group — see "Stopping preterm labor" later in this chapter) as a preventive step to keep it from starting

✔ Taking antibiotics unnecessarily

While studies show these things have not been shown to be beneficial, they are still sometimes prescribed in individual situations in the hope that they may help.

Checking for signs of preterm labor

Practitioners have various ways of detecting preterm labor, although the techniques aren't always effective. The most common methods are for your practitioner to check your cervix by performing an internal exam and to monitor you for contractions.

Some practitioners look for symptoms of preterm labor using transvaginal ultrasound. A small ultrasound probe is placed into the vagina next to the cervix in order to measure the length of the cervix. Measuring cervical length can help predict whether you are at an increased risk of delivering prematurely. If you are found to have a shortened cervix and are considered high risk for preterm birth, vaginal progesterone may be helpful in decreasing the chance of delivering prematurely. The routine use of cervical ultrasound for the prediction of preterm birth in women without any symptoms or risk factors is controversial. More studies are needed to show doctors how best to use transvaginal ultrasound.

Expectant mothers ask . . .

Q: "Is monitoring contractions from home an effective way to detect preterm labor?"

A: Home-contraction monitoring is a technology rarely used anymore because studies haven't proven that it's beneficial. Your practitioner gives you a device that you strap to your abdomen for a period of a half-hour to an hour each day (or sometimes twice a day). This device can sense contractions you may not be able to feel. The information that the device receives is then transmitted through a telephone modem to a nursing station. If it appears you're contracting more frequently than you should be, the device alerts your doctor. In this way, you may pick up preterm labor at an early stage. However, recent studies suggest that this kind of monitoring is no more useful than having the patient keep in close contact with nurses or teaching her to be aware of preterm labor's symptoms.

Interestingly, some researchers found that a specific type of pessary, which is a device placed into the vagina and around the cervix, may also help to decrease preterm delivery in singletons.

 A test called *fetal fibronectin* is probably the best available predictor of who is *not* likely to have preterm delivery. The test involves swabbing the back of the vagina with a cotton swab. A negative result on this test is a good indicator that preterm delivery is unlikely within the next few weeks. A positive result, however, does not necessarily mean that you are going to deliver prematurely.

Stopping preterm labor

Depending on how far along you are when you develop preterm labor, your doctor may attempt to stop your contractions (assuming he believes in this practice), and you may be admitted to the hospital. Your doctor may use several medications (called *tocolytics*) to block preterm labor.

 Doctors have never come to widespread agreement that these medications are useful in the long run, although they have been shown to help for a few days to a week. Most tocolytics have side effects on the mother. Terbutaline is a medication that

was commonly used until 2011, when the U.S. Food and Drug Administration (FDA) issued a warning regarding its use to treat preterm labor. The side effects of terbutaline include flushing and a feeling that your heart is racing. It can also make it easier for you to develop a serious condition known as pulmonary edema, where water accumulates in your lungs. The data suggest that the use of terbutaline should be limited to only short-term in-patient use to stop preterm labor. Two other types of medications have side effects as well: Magnesium sulfate may cause nausea, flushing, or drowsiness; and Indomethacin is well-tolerated, but can't be used for too long because of some effects on the fetus with long-term use. Nifedipine has recently become the first line of treatment for many doctors because it appears to have few side effects, and there are no restrictions on the length of use.

If your doctor thinks your preterm labor may lead to premature delivery prior to 34 weeks, he will probably recommend you receive an injection of steroids, which have been shown to decrease the risk of respiratory problems and other complications in the premature newborn. The risks to the mother of taking these drugs are negligible, and large studies have shown that the steroids are beneficial to the baby for about a week. Patients who continue to be at risk for preterm delivery a week after the steroids were first administered may be given a second course of steroids under certain circumstances. In particular, if you are less than 28 weeks and still at risk for preterm birth, a repeat course may be beneficial to the baby. Recent data suggests that using a lower dose of steroids for the second course is still beneficial and may have fewer long-term side effects.

Recently magnesium sulfate has been used, not for its anti-contractive effect, but for its effectiveness to protect the preterm fetal brain. Studies have shown that magnesium sulfate given to mothers shortly before delivering infants prior to 32 weeks reduces the chance of infant death as well as cerebral palsy.

Preventing preterm labor

Several recent studies indicate that women who are at an increased risk for a preterm delivery (see the "Dealing with Preterm Labor" section earlier in this chapter) may have a

reduced chance of delivering preterm if they take a specific type of progesterone during their pregnancies. The studies looked at both progesterone injections and progesterone vaginal suppositories.

The injections involve weekly doses of a medication called 17-hydroxyprogesterone caproate (17-P) starting at 16 to 20 weeks and continuing until about 36 weeks. The suppositories involve placement of a tablet or gel into the vagina nightly starting at 16 to 24 weeks and continuing until 36 weeks.

At this time, progesterone injections seem effective for women with a history of a prior preterm birth, and possibly for women with abnormally shaped uteruses or cervical insufficiency. Recent studies suggest that high-risk women diagnosed with a shortened cervix may also benefit from progesterone therapy. Also in women with singleton gestations but without a history of a prior preterm birth, and a short cervix found on ultrasound prior to 24 weeks, vaginal progesterone, either 90-mg gel or 200-mg suppository, can help reduce preterm birth. There is currently not good enough data to recommend progesterone to women carrying twins or more, and further research is needed.

Delivering the baby early

Sometimes delivering a baby early makes sense. When a woman experiences preterm labor at 35 or 36 weeks, for example, letting her go ahead and deliver is usually wise because the outlook for the baby is so good that there's no reason to subject the mother to the side effects of medications to forestall labor. Regardless of the gestational age, premature delivery may also be the best option in some cases where the baby has a condition that doctors can't treat inside the uterus or when the mother has a condition that is worsening, such as preeclampsia (see the next section), and continuing the pregnancy would be risky.

Handling Preeclampsia

Also known as *toxemia,* or *pregnancy-induced hypertension (PIH), preeclampsia* results when a woman experiences elevated blood pressure along with some other laboratory abnormalities or symptoms after about 20 weeks of gestation.

This condition isn't all that uncommon, occurring in about 7 percent of pregnancies. Women having their first child are especially susceptible. Preeclampsia usually occurs late in pregnancy, but it can develop in the late second or early third trimester. The condition goes away after delivery.

Doctors have different criteria for diagnosing the condition, but, in general, blood pressure that stays above 140/90 is considered elevated if you have no history of blood pressure problems prior to pregnancy.

Recently, the criteria to diagnose preeclampsia has changed. Following is a list of the criteria for the diagnosis of preeclampsia:

- **Recurring high blood pressure.** Systolic blood pressure ≥ 140 mm Hg or diastolic blood pressure ≥ 90 mm Hg on two occasions at least 4 hours apart after 20 weeks in a patient without any history of chronic hypertension

- **Protein in the urine (proteinuria).** Protein in the urine of ≥ 0.3 grams in a 24-hour urine specimen or protein/creatinine ratio of ≥ 0.3 mg/dl or a dipstick urine protein of 1+.

- **Other factors.** In a patient with new onset hypertension without proteinuria, the new onset of any of the following is also diagnostic of preeclampsia:

  - Platelet count < 100,000/microliter

  - Serum creatinine > 1.1 mg/dl or doubling of serum creatinine in the absence of other renal disease

  - Certain liver enzymes at least twice normal

  - Pulmonary edema (fluid in the lungs)

  - Cerebral or visual symptoms

The presence of one or more of the following criteria are features of severe preeclampsia:

- Symptoms of central nervous system dysfunction

- New onset cerebral or visual disturbances, severe headache, or altered mental status

- Liver abnormalities

- Severe persistent pain just under your rib cage on the right or in the middle just under your breast bone (sternum)

Many of these symptoms can occur harmlessly during any pregnancy. Unless they happen in combination with elevated blood pressure or protein spillage in the urine, they're quite normal. If one day you have a headache, or if for a second you see spots, don't jump to the conclusion that you have preeclampsia. If the symptoms persist, though, tell your doctor.

No one knows exactly what causes preeclampsia, but it probably involves a combination of maternal, fetal, and placental factors. We do know that some women are at a higher risk for developing it than others. The following are risk factors for preeclampsia:

- ✔ Existing chronic hypertension

- ✔ First pregnancy

- ✔ History of preeclampsia in a prior pregnancy

- ✔ Long-standing diabetes

- ✔ Mother older than 40

- ✔ Significant obesity

- ✔ Some medical problems, such as serious kidney or liver disease, lupus, or other vascular diseases

- ✔ Triplets or more (twins, also, but to a much lesser extent)

Despite extensive ongoing medical research on preeclampsia, no one knows exactly how to prevent it. Some data suggest that taking a low dose of aspirin daily starting at 12 to 14 weeks may help reduce the incidence of preeclampsia or delay its onset for women at moderate to high risk of developing the condition. Other treatments have been tried with varying degrees of success, including

- ✔ **Calcium supplementation and antioxidant therapy:** Like low-dose aspirin, calcium has not been shown to prevent preeclampsia in low-risk women; however, there may be some benefit to women at high risk.

- ✔ **A combination of vitamins C and E:** Although initial studies suggested a benefit, more recent data show not only no benefit, but a higher risk of certain complications.

- ✔ **Fish oil:** This has been investigated, but it hasn't been shown to be helpful in lowering the incidence of preeclampsia.

Ultimately, the only real treatment for preeclampsia is delivering the baby. When to deliver depends on how severe the condition is and how far along you are in your pregnancy. If you're close to your due date, induced delivery may be the wisest approach. If you're only 28 weeks along, your doctor may try close observation of you and the baby, either at home or in the hospital. Doctors weigh the risks to the mother's health against the risks to the baby of preterm delivery.

Understanding Placental Conditions

Two different problems with the baby's placenta can sometimes occur in the latter part of pregnancy: placenta previa and placental abruption. In this section, we describe both.

Placenta previa

Placenta previa is when the placenta partially or completely covers the cervix, as shown in Figure 14-1. Doctors typically diagnose patients with placenta previa during a routine ultrasound exam, but sometimes women find out about the problem only when they begin bleeding late in the second trimester or early in the third.

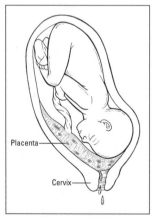

Placenta

Cervix

Kathryn Born, MA

Figure 14-1: Placenta previa.

In early pregnancy, having the placenta positioned near the cervix or even partially covering it is common and usually poses no danger to the mother or the baby. In fact, this condition occurs in as many as one out of five pregnancies. In the vast majority of women (95 percent), the placenta rises as the uterus enlarges with the growing baby, which is why you have no reason to worry about the placenta covering the cervix early in pregnancy.

Even if the situation persists through the late second trimester and into the third, it can be harmless. Many women who have placenta previa never bleed at all. However, the possibility of heavy bleeding is the main concern with placenta previa. Sometimes bleeding leads to preterm labor. In this case, your practitioner attempts to stop the contractions, which often stops the bleeding. If bleeding is severe and can't be stopped, the baby may have to be delivered.

If you're in your third trimester and you have placenta previa, your practitioner may want you to have regular ultrasound examinations to see whether the placenta will eventually move out of the way. These are usually transvaginal ultrasounds and are safe to use with a placenta previa in experienced hands. He may tell you to avoid intercourse and not undergo internal (digital) examinations in order to lower the risk of any bleeding. If the condition persists until 36 weeks, your doctor most likely will recommend a cesarean delivery because the baby can't come through the birth canal without disrupting the placenta, and this can lead to heavy bleeding.

Placental abruption

In some women, the placenta separates from the uterine wall before pregnancy is over. This condition is called *placental abruption* (it's sometimes also called *abruptio placentae* or *placental separation*). Figure 14-2 shows you what it looks like.

Placental abruption is a common cause of third-trimester bleeding. Because blood is an irritant to the uterine muscle, it can also cause premature labor and abdominal pain. An abruption is difficult to see on an ultrasound exam unless it is quite large. So in many cases, doctors can make the diagnosis only after they rule out every other possible cause of bleeding. Rarely, a placental abruption occurs suddenly, and if the separation is large enough, it may necessitate rapid delivery. See Chapter 7 for other causes of third-trimester bleeding.

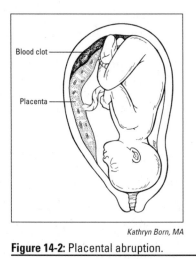

Kathryn Born, MA

Figure 14-2: Placental abruption.

If you experience a small placental abruption, your practitioner may recommend you try bed rest. He will also start to observe your pregnancy more closely to make sure the problem has no harmful side effects on the fetus.

Recognizing Problems with the Amniotic Fluid and Sac

As you know, the fetus grows within a "bag of water" known as the *amniotic sac,* which contains the amniotic fluid. This fluid increases in volume throughout the first part of pregnancy and reaches its maximum level at 34 weeks. After that, the volume gradually declines. Medical science hasn't yet discovered exactly what mechanism regulates the amniotic fluid volume, although we do know that the fetus plays some role in how much fluid the sac contains. During the second half of pregnancy, the amniotic fluid comprises mainly fetal urine. The fetus urinates into the sac and then swallows the fluid. The fluid circulating around the fetal lungs aids in lung development.

Sometimes, a practitioner may suspect that the amount of amniotic fluid is above or below average, and he may do an ultrasound examination to see what's happening. Minor increases or decreases in the amount of amniotic fluid usually

aren't a problem. But large variations in amniotic fluid volume may be a symptom of some other problem. This section describes what happens when problems with the amniotic fluid or sac occur.

Too much amniotic fluid

The medical term for too much fluid is *polyhydramnios* or *hydramnios*. This situation occurs quite frequently, in about 1 to 10 percent of pregnancies. Often the increase in volume is small. Doctors don't always know what causes it, but they do know that a small increase usually isn't a problem. Larger increases may be associated with a medical condition in the mother — diabetes or certain viral illnesses, for example. In some rare cases, the excess fluid may be due to certain fetal problems. The fetus may be having difficulty swallowing the fluid, for example, so more of it accumulates inside the sac.

Usually the fluid isn't increased to the point where it causes significant problems, but on rare occasions there can be massive accumulations of fluid to the point that it becomes difficult for the mom to breathe and causes the uterus to contract prematurely (premature labor). If this happens and mom is near her due date, then her doctor will most likely recommend delivery to relieve the discomfort. If, however, she is remote from her due date, then doctors can remove some of the fluid during an amniocentesis to make mom more comfortable. Also, indomethacin has occasionally been used in this setting because one of the side effects of indomethacin is that it causes amniotic fluid volume to decrease.

Expectant mothers ask . . .

Q: "Is the amount of amniotic fluid determined to any extent by the amount of water I drink?"

A: No. The mother's fluid intake has little to do with it. Some recent studies suggest a mother can cause small increases in the amount of amniotic fluid by drinking plenty of liquids, but the effect isn't that great. Nevertheless, stay well hydrated.

Too little amniotic fluid

A woman who has too little amniotic fluid has *oligohydramnios*. As we mention earlier, amniotic fluid volume normally decreases after 34 to 36 weeks. If yours starts to fall below a specific range, however, your practitioner may want to observe the fetus more closely by performing certain tests. One common cause of low amniotic fluid is a rupture of the membranes, which allows fluid to leak out.

A fluid level that drops significantly prior to 34 weeks may indicate a problem with the mother or the baby. For example, some women with hypertension or lupus may have less blood flow to the uterus and, consequently, less blood flow to the placenta and the baby. When the baby receives less blood, the baby's kidneys make less urine, and that results in lower levels of amniotic fluid.

If the reduction in fluid is mild or moderate, the baby is watched carefully and undergoes tests of fetal well-being. Sometimes, oligohydramnios is a sign the baby's growth is restricted (see the "Describing Problems with Fetal Growth" section later in this chapter) or, rarely, that there are abnormalities in the baby's urinary tract. Sometimes it's a sign the placenta isn't functioning optimally.

If you have decreased amniotic fluid, your doctor may suggest you get more rest and try to stay off your feet. By doing so, you may promote more blood flow to the uterus and placenta and thus increase the baby's urine output. (Just be glad you don't have to change all the diapers yet!)

Rupture of the amniotic sac

Premature rupture of the membranes or amniotic sac, sometimes called PROM (don't worry, no bad tuxedos, gaudy dresses, or ugly corsages involved here), is when a woman's water breaks sometime before labor starts. When it happens close to your due date, it's referred to as *term PROM*. If you're less than 37 weeks at the time, it's called *preterm PROM*.

✔ If you experience term PROM, your practitioner may simply wait until you go into labor on your own. Or, he may induce labor in order to avoid the risk of an infection developing inside the uterus.

✔ If you experience preterm PROM, you may or may not go into labor, depending on how far along you are. If you're very far from your due date and don't appear to have an infection in your uterus, your doctor may use some medications (antibiotics, tocolytics, and steroids) to prolong the pregnancy as long as possible and to help your baby's chance of lung development. Your doctor will probably perform frequent ultrasound exams and monitor the fetal heart rate to ensure the baby is managing okay.

If you think your membranes may have ruptured and you're preterm, let your practitioner know immediately or go to the hospital. He can perform tests to definitively let you know whether the membranes have actually ruptured.

Describing Problems with Fetal Growth

One of the main reasons to get prenatal care is to ensure that your baby is growing well. A practitioner typically gauges growth by measuring the fundal height (see Chapter 3). As a general rule (in a singleton pregnancy), the measurement in centimeters from the top of the pubic bone to the top of the uterus roughly equals the number of weeks gestation. If your practitioner finds this measurement is greater or less than expected, he may recommend you have an ultrasound exam to more precisely assess the baby's growth. During the exam, the technician measures various fetal body parts to come up with an approximate fetal weight. That estimate is then compared with the average weight for fetuses at the same gestational age and assigned to a certain percentile. The 50th percentile is average. But because fetuses (like babies, toddlers, children, teenagers, and grown-ups) come in different sizes, there is a range of normal weights. Anything between the 10th and the 90th percentiles is considered normal (see Chapter 7 for more information about fetal weight).

These upper and lower limits are somewhat arbitrary. They do imply that 10 percent of the population is larger than normal and that 10 percent is smaller, but this statement isn't exactly true. Most fetuses below the 10th percentile or above the 90th percentile are completely normal. On the other hand, some of them may not be growing normally and may need extra surveillance.

Smaller-than-average babies

A fetus whose estimated weight falls below the 10th percentile may have *intrauterine growth restriction (IUGR)*. IUGR can lead to the birth of a baby who is small for gestational age (SGA). IUGR has many possible causes, including the following:

- ✔ **The baby is measuring small, but is otherwise normal.** Just as healthy adults come in all sizes, so do fetuses.

- ✔ **Chromosomal abnormalities.** This cause is most common with early-onset IUGR, which occurs in the second trimester.

- ✔ **Environmental toxins.** Cigarette smoking causes a decrease in birth weight between one-fourth and one-half of a pound, on average. Chronic alcohol consumption (at least one to two drinks a day) and cocaine use also can cause low birth weight.

- ✔ **Genetic factors.** Some genetic factors cause the fetus to grow less than average.

- ✔ **Heart and circulatory abnormalities in the fetus.** Examples include a congenital heart defect or umbilical cord abnormalities.

- ✔ **Inadequate nutrition for the mother.** Proper nutrition is especially important in the third trimester.

- ✔ **Infection such as cytomegalovirus (CMV), rubella, or toxoplasmosis.** Chapter 15 provides more information.

- ✔ **Multiple gestation.** Fifteen to 25 percent of twins, and an even higher percentage of triplets, have IUGR. Twins grow at the same rate as singletons until 28 to 32 weeks, when the twin growth curve drops off.

- ✔ **Placental factors and uterine-placental problems.** Because the placenta provides nutrition and oxygen to the fetus, if it's functioning poorly or if the blood isn't flowing smoothly from the uterus to the placenta, the fetus may not grow properly. Women with antiphospholipid antibody syndrome (a blood-clotting problem), recurrent bleeding, vascular diseases, or chronic hypertension are at risk for IUGR because those conditions cause poor placental function. Preeclampsia may also impair placental function and lead to IUGR.

Expectant mothers ask . . .

Q: "If I eat more, will my baby grow into the normal range?"

A: Unfortunately, the answer is no. Eating more doesn't correct the problem unless you're significantly malnourished.

The way your practitioner responds to IUGR depends on your individual situation. Fetuses with mild IUGR, normal chromosomes, and no evidence of infection are likely to be fine. Sometimes early delivery is warranted, however, because the fetus may grow better in the nursery than inside the uterus. The way your practitioner responds to signs of IUGR depends on both the cause of the problem and the gestational age at which it is diagnosed. He may recommend more frequent office visits, periodic ultrasound examinations, fetal heart rate exams (known as NSTs — see Chapter 7), or other tests such as a biophysical profile (an ultrasound assessment of fetal well-being) and measurement of blood flow through the umbilical cord called Dopplers. If the problem is severe but the pregnancy is far enough along, your doctor may recommend delivery.

In many cases, SGA babies turn out to be perfectly normal. Unfortunately, though, severe cases have been associated with learning difficulties later in life and even fetal death, which is why having your practitioner conduct some form of fetal surveillance is important.

Larger-than-average babies

A baby whose estimated weight is above the 90th percentile may have *macrosomia* ("big body") and end up being large for gestational age, or LGA. Many different reasons can explain why a woman may have an exceptionally large baby, including the following:

✓ The mother has previously delivered a large baby.

✓ The mother has gained an excessive amount of weight during the pregnancy.

✓ The mother is obese.

✔ One (or both) of the parents was born very large.

✔ The pregnancy lasts longer than 40 weeks.

✔ The mother has poorly controlled diabetes.

The mother's main risk, naturally, is that the delivery is more difficult. If she delivers vaginally, she may suffer increased trauma to the birth canal, and she has an increased chance of needing a cesarean delivery. The main risk to the baby, likewise, is injury during delivery. Birth injury is more likely when a large baby is delivered vaginally, but it can also occur during a cesarean delivery. Most commonly, birth injury involves excessive stretching of the nerves in the baby's upper arm and neck resulting from a shoulder dystocia (see Chapter 9) during delivery.

If your practitioner thinks your baby may be exceptionally large, based on either an ultrasound estimate of fetal weight or an abdominal exam, and it appears your pelvic bones may make for a tight fit, he will discuss your delivery options with you.

Looking at Blood Incompatibilities

If a baby's parents have two different blood types, the baby's blood type can be different from the mother's. Usually this situation creates absolutely no problem for the mother or the baby. In some rare cases, these blood-type mismatches warrant special consideration. Even then, however, there is hardly ever a significant problem.

The Rh factor

Most people are Rh-positive, which means they carry the Rh factor on their red blood cells. Those who don't carry the Rh factor are considered Rh-negative. If an Rh-positive man and an Rh-negative woman conceive, the fetus may be Rh-positive, thereby creating a mismatch between baby and mother.

This kind of mismatch usually isn't a problem and is almost never a problem in a first pregnancy. If, however, any of the baby's blood leaks into the mother's circulation, her immune

system may form antibodies to the Rh factor. And if any such antibodies reach a significant level in a future pregnancy, they can cross through the placenta into the baby's circulation and begin to destroy the baby's red blood cells. It sounds scary, we know. But the problem isn't insurmountable. In order to prevent it, the doctor usually gives the mother an injection of anti-D immune globulin at certain times to prevent the formation of antibodies. Rhogam and Rhophylac are two common preparations of anti-D globulin. If your baby's father is Rh-positive and you're Rh-negative, your doctor may recommend that you receive anti-D immune globulin at the following times:

✔ Within 72 hours of delivery (either vaginal or cesarean). A nurse gives the injection after delivery in order to prevent problems in future pregnancies.

✔ Routinely at about 28 weeks gestation (as a precaution, just in case any passage of blood across the placenta has already occurred) and again 12 to 13 weeks later, if you haven't already delivered.

✔ After amniocentesis, CVS (chorionic villus sampling), or any invasive procedure (see Chapters 6 and 7).

✔ After a miscarriage, abortion, or ectopic pregnancy (see Chapter 5 for more on ectopic pregnancy).

✔ After significant trauma to your abdomen during pregnancy, if your doctor thinks that some of the baby's blood may have leaked into your circulation.

✔ After significant bleeding during pregnancy.

In unusual circumstances — either when the anti-D immune globulin wasn't given but should have been (very rare) or when it didn't work effectively (exceedingly rare) — a mother produces antibodies to the Rh factor. Then, if she ever becomes pregnant again, an Rh-positive fetus may be at risk of developing anemia (not enough red blood cells), depending on the levels of antibodies in the mother's blood and how they interact with the baby's blood. The anemia may be mild, requiring only that the baby be placed under special lights in the nursery to clear any extra *bilirubin* (a pigment that is released from red blood cells that are destroyed). If you have been sensitized and have developed these antibodies, your doctor can perform tests on amniotic fluid to check the baby's Rh status. If the fetus is Rh(D)-negative, he is not at risk of anemia, even though the mother has the antibodies.

In moderate cases, frequent ultrasound exams may be necessary to assess the situation's severity. Recently, a new technique using ultrasound to measure the blood flow through one of the blood vessels in the fetus's brain (the middle cerebral artery, or MCA) has emerged as the best method for predicting fetal anemia in at-risk pregnancies. If the mother is close to her due date, her practitioner may recommend an early delivery. In the most severe cases, the baby may need to have a blood transfusion while he is still inside the uterus. The procedure is called a fetal blood transfusion (see Chapter 6), and a maternal-fetal medicine specialist performs it. A transfusion is the worst-case scenario, but even if things become this severe, a baby who has transfusions in a timely fashion can be born healthy. However, this procedure is associated with some risks.

 Determining the baby's Rh(D) status by detecting fetal DNA in the mother's blood is now possible. Practitioners in Europe routinely use this method, and it will probably become part of the routine prenatal care of Rh(D)-negative women in the future in the United States. This test allows sensitized women to avoid invasive procedures for determining the fetal blood type, and it allows some women who aren't sensitized to avoid the anti-D immune globulin injection.

Other blood mismatches

Other kinds of blood mismatches are possible. Kell, Duffy, and Kidd are a few examples of blood factors that can differ between mother and baby. Fortunately, all these factors are very rare. No Rhogam-like medications are available to treat these mismatches. But in the very few cases where a problem does occur, your practitioner can provide care for the babies in the other ways we describe previously for Rh incompatibility (special lights, early delivery, or blood transfusion). And these babies, too, are usually born healthy.

Finally, some blood group antibodies — Le, Lu, and P, for example — can be mismatched but have no harmful effects on the fetus. Usually, no special action is needed.

Dealing with Breech Presentation

A baby is in a so-called *breech* position when its buttocks or legs are down, closest to the cervix. Breech presentation happens in 3 to 4 percent of all singleton deliveries. A woman's risk of having a breech baby decreases the further along she goes in her pregnancy. The fetus is more likely to assume a breech position for one of the following reasons:

- ✔ The fetus is preterm or especially small.

- ✔ An increased amount of amniotic fluid exists (all the more room to turn around in).

- ✔ A congenital malformation of the uterus is present (for example, a bicornuate, or T-shaped, uterus).

- ✔ Fibroids that impinge on the uterine cavity are present.

- ✔ You have placenta previa (see the "Placenta previa" section earlier in this chapter).

- ✔ You're having twins or more.

- ✔ Your uterus is relaxed from having had several babies already.

If your baby is in a breech position, your will doctor talk with you about the potential risks and benefits of a vaginal breech delivery versus version (turning the baby) or cesarean section. Special concerns about a breech delivery include the following:

- ✔ Trapping the baby's head (which comes out last in a breech delivery) in a cervix that has been incompletely dilated by the passage of the baby's body, which is smaller than the head. (This situation is especially troublesome if the baby is very small or premature.)

- ✔ Trauma resulting from an *extended fetal head* (meaning the head is tilted back).

- ✔ Difficulty delivering the arms, which can lead to potential arm injuries.

Because of these potential problems, many practitioners recommend that all breech babies be delivered by cesarean section. However, some fetuses in breech position are actually good candidates for vaginal delivery. Conditions that should be present for you and your doctor to consider a vaginal breech delivery include the following:

- ✔ Estimated fetal weight is between 4 and 8 pounds.

- ✔ The baby is in a *frank* breech position, which means the buttocks, not the feet, are positioned to come out first.

- ✔ The buttocks are engaged in the pelvis.

- ✔ Your doctor doesn't detect (by physical exam or by X-ray) any problem with the baby's head fitting through the birth canal.

- ✔ Ultrasound shows the fetal head is either flexed (chin to chest) or in the *military* position (looking straight ahead, not tilted back).

- ✔ Immediate anesthesia is available so that cesarean delivery can be done in an emergency.

- ✔ The doctor is experienced in vaginal breech deliveries.

A few recent large studies have shown that breech babies delivered vaginally are at a higher risk for certain complications. In fact, the information is so compelling that most obstetricians have stopped performing vaginal breech deliveries. However, studies show that while the short-term complications were higher in the babies born vaginally, there was no difference in long-term problems (combined death and neurodevelopmental delays) at 2 years of age.

If you and your practitioner decide that a vaginal breech delivery isn't right for you, another option is *external cephalic version,* a procedure in which the doctor tries to turn the baby into normal delivery position by externally manipulating the mother's abdomen, which is a common and usually safe procedure. Sometimes it's fairly uncomfortable, but it works in about 50 to 70 percent of cases. The use of spinal or epidural anesthesia for the version may decrease the discomfort for the mother and improve the chances of successfully turning the baby.

There are certain conditions in which external cephalic version isn't advisable, such as bleeding, low amniotic fluid level, or in multiple gestations.

Pondering Post-Term Pregnancy

The average pregnancy lasts about 40 weeks (or 280 days) after the last menstrual period, but only about 5 percent of women deliver on their due date. Some deliver a couple of weeks earlier and some a couple of weeks later, and all are considered to be "at term." Recently, there are new definitions of term pregnancy:

- **Early term:** 37 0/7 weeks through 38 6/7 weeks
- **Full-term:** 39 0/7 weeks through 40 6/7 weeks
- **Late term:** 41 0/7 weeks through 41 6/7 weeks
- **Post-term:** 42 0/7 weeks and beyond

Why should you or your practitioner care whether you go past your due date? We care because the chance of certain complications rises as time goes on. From 40 to 42 weeks, the increased risks are small, but after 42 weeks, they climb into a range that is more worrisome. The worst complication is perinatal death (also called perinatal mortality). The chances of perinatal death start to increase after 41 to 42 weeks and double by 43 weeks.

This situation isn't as scary as it may sound, though, because the actual number of deaths is so low. The vast majority of late babies are born healthy. Even at 44 weeks, the point at which perinatal mortality rates quadruple, 95 percent of babies are fine if appropriate testing is done. Your doctor can help you make the best decision for you as to the safe timing of delivery.

The increase in mortality rates in post-date pregnancies involves several factors, including

- **The placenta can function efficiently for only a finite length of time — about 40 weeks.** Fortunately, most placentas have some amount of "reserve," and they still work well beyond 40 weeks. But in a few rare cases, they don't last as well. If a placenta can't get enough nutrients to the baby, the baby may actually lose some weight by remaining inside the uterus.

- **In a post-term pregnancy, the volume of amniotic fluid may decrease.** As we mention earlier in this chapter, amniotic fluid volume peaks at about 34 to 36 weeks gestation and starts to slowly drop after that. Most of the

time, adequate fluid is left after 40 weeks. Sometimes, however, the fluid level drops into a range doctors consider too low. In this situation, the umbilical cord has a chance of becoming compressed, and doctors may recommend that labor be induced.

✔ **Babies can sometimes pass their first bowel movement while they're still inside the uterus.** The longer a pregnancy lasts, the more likely this is to happen. In rare instances, the baby may breathe in this thick *meconium,* either before or during birth, which can cause problems with breathing in the first few days or weeks after birth (for more information, see Chapter 10).

✔ **In a post-term pregnancy in which the placenta continues to function normally, the baby keeps growing.** These late babies are more likely to be very large (macrosomic; see the "Describing Problems with Fetal Growth" section earlier in this chapter), or large for gestational age. So they may be at risk for all the problems that come with being extra-large.

Practitioners use various strategies to manage post-date pregnancies, none of which is inherently better than another. Some want to be sure all babies are delivered as soon after 40 weeks as feasible and induce labor to ensure that they are. (See Chapter 8 for more information on labor induction.) Others are willing to wait longer for spontaneous labor. The argument for the first approach is that you don't have to worry about any of the aforementioned complications. With the second approach, on the other hand, you may have less chance of needing a cesarean delivery.

Chapter 15

Pregnancy in Sickness and in Health

. . . .

In This Chapter

▶ Treating infections from the common cold to bladder infections

▶ Handling asthma, diabetes, and other preexisting health problems

. . . .

*P*regnancy may give you a "maternal glow" and make you feel as if something magical is happening to your body. But face it: Pregnancy doesn't make you superhuman. You're still susceptible to all the illnesses and other health problems that can affect anyone who's not expecting a baby. When illnesses arise during pregnancy, they can have special consequences. In this chapter, we talk about how a variety of medical conditions affect pregnant women.

Getting an Infection While Pregnant

Try as you may, avoiding every person who's carrying an infection during your pregnancy may be impossible. Keep in mind that most infections don't hurt the baby at all; they just make life more uncomfortable for you for a while. In this section, we cover the most common infections as well as some of the more unusual ones.

Bladder and kidney infections

Bladder infections come in two basic types: with and without symptoms. *Silent* (symptom-free) bladder infections are

common, occurring in about 6 percent of pregnant women. The other kind, called *cystitis,* comes with symptoms that include

- ✔ Constantly feeling that you need to urinate
- ✔ Discomfort above your pubic bone (where the bladder is)
- ✔ More frequent urination
- ✔ Pain with urination

If you develop either type of bladder infection, your doctor treats it with antibiotics.

If left untreated, a bladder infection can progress into a kidney infection, also known as *pyelonephritis.* A kidney infection produces the same symptoms as cystitis, plus a high fever and *flank pain* — pain over one or both kidneys (see Figure 15-1). Flank pain also can occur in someone who has kidney stones. The difference: A kidney infection causes a constant pain, whereas kidney stones produce more severe, but intermittent, pain. Also, kidney stones are more often accompanied by small quantities of blood in the urine.

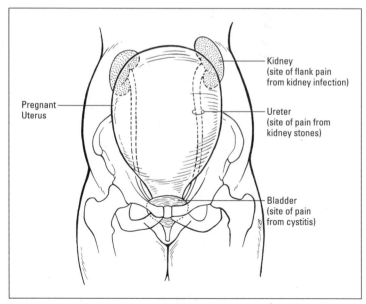

Kidney
(site of flank pain
from kidney infection)

Pregnant
Uterus

Ureter
(site of pain from
kidney stones)

Bladder
(site of pain
from cystitis)

Kathryn Born, MA

Figure 15-1: Bladder infections, kidney infections, and kidney stones have their own unique symptoms.

If your practitioner diagnoses you with pyelonephritis, she may want to admit you to the hospital for a few days so that you can get intravenous antibiotics. Because kidney infections tend to recur during pregnancy, your practitioner may also want to keep you on a daily antibiotic for the remainder of your pregnancy.

Chickenpox

The varicella zoster virus causes chickenpox. The first time someone comes down with an infection caused by this virus, usually in childhood, she gets chickenpox. Chickenpox is pretty rare in adults, and pregnant women stand no greater risk of contracting this virus than women who are not pregnant.

If you have already had chickenpox, you aren't likely to get it again because your body has produced antibodies that make you immune. Even if you've never had chickenpox, you have a good chance of having these protective antibodies in your blood because you've probably had some exposure to the virus in the past, even though it didn't produce any illness. However, if you know that you've never been exposed to chickenpox and you haven't recently been vaccinated (a vaccine against this virus now exists), or if you're unsure about your prior exposure, have your blood checked to see whether you're immune. Most of the time antibodies to the varicella virus are checked at the first prenatal visit with all of the rest of the routine prenatal labs.

Because the chickenpox vaccine is relatively new, we have very little information about how safe it is for pregnant women, which is why the vaccine's manufacturer recommends that pregnant women be given it after delivery. The recommendation is that women wait three months after receiving the vaccine before they get pregnant. If you get the vaccine and then suddenly find out you were pregnant at the time, let your doctor know. The little experience that pregnant women have had with the vaccine suggests that it probably doesn't increase the chances of birth defects, nor has it led to any cases of congenital varicella syndrome (see the bulleted list that follows) in the baby.

If you aren't immune to chickenpox and you're exposed to someone with the infection while you're pregnant, let your practitioner know immediately so that you can receive an injection known as VZIG *(varicella zoster immune globulin)*,

which may reduce the risk of infection to you and the baby. Get this injection within three days of exposure, if possible. If you contract chickenpox within several days of giving birth (before or after), your baby should receive VZIG.

Chickenpox can cause three potential problems during pregnancy:

✔ It can make the mother ill with flu-like symptoms, plus produce the infamous skin rash (lots of little red blemishes). In rare circumstances, pneumonia develops two to six days after the rash appears. If you have chickenpox and you develop symptoms like shortness of breath or a dry cough, let your doctor know right away.

✔ If you contract chickenpox during the first four months of pregnancy, the fetus has a small chance of developing the infection, too, leading to congenital varicella syndrome. With this syndrome, the fetus can have scarring (the same kinds of scars that little kids get on their bodies from chickenpox), some abnormal development of the limbs, problems with growth, and developmental delays.

Fortunately, congenital varicella syndrome is very rare. (It happens in less than 1 percent of cases in which the infection occurs in the first trimester, 2 percent if in the early second trimester.)

✔ If you contract chickenpox within the interval from five days before to five days after giving birth, the baby is at risk for developing a serious varicella infection in the newborn period. You can greatly reduce this chance by giving the baby VZIG.

The same varicella zoster virus that causes chickenpox can also produce a recurrent form of the infection called shingles or herpes zoster. Most babies born to pregnant women who develop shingles are completely normal. Because shingles is much less common than chickenpox in pregnancy, doctors don't really know how common birth defects are after a pregnant woman develops this condition, although the incidence is thought to be less than the 1 to 2 percent seen with chickenpox.

If you know that you're susceptible to chickenpox, avoid direct contact with anyone who has shingles or herpes zoster because the lesions contain the varicella zoster virus and can cause a chickenpox infection in susceptible women.

Expectant mothers ask . . .

Q: "Is getting the flu vaccine safe while I'm pregnant?"

A: Yes: The vaccine is completely safe. In fact, not only is it safe, but it is recommended that pregnant women get vaccinated during pregnancy when it is flu season. This is because pregnant women who get the flu can become much sicker than nonpregnant women. There is no evidence that additives in the vaccine cause any problems for the baby (like birth defects or autism). Remember, the vaccine doesn't protect against all flu viruses, only the ones that researchers believe will be common in your area.

Colds and flu

Most people get a cold about once a year, so the fact that most women get one during pregnancy isn't surprising. Nothing about pregnancy makes you more vulnerable to a cold virus, but the fatigue and congestion that go along with pregnancy can make a cold seem worse. In any case, the common cold is perfectly harmless to the developing fetus. As we all know, there is no cure for a cold, so the only option is to treat the symptoms. Contrary to popular belief, most cold medications — antihistamines, cough suppressants, and the like — are safe for pregnant women when taken in the recommended doses.

Following are a few suggestions for dealing with cold and flu symptoms:

> ✔ **Drink fluids, fluids, and more fluids.** All viral illnesses promote dehydration, and being pregnant only makes the problem more extreme. If you are normally hydrated, your urine will be a pale yellow color or colorless and you will typically urinate every 4 to 6 hours. If you go for hours without urinating or notice dark yellow or orange urine, then you are probably dehydrated. To keep from getting dehydrated when you have a cold or the flu, drink plenty of water, juice, or soda. We recommend staying away from milk because many pregnant women complain that it makes the nausea often associated with the flu feel worse. If you think you may be dehydrated, you can try some of the over-the-counter oral rehydrating electrolyte solutions sold at your drugstore (like Rehydralyte or CeraLyte) but

if you don't notice your urine turning lighter quickly or that you're going to the toilet at more typical intervals, then you should contact your provider for advice.

✔ **Take a fever reducer.** Taking acetaminophen (Tylenol) in the recommended doses is okay to help bring a fever down. This action alone helps some people feel better. If your fever persists for more than a few days, however, call your doctor.

✔ **Take a decongestant.** Pseudoephedrine (Sudafed) is the decongestant of choice during pregnancy. No evidence suggests that Sudafed taken in normal doses after the first trimester has any harmful effects.

✔ **Try nasal spray, but not for long.** Nasal spray decongestants are okay if you use them only short-term (the same is true for people who aren't pregnant). Used intermittently, decongestant sprays may allow you to breathe more comfortably. Used day after day, they may only make the problem last longer. Saline nasal sprays are fine long-term, but they often aren't as effective in reducing congestion.

✔ **Eat some comfort food.** Last, but certainly not least, eat some chicken soup. Scientific studies have shown that chicken soup has properties that help cold sufferers feel better, even though no one knows exactly what those properties are. (See Joanne's mother's recipe in the nearby sidebar.)

You can use the same treatments for the common cold and for influenza infections. If you get the flu while you're pregnant, you're likely to have the same experience as when you're not pregnant.

Many of our patients ask about the use of echinacea during pregnancy. People in Asia have used this herb for centuries to fight inflammation and the common cold. Typically, people use a preparation or supplement containing echinacea when they feel the first signs of a cold coming on. No evidence suggests that echinacea causes a problem during pregnancy. The only study we found was one that included only a small number of patients. Although no adverse effects were found, drawing any conclusions from such a limited study is difficult.

If your fever persists for more than a few days, or if you develop a cough with greenish or yellow phlegm or have difficulty breathing, call your doctor to make sure that you're not developing pneumonia.

Mother Regina's chicken soup recipe

Rely on this classic pick-me-up to help you through a cold or the flu.

4 quarts water

1 chicken, cut in large pieces

3 onions, peeled and quartered

4 parsnips, peeled and halved

6 celery stalks, halved

6 carrots, peeled and halved

Salt and pepper to taste

2 to 4 chicken bouillon cubes to taste

4 tablespoons fresh parsley

4 tablespoons fresh dill

1. Put water and chicken in a large stockpot and bring to a boil. Skim off froth.

2. Add onions, parsnips, celery, carrots, and salt and pepper.

3. Cover and simmer for 2 hours.

4. Add bouillon cubes.

5. Add parsley and dill.

6. Simmer for another hour.

7. Strain broth into another container, reserving the chicken and discarding the vegetables.

8. When cool enough to handle, cut up the chicken meat and use for chicken salad or whatever you want.

9. Eat right away or, if possible, refrigerate overnight and then strain off the solidified fat that accumulates on top of the broth.

Tip: Add cooked noodles to make chicken noodle soup.

Seasonal allergies and hay fever

People commonly take antihistamines to treat seasonal allergies. The older, first-generation medications, such as chlorpheniramine (Chlor-Trimeton or Sinutab), have been around for a long time, and most obstetricians are comfortable with their use in pregnancy. The newer antihistamines, such as Claritin or Zyrtec, have an additional benefit of not causing as much drowsiness. Although researchers haven't studied these newer medications as much in pregnancy, we know of no reports of an increased risk for fetal malformations or adverse effects. A third, very effective option is a nasal spray containing cromolyn or low-dose steroids.

Cytomegalovirus (CMV) infections

Cytomegalovirus (CMV) is a viral illness that's common among preschool-age children. The symptoms are very similar to the ones you get with the flu — fatigue, malaise, and aches. In most cases, though, an infection produces no symptoms at all. By the time they're old enough to have children, more than half of women have already had a CMV infection at some time in their lives, as evidenced by antibodies present in their blood.

Most practitioners don't routinely test for antibodies because of the very small chance that a woman would acquire the infection during pregnancy. Also, the infection doesn't usually cause any symptoms, so a woman would have to be repeatedly tested to see whether she develops the infection during her pregnancy. However, checking for susceptibility to the infection (that is, checking for antibodies) in women who are at higher risk — for example, women in close contact with preschool-age children — may be useful.

The importance of CMV infection during pregnancy is that the virus can pass to the fetus and cause a congenital infection. Actually, congenital CMV is the most common cause of an infection inside the uterus, and it occurs in 0.5 to 2.5 percent of all newborns. However, most of the time, babies born with this infection are healthy at birth.

If you do develop CMV during pregnancy (and only 2 percent of susceptible pregnant women do), only about one-third of the time is the infection transmitted to the fetus. Options for diagnosing the fetal infection include undergoing amniocentesis to check for evidence of infection in the amniotic fluid and having ultrasound exams. Even in those babies who contract CMV, 90 percent have no symptoms of the infection at birth (although a small percentage experience symptoms later in life, such as hearing loss or developmental problems).

If your baby contracts CMV in utero, the chances of the baby having serious problems vary according to the following:

✔ The baby's gestational age when the infection occurs

✔ Whether the mother comes down with CMV for the first time during pregnancy (a primary infection) or whether she ever had it in the past (a recurrent infection)

If the mother comes down with the infection after the second trimester or if it is a recurrent infection, the chance of serious problems in the newborn is much less.

Severe symptomatic congenital CMV is rare and occurs in only about 1 in 10,000 to 20,000 newborns. It can lead to hearing impairment, visual problems, and even some mental deficiencies. Because CMV is a virus, antibiotics don't help.

German measles (rubella)

The rubella virus causes German measles, which are the only kind that have any significant impact on pregnancy. If you contract rubella within the first trimester, the baby has about a 20 percent chance of developing congenital rubella syndrome. The chance of this, however, varies even within the first trimester from the first month to the third month. Fortunately, acute rubella infection during pregnancy is extremely uncommon because most people in the United States are vaccinated at childhood.

Hepatitis

Various types of hepatitis affect the mother and baby in different ways:

- **Hepatitis A** is transmitted by person-to-person contact or by exposure to contaminated food and water. Serious complications from hepatitis A in pregnancy are rare. The virus isn't passed to the developing baby. If you're exposed during pregnancy, take immune globulin within two weeks after exposure. Hepatitis A isn't transmitted in breast milk, so it's okay to breast-feed after you have had hepatitis A.

- **Hepatitis B** virus is transmitted through sexual contact, intravenous drug use, or through a blood transfusion. A small percentage of women with hepatitis B infection have a chronic condition, which can lead to liver damage. The use of antiviral therapy for women with high amounts of virus in their blood, or continued use for those women who became pregnant while on therapy, should be discussed with their doctors. Although not that common, hepatitis B infection can be transmitted to the fetus. If you're positive for hepatitis B infection, inform the baby's pediatrician after delivery, so that the baby can receive the appropriate immunizations and be a candidate for breast-feeding.

✔ **Hepatitis C** is transmitted in the same way as hepatitis B. Less than 5 percent of hepatitis C–positive women transmit the infection to their baby. If you're positive for this virus, you should not breast-feed. The CDC, ACOG, and the American Academy of Pediatrics all support breast-feeding in a mom who hepatitis C. The only time they recommend not breast-feeding is when mom's nipples become sore and cracked to the point that they bleed.

✔ **Hepatitis D, E, and G** are much less common. Ask your practitioner if you want more information.

Herpes infections

Herpes is a common virus that infects the mouth, the throat, the skin, and the genital tract. If you have a history of herpes, rest assured that the infection poses no risk to the developing fetus. The main concern is that you may have an active genital herpes lesion when you go into labor or when your water breaks. If you do, there is a small risk of transmitting the infection to the baby as she passes through the birth canal. If it's your first herpes infection, the chance of the fetus contracting the virus is greater because you have no antibodies to the virus. Studies show that women with a history of recurrent herpes may lower the chance of having an active herpes infection at delivery by taking a medication called *acyclovir* or *valcyclovir* in the last month of pregnancy.

If you have active genital herpes lesions at the time of labor or ruptured membranes, let your practitioner know. She is likely to perform a cesarean delivery to avoid infecting the baby. If you see no lesions, but you feel as if you may be developing them, also tell your doctor. In this case, having a cesarean may also be advisable.

Human immunodeficiency virus (HIV)

Over the past few years, studies have shown that some of the medications used to treat HIV infection can dramatically reduce the chance of the virus being transmitted from a mother to her baby. For this reason, doctors recommend that women undergo HIV testing early in pregnancy, and that if a woman is

HIV-positive, she receives these medications during pregnancy as well as during labor. Some states even require that every pregnant woman be tested, and if the testing hasn't been performed, that her newborn be tested prior to discharge from the hospital. HIV testing is often repeated at about 35 weeks to see if the infection was contracted during the pregnancy, so that treatment during labor can be initiated.

In order to decrease the chance of your baby becoming infected with HIV, avoid any invasive procedures that can cause bleeding, such as amniocentesis or CVS, unless they're absolutely required. If your doctor performs these procedures, most doctors recommend the mother receive IV doses of antiviral medications immediately beforehand to minimize the chance of infecting the fetus.

Depending on your individual situation, most experts recommend that you not breast-feed if you're infected with HIV because you may transmit the virus to your baby. Whatever form of birth control you choose, the additional use of condoms is absolutely necessary.

If you're HIV-positive, maintain close contact with HIV specialists so that you may benefit from the ever-improving treatments.

Listeria

Many women ask us about whether they can eat "soft" cheese. What they're usually concerned about is an infection called listeriosis that is caused by eating food contaminated with the bacterium *Listeria monocytogenes*. Listeria is a cause for concern because it can lead to fetal infection, miscarriage, or preterm birth. When infection occurs during pregnancy, antibiotics given promptly can often prevent infection of the fetus or newborn.

Listeria can be found in a variety of different foods — packaged salads, hot dogs, luncheon meats, cheeses, and raw fruits and vegetables. Cheese is a concern because some outbreaks of listeria have been reported with certain unpasteurized cheeses. In the United States, all cheese that is sold is supposed to be either pasteurized or, if it's raw, aged for 60 days (the aging process prevents the growth of the bacteria). The good news is that it really is quite uncommon. The chance of contracting listeria during pregnancy is about 0.12 percent.

Because of the rarity of infection and the ubiquity of the bacteria — and because you can't avoid eating everything! — we advise patients to limit their exposure to the highest-risk foods only:

- ✔ Don't eat hot dogs from the fridge without heating them completely.

- ✔ Make sure the cheese you eat is either pasteurized or aged.

- ✔ Wash all raw fruits and vegetables well.

Lyme disease

Lyme disease is an infection transmitted through a deer tick bite. Pregnancy doesn't predispose you to getting Lyme disease or make it any worse if you get it. The great news is that no evidence suggests that Lyme disease causes any harm to the fetus. The main problem is that it may make you sick.

If you think a deer tick has bitten you, let your practitioner know. She may want to draw blood to see whether you have contracted Lyme disease and possibly start you on antibiotics to prevent long-term effects.

Parvovirus infection (fifth disease)

Parvovirus is a common childhood infection that comes with a fever and a characteristic "slapped cheek" rash. In adults, the infection can bring on flu-like symptoms — fever, aches, sore throat, runny nose, and joint pain, but may not cause a rash at all. Or it may come without any symptoms whatsoever. Three-fourths of all pregnant women are immune to parvovirus, so even if they're exposed to someone who has it, no problems come of it.

If you aren't immune to parvovirus or don't know whether you are and you come in contact with an infected person, let your practitioner know so that you can be tested. Pregnant women who spend a great deal of time around school-age children (teachers or daycare workers, for example) may undergo routine testing before pregnancy or in the early first trimester.

Even if you contract this illness, chances are very good that your baby will be born healthy. No evidence indicates that parvovirus causes any birth defects. However, in rare cases, it can increase the risk of early miscarriage or the development of anemia in the fetus. For this reason, your practitioner may recommend that you have periodic ultrasound exams to look for signs of fetal anemia and to measure blood flow in a particular blood vessel in the brain, which can also indicate fetal anemia. (These are called *MCA* or *middle cerebral artery* Dopplers and are usually done on a weekly basis for 12 weeks after exposure.) If anemia does occur, doctors can perform a fetal blood transfusion (see Chapter 6) while the baby is still inside you or suggest that the baby be delivered, if you're nearing the end of pregnancy.

The ultimate good news: Recent studies show that babies infected with parvovirus during pregnancy, even if they develop anemia, are likely to be born as healthy as any other baby if they're adequately treated.

Stomach viruses (gastroenteritis)

A bout of stomach flu can occur any time, regardless of whether you're pregnant. Symptoms include stomach cramps, fever, diarrhea, and nausea, with or without vomiting, and they last anywhere from 24 to 72 hours. The viruses that cause gastroenteritis usually don't harm your baby.

 Don't worry that your baby won't get adequate nutrition if you can't eat for a few days. Fetuses do just fine even when their mothers miss a few meals.

 If you get a stomach virus, make sure that you drink plenty of liquids. Dehydration can lead to premature contractions and can contribute to fatigue and dizziness. Try the chicken soup we mention earlier, as well as other liquids — water, ginger ale, tea, or broth. Take care of yourself in the same way you would if you weren't pregnant. If your symptoms persist for more than 72 hours, call your doctor.

Toxoplasmosis

Toxoplasmosis is an infection caused by a parasite that lives in raw meat and in cat feces. If the parasite enters a person's bloodstream, it may lead to flu-like symptoms or, in some

cases, no symptoms at all. This type of infection is very rare in the United States, and infections in pregnant women are rarer still, occurring in only 2 out of every 1,000 women, whereas in France, infection is more common.

If a pregnant woman is infected, the chance that she will transmit the infection to her baby, and the possible effects it may have, depend largely on when she contracts it. If she contracts it during the first trimester, the chance of the baby becoming infected is less than 2 percent. Later on in pregnancy, the chance of the baby being infected is greater, but the effects of infection are less severe. In a fetus, early toxoplasmosis infection can cause abnormalities of the central nervous system and in vision.

If you've had the infection in the past and therefore have antibodies in your blood, you're highly unlikely to get the infection again. If a screening indicates that you may have been recently infected, your practitioner is likely to have your blood tested by a special laboratory to confirm that the positive test result was real. (Many initial tests produce false positives.) If the result still comes back positive, and you appear to have contracted the infection after you became pregnant, your practitioner can give you special antibiotics to reduce the chance of the fetus becoming infected. Then, in the second trimester, your practitioner may perform an amniocentesis to find out whether the fetus has been infected. If so, taking additional antibiotics for the rest of the pregnancy is necessary. Your practitioner may advise you to consult a maternal-fetal medicine specialist to discuss all your options.

If you get toxoplasmosis, keep in mind that recent studies from France indicate that the vast majority of fetuses infected with the parasite and are treated with appropriate antibiotics have an excellent prognosis.

No vaccine exists to prevent toxoplasmosis. The best way to avoid the disease is to minimize your exposure to raw or undercooked meat. Skip the carpaccio. Order your steaks cooked at least medium. Also avoid cat feces. If you have an outdoor cat, ask someone else to change the litter. (Indoor cats that have never been outdoors and never come in contact with mice or rats are extremely unlikely to have the parasite.) If no one else can do it, wear rubber gloves when you change the litter. Also wear gloves if you work in a garden that neighborhood cats may play in.

Vaginal infections

Bacteria and other organisms, when given half a chance, readily make themselves at home in a vagina, where the conditions — warm and moist — are perfect for them to grow and reproduce. A woman can get an infection at any time, even when she's pregnant.

Bacterial vaginosis

Bacterial vaginosis (BV) is a common vaginal infection. Symptoms include a whitish-yellow, odorous discharge that gets worse after sexual intercourse. Research has linked BV to a slightly higher risk for premature delivery, which is why some practitioners screen for BV in patients known to be at risk for preterm delivery. Treatment includes oral antibiotics or vaginal antibiotic creams.

Chlamydia

Chlamydia is one of the more common sexually transmitted diseases. It often comes with no symptoms. Some practitioners routinely perform a culture from the cervix to check for chlamydia at the same time they do a Pap smear. If you have a positive culture, your doctor will prescribe a medication to treat the infection. Chlamydia can be passed to your newborn during vaginal delivery, increasing the chance of the baby developing conjunctivitis (an eye infection) or, less likely, pneumonia. Most hospitals routinely place an ointment in a newborn's eyes shortly after delivery to prevent conjunctivitis, regardless of whether the mother is infected with chlamydia.

Yeast infections

Yeast infections are very common in pregnancy. The large amounts of estrogen that circulate in the bloodstream during pregnancy promote the growth of yeast in the vagina. Symptoms of an infection are vaginal itching and a thick, whitish-yellow discharge. However, many women get infections without any symptoms. Often the only treatment needed is a short course of vaginal suppositories or creams. For stubborn infections, your doctor can prescribe oral medications.

Yeast infections usually don't cause problems for the fetus or newborn.

Handling Pre-Pregnancy Conditions

The following sections detail conditions that you may have before you get pregnant and how those conditions may affect your pregnancy and vice versa.

Asthma

Predicting how pregnancy can affect a woman's asthma is difficult. Some women find that their condition improves when they're expecting. Some find it gets worse, and about half notice no difference at all.

The main concern that women with asthma have is whether they can safely continue taking their medications during pregnancy. Remember, the biggest problem with asthma isn't the medications, but the possibility of pregnant women with asthma under-treating themselves. If you're having trouble breathing, you may not be getting enough oxygen to the baby. Most commonly used asthma treatments are quite safe for the baby, including the following:

✔ Beta-agonists (serevent, albuterol, metaproterenol, terbutaline, Proventil, Allupent)

✔ Corticosteroids (Prednisone)

✔ Cromolyn sodium

✔ Theophylline (Theodur)

✔ Inhaled steroids (Flovent, Vanceril, Beclavent, Azmacort, and so on)

You can take preventive measures to control acute attacks. Predicting attacks by self-monitoring is useful for asthmatic patients with peak expiratory flow rates (most asthma patients know what these are — if you don't, ask your lung specialist). Naturally, it helps to avoid situations that trigger attacks.

Expectant mothers ask . . .

Q: "Are blood pressure medications safe?"

A: Most medications are safe, but many haven't been well-studied during pregnancy. Discuss this important question with your doctor. Certain medications, however, should be avoided. Angiotensin converting enzyme inhibitors (known as ACE inhibitors) pose some risk for kidney problems in the fetus. Beta-blockers and certain calcium channel blockers are generally considered safe in pregnancy. Commonly used antihypertensive medications include labetolol, nifedipine, and Aldomet. Also, diuretics are best avoided, unless this is the only way of treating the high blood pressure.

Chronic hypertension

Chronic hypertension refers to high blood pressure that occurs independently of pregnancy. Although many women who have this condition are aware that they have it before they conceive, doctors occasionally diagnose it during pregnancy. If you have mild or moderate chronic hypertension, chances are good that you'll have an uneventful pregnancy. However, your doctor will be on the lookout for certain conditions that can affect you or the baby.

Women with chronic hypertension stand an increased risk of developing preeclampsia, so your doctor looks for any signs that you're developing this condition. The main risk for the baby is intrauterine growth restriction (IUGR) or placental abruption (see Chapter 14). Your doctor may use repeated sonograms to check on the baby's growth and to make sure that you have adequate amniotic fluid. She may also suggest that you undergo some tests later during your pregnancy for fetal well-being, such as non-stress tests (see Chapter 7). The overall management of your pregnancy depends on how well-controlled your blood pressure is, your overall health, and how the baby grows.

Deep vein thrombosis and pulmonary embolus

A deep vein thrombosis (DVT) is a blood clot that develops within a deep vein, most commonly in the leg. A pulmonary embolus is a blood clot within the lung, which is often a clot that has dislodged from one of the deep veins of the leg and made its way to the lung. Both of these conditions are rare, affecting far less than 1 percent of pregnant women.

Symptoms of a DVT include pain, swelling, and tenderness, usually in the calf, and a rope-like hardness running down the back of the lower leg. Diagnosing DVT before it has the chance to lead to a pulmonary embolus is important.

Keep in mind that muscle pain, cramping, and swelling are common symptoms of a normal pregnancy, and a DVT is quite unusual. Let your doctor know when you're experiencing the sudden onset of these symptoms, but don't panic about them.

Diabetes

Diabetes comes up as a problem in pregnancy in two ways:

- ✔ You already have the condition before you become pregnant.

- ✔ You develop what's called *gestational diabetes,* which is unique to pregnancy and usually goes away after pregnancy.

Diabetes before pregnancy

If you have a history of diabetes, talk to your doctor about it before you get pregnant. If you have your blood sugar level under good control before you conceive, your pregnancy is more likely to proceed smoothly. Women with pregestational diabetes stand a higher-than-average risk of having a fetus with certain birth defects, but you can reduce this risk down to the normal range if you achieve excellent glucose control.

Some doctors suggest that you have a blood test called a hemoglobin A1C to check how well your sugar has been controlled over the past few months. Your doctor may also suggest that you have a special sonogram, called a *fetal echocardiogram*

(see Chapter 6), to make sure that the baby's heart is okay. If you take an oral medication to control your blood sugar, your practitioner may suggest you switch to insulin injections for better control. Some women with diabetes suffer kidney complications, but this kind of problem isn't likely to worsen during pregnancy. If you have eye problems related to diabetes (proliferative retinopathy), have your doctor closely monitor and possibly treat your eyes during pregnancy.

The vast majority of diabetic women proceed through pregnancy without a hitch. However, your doctor may need to adjust your insulin dose. Your doctor also follows the baby's growth with periodic ultrasound exams and is on the lookout to see that you don't develop high blood pressure. In the third trimester, your doctor probably begins to monitor the fetus closely, performing certain tests for fetal well-being (periodic NSTs, for example — see Chapter 7).

When you're in labor, your doctor keeps a close eye on your glucose level and may give you insulin. With optimal glucose control and close monitoring of the baby and mother-to-be, most women with diabetes have an excellent outlook for pregnancy.

Gestational diabetes

Gestational diabetes is one of the most common medical complications in pregnancy, occurring in 2 to 3 percent of all pregnant women. Your practitioner can diagnose gestational diabetes by giving you a special blood test. (See Chapter 6 for more information about this test.)

If you have gestational diabetes and you don't control your glucose levels, your baby may be at higher risk for certain problems. If your blood sugar levels are high, the fetus's are, too. And high blood sugar levels cause the fetus to produce certain hormones that stimulate fetal growth, which may cause her to grow too large (see Chapter 14). Furthermore, if the fetus has high blood sugar levels while still in the uterus, once born she may have temporary problems with sugar regulation. If the mother's (and fetus's) glucose levels are controlled during pregnancy, the risk of these complications drops dramatically.

Expectant mothers ask . . .

Q: "If I develop gestational diabetes, will I recover when my pregnancy ends?"

A: Most women do recover completely, but a minority remains diabetic. In these cases, pregnancy itself didn't cause the diabetes. Instead, the women were already at risk for developing the condition. If you develop gestational diabetes, being tested for diabetes within a few months after you deliver is important. Also, keep in mind that your risk for developing diabetes at some point later in your life increases.

You need to control your sugar levels if you have gestational diabetes. Most of the time, altering your diet is enough. (Most women have a consultation with a nurse and/or a nutritionist to come up with a specific diet plan.) Exercise also helps. Only in rare cases do women need to resort to taking medication to keep their sugar level under control. Traditionally, doctors have prescribed insulin injections to control blood glucose levels, but recent research suggests that an oral agent called glyburide is safe and effective. If you develop gestational diabetes, your doctor may ask you to check your sugar level several times during the day or on a weekly basis. You do this by pricking your finger (called a fingerstick) and placing the drop of blood onto a test strip, which you then insert into a small meter that gives immediate results.

Fibroids

Fibroids (also called *uterine myomas*) are benign growths of the muscle cells that make up the uterus. They're extremely common, and your practitioner often diagnoses them during routine sonograms. The high levels of estrogen in a pregnant woman's bloodstream can encourage fibroids to grow larger. Yet, predicting whether any woman's fibroids will grow, stay the same, or shrink during pregnancy is difficult. Most of the time, fibroids cause no problems for a pregnancy.

In extreme cases, fibroids can cause difficulties, such as the following:

✔ Fibroids may grow so fast that they outgrow their blood supply and begin to degenerate, which sometimes causes pain, uterine contractions, and even preterm labor.

Symptoms of degeneration include pain and tenderness directly over the fibroid (in the lower abdomen). Short-term treatment with anti-inflammatory medications (Motrin or Indocin, for example) may help.

✔ Very large fibroids in the lower portion of the uterus or near the cervix may interfere with the baby's ability to make its way through the birth canal. Thus, they may increase the risk for cesarean delivery, although this situation is quite unusual.

✔ Large fibroids within the uterus can sometimes increase the likelihood that the baby will be in the breech or transverse position. But this possibility, too, is rare. Most commonly, fibroids cause no problem at all. And most often, they shrink after delivery.

Immunological problems

Immunological problems are conditions in which a person's immune system produces atypical antibodies, which can lead to a variety of problems. In most cases, women who have immunological problems already know they have them before they become pregnant. If you're one of those women, discuss your problem with your doctor before you become pregnant or as early in your pregnancy as possible.

Antiphospholipid antibodies

Antiphospholipid antibodies are a class of antibodies that circulate in some women's blood. The two most common kinds are lupus anticoagulant and anticardiolipin antibodies. They may be found in some women with collagen vascular diseases (such as lupus), in women who have had blood clots, and in some women with no known medical problems. They're significant in pregnancy because they have been associated with recurrent miscarriages, unexplained fetal death, early onset of preeclampsia, and intrauterine growth restriction. Doctors don't routinely screen for these antibodies because many women who have them experience no resulting problems. But if you have one of the following conditions, your doctor will probably want to test you:

✔ Autoimmune platelet conditions

✔ A false positive test for syphilis

✔ A history of spontaneous blood clots in the legs or lungs

✔ A history of stroke or transient ischemic attacks (a "temporary" kind of stroke)

✔ Lupus (or other collagen vascular disease)

Your doctor may also want to test you if you have had any of the following obstetrical problems in the past:

✔ Early-onset preeclampsia

✔ Problems with fetal growth (intrauterine growth restriction)

✔ Recurrent miscarriages

✔ Unexplained stillbirth or fetal death

Antiphospholipid antibody syndrome is diagnosed when a woman has antiphospholipid antibodies in her bloodstream plus one of the listed risk factors. If you have the syndrome, depending on its severity, your doctor may recommend that you take baby aspirin, heparin, oral steroids, or some combination of these medications. She probably will also recommend that you have periodic ultrasound exams to make sure the baby is growing appropriately, and that you undergo tests for fetal well-being (see Chapter 7).

We realize that this syndrome may sound scary, but the good news is that most women who receive adequate medical care have normal pregnancies and healthy babies.

Lupus

Systemic lupus erythematosus (SLE, or lupus) is one of several so-called *collagen vascular diseases.* Pregnancy doesn't make the disease worse, but some women do experience more flare-ups during pregnancy.

On the other hand, lupus can affect pregnancy in some cases, depending on the problem's severity going into pregnancy. If you have a mild form of lupus, chances are it will have little effect on your pregnancy. Some women with more severe lupus stand an increased risk of miscarriage, problems with fetal growth, and preeclampsia (see Chapter 14). Depending on your medical history, your doctor may recommend certain medications such as heparin, baby aspirin, or oral steroids. She may also recommend more frequent sonograms and other measures of fetal well-being. Your best bet for a successful

pregnancy is to have the disorder under control as much as possible before you become pregnant.

Inflammatory bowel disease

The two kinds of inflammatory bowel disease are Crohn's disease and ulcerative colitis. Fortunately, pregnancy does nothing to exacerbate either condition. If you have inflammatory bowel disease, but your symptoms were minor or nonexistent during the months before you became pregnant, chances are good that they will remain at bay during your pregnancy. Doctors often recommend that women whose symptoms are frequent and severe postpone pregnancy until the disease abates or is brought under control. Most medications to control symptoms are considered to be safe and effective during pregnancy.

Seizure disorders (epilepsy)

Most women who have epilepsy can have an uneventful pregnancy and give birth to a perfectly healthy baby. However, epilepsy does require that a woman's obstetrician and her neurologist work together to come up with the right strategy for controlling seizures. If you have epilepsy, make an effort before you get pregnant to control your seizures with the lowest possible dose of medication. Studies show that women whose seizures are well-controlled on a minimal dose of a single medication before they get pregnant have the best pregnancy outcomes. So by all means, consult your neurologist before you get pregnant, and don't stop taking your medications unless your doctor advises you to.

All medications used to treat seizures pose some risk of birth defects. The problems they can cause vary, depending on the particular medication, but they include facial abnormalities, cleft lip and cleft palate, congenital heart defects, and neural tube defects. For this reason, women who take seizure medications need to have an ultrasound to evaluate fetal anatomy and a fetal echocardiogram (see Chapter 6) to look for abnormalities in the baby's heart.

 Women with seizure disorders should begin taking extra folic acid about three months before trying to conceive, because some seizure medications can affect folic acid levels.

Don't adjust or stop your medications on your own, especially after you become pregnant. Your seizure activity could increase, which would probably be worse for the developing baby than the medications themselves.

Thyroid problems

Problems with thyroid function are relatively common in women of reproductive age; we see many women with over-active or underactive thyroids during pregnancy. Although these conditions require extra testing, they usually don't cause significant problems for pregnancy.

Hyperthyroidism (overactive thyroid)

There are many different causes of hyperthyroidism, but the most common by far is Grave's disease, which is associated with its own special set of antibodies (thyroid-stimulating immunoglobulins, or TSIs) in the blood. These antibodies cause the thyroid to make too much thyroid hormone. Women with an overactive thyroid must receive adequate treatment during pregnancy (ideally, beginning before conception) in order to reduce their risk of such complications as miscar-riage, preterm delivery, and low birth weight.

If you have an overactive thyroid, unless your condition is extremely mild, your doctor is most likely to recommend that you take certain medications to lower the amount of thyroid hormone circulating in your blood. Some of these medications may cross the placenta, so your doctor watches the fetus closely, usually by performing regular sonograms, to look for any evidence that the medications are lowering the baby's thyroid levels too much. Specifically, she monitors the baby's growth and heart rate to see that they're normal and checks for any evidence that the fetus has developed a goiter (an enlarged thyroid).

Your doctor probably also will monitor the levels of thyroid-stimulating antibodies in your blood because these antibodies may, in some rare cases, cross the placenta and stimulate the baby's thyroid as well. After delivery, your baby's pediatri-cian watches the baby carefully for any evidence of thyroid problems.

Some women develop hyperthyroidism in the first trimester due to high levels of the pregnancy hormone hCG. This is usually self-limited and resolves without treatment.

Hypothyroidism (underactive thyroid)

A woman with an underactive thyroid (hypothyroidism) can have a healthy pregnancy as long as her condition is adequately treated. If it's not, she stands a higher risk of developing certain complications, such as a low birth-weight baby. The condition is treated with a thyroid replacement hormone (Synthroid, for example). This medication is safe for the baby because very little of it crosses the placenta. If you have an underactive thyroid, your doctor may want to periodically check your hormone levels to see whether your medication needs to be adjusted. While some doctors recommend routine testing (and possibly treatment) for hypothyroidism in the first trimester in women *without* a history of thyroid disease, this is not actually recommended by major obstetrical organizations such as the American Congress of Obstetricians and Gynecologists (ACOG).

Chapter 16

Coping with the Unexpected

*W*e wish we had no reason to include this chapter. We wish every pregnant couple could end up delivering a healthy baby. Most do, but not everyone is so fortunate. Those who suffer the loss of a fetus or discover that their baby has a significant abnormality need to understand what happens and figure out how to respond when things go wrong. If you're experiencing any of the problems we cover in this chapter, we hope you find some of this information helpful.

Perhaps you're drawn to this chapter because you've had an unsuccessful pregnancy in the past. If so, you may be anxious about your current pregnancy. That's entirely normal. We take care of many women who have had poor outcomes in the past, and we realize the only thing that can truly alleviate their anxiety is to hold a healthy baby.

One way to at least minimize your worry is to sit down with your doctor and discuss the situation. Ask him to map out a plan for your current pregnancy that maximizes your chances for a favorable outcome and helps you cope with your concerns. When you feel certain you're doing everything you possibly can do to avoid a recurring problem, you may rest a little easier. Your worry probably won't entirely disappear, but remember

that although a certain part of the process is in Mother Nature's hands, you can take medical steps to maximize your chances of having a healthy baby.

Surviving Recurrent Miscarriages

Unfortunately, a first-trimester miscarriage is a fairly common occurrence. Doctors estimate that about 15 to 20 percent of recognized pregnancies — those that have yielded a positive pregnancy test — end up in miscarriage. Still more early embryos (also called *conceptuses*) are lost before they're actually known to exist — that is, before a woman takes a pregnancy test. More than half the time, the cause of first-trimester miscarriage is the presence of some chromosomal abnormality in the embryo or fetus. Another 20 percent of early miscarriages are due to structural abnormalities in the embryo. Usually they're spontaneous events with low chances of recurrence.

Fortunately, 80 to 90 percent of women who experience a single early miscarriage subsequently deliver a normal baby.

Recurrent miscarriage — technically, the loss of three consecutive pregnancies — is far less common. This problem occurs in only ½ to 1 percent of women. A variety of causes contribute to recurrent miscarriage, including the following:

- ✔ Genetic causes

- ✔ Uterine abnormalities

- ✔ Immunologic causes (though not all physicians agree that this is a factor)

- ✔ Inadequate progesterone secretion

- ✔ Certain infections (although this cause is also controversial)

- ✔ Antiphospholipid antibody syndrome (lupus anticoagulant or anti-cardiolipin antibodies, see Chapter 14)

- ✔ Certain environmental toxins or drugs (such as antimalarials and some anesthetic agents)

Most doctors suggest that women undergo certain tests after having three miscarriages; some begin testing even sooner. Because chromosomal abnormalities are the most common cause of miscarriage, an important first diagnostic step is to run tests on the chromosomes of the fetal tissue, when possible.

Various strategies for treating recurrent miscarriage are available, but doctors may disagree about which one, if any, is best. Choosing a strategy is easier if you know what the problem is. For example, your doctor may be able to surgically repair an abnormally shaped uterus. If doctors can't find a cause for recurrent miscarriage, knowing which treatment is best may be difficult. Note, however, that even if no treatment is attempted, women who have had three consecutive miscarriages still have a greater than 50 percent chance of having a normal, successful pregnancy.

Coping with Late-Pregnancy Loss

Late-pregnancy loss refers to a fetal death, stillbirth, or death of an infant in the immediate newborn period. Fortunately, these losses are infrequent and rarely occur more than once. Some causes of late losses include

- ✔ Chromosomal abnormalities

- ✔ Other genetic syndromes

- ✔ Structural defects

- ✔ A massive placental abruption or separation (see Chapter 14)

- ✔ Antiphospholipid antibodies or clotting disorders (see Chapter 14)

- ✔ Umbilical cord compression

- ✔ Unexplained reasons, which are, unfortunately, very common

Women who suffer a loss of pregnancy often ask, "Did I do something to cause this?" The answer is almost always no. So you have no reason to add to your grief by mixing in guilt.

Many patients find it helpful, after the initial hurt has begun to subside, to gather all their pregnancy records, including any pathology reports, and consult with their doctor or a specialist. Sometimes your doctor can identify a cause, and sometimes not. Either way, most patients benefit from sitting down with their doctor and mapping out a strategy for trying to prevent a loss in future pregnancies. Having a plan to focus on makes many patients feel less helpless. Support groups are also very helpful (see the "Finding Help" section later in this chapter).

In subsequent pregnancies, your doctor may recommend you undergo blood tests to check for certain abnormalities that have been associated with fetal loss. Often, if you have experienced a prior late-pregnancy loss, doctors follow your progress with regular ultrasound examinations and tests of fetal well-being. Your doctor may recommend you deliver somewhat early, before you go into labor. You're likely to feel anxious during subsequent pregnancies, which is completely normal. But keep in mind, suffering a pregnancy loss a second time is quite unlikely.

A good Internet source for pregnancy loss is www.marchof dimes.com.

Dealing with Fetal Abnormalities

All prospective parents wonder whether their baby will be "normal." And, for most, the answer is yes. Still, 2 to 3 percent of babies end up having a significant abnormality. Some of these abnormalities can be repaired and have very little impact on the baby's overall quality of life. Occasionally, however, the condition can have a bigger impact, whether it is a structural, chromosomal, or genetic abnormality.

When an abnormality occurs, the first question many women ask us is, "Is this my fault?" And the answer, most often, is no. From what is known about fetal abnormalities, most are what are called *sporadic,* meaning they occur randomly and have no identifiable cause. If your doctor can't identify a cause, chances are low that the same kind of abnormality will recur in a subsequent pregnancy. (If the cause is genetic, there may be some chance that the abnormality could occur again.)

If your fetus is diagnosed with a birth defect or genetic disorder by ultrasound or some other test, your doctor may recommend you have additional tests to look for other factors that have been associated with that particular problem. He may

recommend you see a genetic counselor to discuss the implications of the abnormality. If the condition is a structural defect that can be surgically repaired or treated, your doctor may recommend you meet with the specialist who can treat the baby after he is born. These discussions help you prepare for what lies ahead during the newborn period and also later on in your child's life.

Nobody wants to get the news that a fetus has an abnormality, but having this information is helpful for several reasons:

- ✔ If you're aware of some disorders, such as fetal anemia or obstructions in the urinary tract, doctors may be able to treat them.

- ✔ The knowledge helps to prepare you for what happens after the baby is born.

- ✔ This information helps you manage your pregnancy and consider all possible options.

- ✔ The information can give you important insights into the management of future pregnancies.

Finding Help

If your pregnancy didn't turn out as you had hoped, the first and most obvious place to look for support is from your partner. Family members, friends, and clergy can also be very helpful. Professional advice or treatment from a psychotherapist or social worker may be useful for many couples. Support groups also can provide understanding and expert insight into your problem. If you have online access, you can find hundreds of support groups on the Internet. Dozens of helpful books are also available, including

- ✔ *How to Go on Living After the Death of a Baby,* by Larry G. Peppers and Ronald J. Knapp (Peachtree Publishers)

- ✔ *Loss During Pregnancy or in the Newborn Period,* by James Woods, Jr., and Jenifer Esposito Woods (Jannetti Publications, Inc.)

- ✔ *Roses in December: Comfort for the Grieving Heart,* by Marilyn Willett Heavilin (Harvest House Publishers)

- ✔ *When Mourning Breaks: Coping with Miscarriage,* by Melissa Sexson Hanson (Morehouse Publishing Co.)

Beginning to Heal

Couples naturally feel a strong emotional attachment to their unborn child, beginning as early as the first trimester. As a result, many couples experience the same grief after the loss of a fetus as they would after the loss of a family member or close friend. The loss of a fetus is no less significant than the loss of a child. Parents who decide to terminate a pregnancy because of an abnormality also go through tremendous grief.

Both parents should acknowledge their need — and their right — to grieve after a pregnancy loss. The emotional response takes time and typically goes through a number of stages, beginning with shock and denial, progressing to anger, and eventually reaching acceptance and the ability to carry on with life. Understand that each of you will grieve in a different way.

After you have gone through the stages of grief and feel you're physically and emotionally strong, you're probably ready to start trying to conceive again. In some couples, one person progresses through the grieving process faster than the other. Make sure both of you are ready before you begin trying to get pregnant again. And remember that a successful pregnancy, while joyful, doesn't replace a lost one — so the grieving process is necessary. From a medical perspective, make sure that you finish looking into possible causes for the loss and have a plan of action for the next pregnancy. Realize that your next pregnancy will be somewhat stressful and that you will need extra attention and compassion from your family, friends, and healthcare professionals.

Part V

The Part of Tens

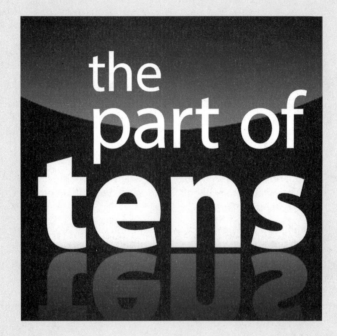

In this part . . .

✔ We put on our best friend hat and explain some of the little details – which many people avoid telling you – that come along with pregnancy.

✔ Feeding yourself healthy snacks is a great way to promote a health pregnancy. We give you 10 terrific recipes.

✔ Through the wonders of ultrasound, we show you some of the fascinating things that you can discover about your baby.

Chapter 17

Ten Things Nobody Tells You

*D*on't worry. We know of no conspiracy keeping you from knowing all there is to know about pregnancy. But your friends, sisters, cousins — whoever tells you what to expect with your pregnancy — often forget the little details, especially the more unpleasant ones. Furthermore, other books often gloss over this stuff, perhaps in the interest of decorum. Well, at the risk of being indecorous, we're going to give it to you straight in this chapter with the ten things nobody else will tell you.

Pregnancy Lasts Longer than Nine Months

Patients always ask, "How many months along am I?" and we have trouble giving them a precise answer. Pregnancy is said to last nine months, but that number isn't exactly accurate. The average pregnancy lasts 280 days, or 40 weeks, starting from the date of the mother's last menstrual period. (You think 40 weeks is a long time? Just be glad you're not an elephant, which has a gestation period of 22 months!) If a month is four weeks, that

calculation comes out to ten months. On the calendar, however, most months contain four weeks plus two or three days, so nine calendar months often do contain close to 40 weeks. Practitioners speak in terms of weeks when measuring gestational age because it's more accurate and less confusing.

Other People Can Drive You Crazy

Friends, relatives, acquaintances, strangers, and even your partner give you unsolicited opinions and advice and want to share with you every pregnancy horror story they've ever heard. They may tell you your rear looks big, you're too fat (or too thin), or you shouldn't be eating whatever you're putting in your mouth.

We realize these people usually have only good intentions when they tell you how their sister's pregnancy ended badly, or about the trouble a friend of a friend had. They don't realize that they're increasing your anxiety. Don't pay attention. Try to politely smile and ignore them. Tell them you really don't want to hear this story right now. If you have any real problems or concerns, talk them over with your practitioner.

You Feel Exhausted in the First Trimester

You may already have heard that you're going to feel tired during the first trimester, but until you go through it, you really have no idea how overwhelming the fatigue can be. You may find yourself looking for every possible opportunity to catch a few winks — on the bus, on the train, at work, or even on the exam table waiting for your practitioner to come into the room. Rest assured this fatigue does go away, usually by the end of the first trimester (at about 13 weeks), and you do get your usual energy back. Look out, though. Around 30 to 34 weeks, the physical stress of pregnancy may overwhelm you again, and you may go back to feeling pretty washed out for several weeks. Frequent naps, either in the first trimester or at any time, are always a good idea if you're feeling tired.

Round Ligament Pain Really Hurts

The round ligaments run from the top of the uterus down into the labia. As the uterus grows, these ligaments stretch, and many women feel discomfort or pain on one or both sides of the groin area, especially at about 16 to 22 weeks. Practitioners tell you this symptom is only round ligament pain and it's nothing to worry about. And they're right — don't worry. But you deserve some sympathy (you have ours) because this pain can be fairly intense.

You can probably ease round ligament pain a bit by getting off your feet or changing positions, thereby taking the pressure off the ligaments. (By the way, if you're having twins or more, the round ligament pain may begin earlier and last longer.) The good news is that round ligament pain usually diminishes by about 24 weeks.

Your Belly Becomes a Hand Magnet

After your stomach protrudes noticeably with pregnancy, you're likely to find that suddenly everyone presumes touching it is okay — not only your friends, family members, and the people you work with, but also the mailman, the cashier at the supermarket, and other people you've never even met. Although some women appreciate the extra attention, many find it an invasion of privacy. You can either grin and bear it or discover how to say, "Hey, hands off!"

Hemorrhoids Are a Royal Pain in the Butt

Your best friend may say she's told you everything about her own pregnancy. But did she mention her hemorrhoids? Believe us, hemorrhoids happen pretty often, and when they do, you're in for some very noticeable pain and discomfort.

Hemorrhoids are dilated veins near the rectum that become engorged because of the pressure on that part of the body or because of pushing during delivery. Some women notice hemorrhoids during pregnancy, others don't have any problem with them until after delivery, and some very lucky women never have them at all.

If your hemorrhoids are significant, be prepared for some discomfort after vaginal delivery (see Chapter 11). Most hemorrhoids go away within a few weeks. If you're fortunate enough not to have them, realize how lucky you are — and have sympathy for all the other new mothers who do have them.

Sometimes Women Poop While Pushing

Our patients frequently ask us about having a bowel movement during labor, so although it may not be the most genteel subject to bring up, we're going to anyway. Pooping while pushing doesn't happen every time; however, it's fairly common. In all likelihood, you and your partner aren't even aware of it happening because your nurse quickly wipes away any mess and keeps you clean throughout the pushing process. In fact, pooping while pushing is actually a good sign, because it means you are pushing effectively — and getting closer to baby time!

The Weight Stays On after the Baby Comes Out

Most women can't wait to weigh themselves after delivering 10 pounds or so of baby, placenta, and fluid. Contain yourself. Wait at least a week. After delivery, many women swell up like dumplings, especially their hands and feet. This extra water retention adds pounds. If you step on the scale right away, you may be very disappointed at the number that comes up. The swelling generally takes about a week or two to go away.

Postpartum Bonding Really Does Happen

Some women worry because they haven't felt attached or bonded to their fetus during pregnancy. We assure you that after you deliver, within 24 hours, an overwhelming sense of love, devotion, and responsibility will happen for the majority of women. If this doesn't happen, speak with your provider to make sure that you aren't developing the postpartum "blues" or postpartum depression (see Chapter 11).

Breast Engorgement Really Sucks, and Breast-Feeding Can Be a Production

Of course you know your breasts fill up with milk after you deliver your baby. But what you may not have heard is how painful and cumbersome this engorgement can be if you aren't breast-feeding, or when you decide to stop breast-feeding. Your breasts may become rock-hard, tender, and warm, and they may seem to grow to the size of blimps. Fortunately, the discomfort is temporary; this intense period of engorgement lasts only a couple of days.

We encourage all of our patients to breast-feed due to the benefits for the baby, but keep in mind it may be harder than you think. Needing some extra help and assistance is very natural. Fortunately, most hospitals have lactation specialists who can help you milk the process along.

Chapter 18

Ten Healthy Snacks for Pregnant Women

● ●

In This Chapter

▶ Getting the extra calories you need in a healthy way

▶ Satisfying your hunger pangs

▶ Using healthy snacks to fulfill your nutritional needs

● ●

*P*regnant women need extra nutrition, but not empty calories, to keep themselves healthy and help their babies grow. Most pregnant women find they're hungry throughout the day, not just at meals. With the busy schedules women have today, finding snacks that are both healthy and satisfying is difficult. Here are some of our recommendations for high-nutrient snacks that are easy to make and yummy.

Recipes in This Chapter

▶ Chunky Dried Fig, Coconut, and Almond Granola

▶ Guilt-Free Oatmeal Cookies

▶ Peanut Butter, Chocolate, and Banana Quesadillas

▶ Double Salmon Dip

▶ Herbed Cottage Cheese Dip with Whole-Grain Bread

▶ Roasted Tomatoes and Mozzarella Bites

▶ Chickpea Parsley Dip with Pita Chips and Celery and Carrot Sticks

▶ Peanut Butter and Dried Fruit Bars

▶ Fruit Smoothie

▶ Sunday Sundae

Chunky Dried Fig, Coconut, and Almond Granola

This recipe uses oats, which are an excellent source of fiber and folic acid, in addition to the nuts and figs. Nuts are a great source of protein, fiber (especially almonds), and heart-healthy unsaturated fats. They're also a cholesterol-free snack. Dried fruits are a great source of quick energy and antioxidants.

Prep time: 25 min • **Baking time:** 30–35 min •
Yield: About 6 cups; serving is ½ cup

Ingredients	Directions
2 cups old-fashioned rolled oats (not instant)	*1* Preheat oven to 300 degrees F.
¾ cup whole raw almonds, roughly chopped	*2* Mix first seven ingredients in a large bowl.
½ cup sweetened flaked coconut	*3* Melt butter and honey in microwave-proof dish about 30 seconds. Pour melted butter mixture over granola mixture and mix well. Spread mixture on baking sheet; bake 20 minutes, stirring occasionally.
½ cup raw cashew pieces	
⅓ cup brown sugar, lightly packed	*4* Add figs and carefully stir to mix. Continue to bake until golden brown, about 10–15 minutes longer.
1½ teaspoons ground allspice	
1 teaspoon ground cinnamon	*5* Eat by the handful or spoon over lowfat yogurt or ice cream.
½ stick (4 tablespoons) unsalted butter	
2 tablespoons honey	
1 cup chopped dried figs	

Per serving: Calories 262 (From Fat 119); Fat 13g (Saturated 4g); Cholesterol 10mg; Sodium 17mg; Carbohydrate 34g (Dietary Fiber 5g); Protein 6g.

Guilt-Free Oatmeal Cookies

Just because you're pregnant doesn't mean you have to deny your sweet tooth an occasional indulgence. Don't feel guilty when you eat these cookies, because they're low in calories and have some protein and fiber.

Prep time: 20 min • **Baking time:** 10–12 min •
Yield: About 30 cookies; 1 cookie per serving

Ingredients	Directions
½ stick (4 tablespoons) unsalted butter, softened	**1** Preheat oven to 375 degrees F.
¼ cup vegetable shortening	**2** Cream butter and shortening with sugar in a mixing bowl. Beat in the egg, baking soda, water, flour, salt, and vanilla. Stir in the remainder of the ingredients.
½ cup brown sugar, lightly packed	
1 egg	**3** Drop rounded spoonfuls of dough onto greased baking sheets.
½ teaspoon baking soda	
1 tablespoon warm water	**4** Bake for 10–12 minutes or until golden.
½ cup + 2 tablespoons flour	
½ teaspoon salt	
½ teaspoon vanilla	
1½ cups old-fashioned rolled oats (not instant)	
½ cup sweetened flaked coconut	
6 ounces semisweet chocolate chips	
⅓ cup roasted cashews or other nuts, chopped	
½ cup raisins	

Per serving: Calories 119 (From Fat 58); Fat 7g (Saturated 3g); Cholesterol 11mg; Sodium 68mg; Carbohydrate 15g (Dietary Fiber 1g); Protein 2g.

Peanut Butter, Chocolate, and Banana Quesadillas

Peanut butter and chocolate is a classic combination. The addition of the banana makes this a heartier snack and adds lots of protein, fiber, and potassium.

Prep time: 10 min • **Baking time:** 12 min •
Yield: 8 pieces or 2 servings

Ingredients	Directions
6 tablespoons peanut butter	*1* Preheat oven to 350 degrees F.
4 10-inch whole-wheat flour tortillas ½ cup semisweet chocolate morsels	*2* Spread half the peanut butter on two tortillas. On top of the peanut butter, sprinkle chocolate morsels. Wrap remaining tortillas in foil to warm in oven.
2 bananas, thinly sliced	*3* Place on baking sheet and bake for 12 minutes or until chocolate begins to melt.
	4 Remove from oven and place sliced bananas on top of peanut butter chocolate spread. Remove foil-wrapped tortillas from oven and place on top.
	5 Let cool slightly, cut into quarters, and enjoy.

Per serving: Calories 742 (From Fat 342); Fat 38g (Saturated 13g); Cholesterol 0mg; Sodium 571mg; Carbohydrate 105g (Dietary Fiber 13g); Protein 21g.

Double Salmon Dip

Salmon is an excellent source of calcium and omega-3 fatty acids. This dip is satisfying, low in saturated fat, and an excellent source of protein. Salmon is also low in mercury and therefore safe to eat in moderation during pregnancy.

Prep time: 15 min • **Yield:** About 3 cups; serving is ½ cup

Ingredients	Directions
2 containers (8 ounces each) whipped, low-fat cream cheese, softened or at room temperature	*1* Mix first four ingredients together. Fold in salmon gently. Season with salt and pepper.
3 tablespoons low-fat milk	*2* Use whole-wheat pita chips for dipping.
2 tablespoons chopped chives	
1 tablespoon horseradish	
4 ounces fresh poached or canned salmon	
4 ounces smoked salmon, cut into pieces	
Salt and pepper to taste	

Per serving: Calories 110 (From Fat 61); Fat 7g (Saturated 4g); Cholesterol 26mg; Sodium 380mg; Carbohydrate 3g (Dietary Fiber 0g); Protein 8g.

Herbed Cottage Cheese Dip with Whole-Grain Bread

If you're worried about adding too many pounds, this recipe is really low in calories, fat, and carbohydrates, but still very satisfying. This recipe has calcium, which is great for fetal bone growth and development, and has the added benefit of some protein.

Prep time: 15 min (additional hour and 15 min for chilling) •
Yield: 4 servings; serving is ½ cup

Ingredients	Directions
1 cup low-fat (1%), small-curd cottage cheese	*1* Blend cottage cheese, lemon juice, and water in a blender or food processor until smooth.
1½ tablespoons fresh lemon juice	
1 tablespoon water	*2* Stir in herbs, chives, salt, and pepper.
¼ cup assorted chopped herbs (such as parsley, dill, thyme)	*3* Serve with toasted whole-grain bread.
3 tablespoons chopped chives	
Salt and pepper to taste	
Whole-grain bread	

Tip: You may want to use the small bowl of a food processor. A blender may require a little scraping down on the sides.

Per serving: Calories 44 (From Fat 6); Fat 1g (Saturated 0g); Cholesterol 2mg; Sodium 232mg; Carbohydrate 2g (Dietary Fiber 0g); Protein 7g.

Roasted Tomatoes and Mozzarella Bites

If you're looking for a savory snack, this one is excellent because it is low-carb and rich in protein and calcium. You can also toss it over some whole-wheat pasta for a nice meal.

Prep time: 15 min • **Roasting time:** 35 min •
Yield: 4 snack-size servings; serving is ½ cup

Ingredients	Directions
1 pint cherry tomatoes, halved	*1* Preheat oven to 400 degrees F.
½ teaspoon dried oregano Salt and pepper to taste	*2* Toss first four ingredients in bowl and spread on baking sheet. Roast for 35 minutes. Let cool.
2 tablespoons olive oil 2–3 mozzarella sticks, sliced into 1-inch cubes	*3* Add sliced mozzarella sticks and basil. Then enjoy this "pizza without the bread" snack.
2 tablespoons fresh basil sliced in a julienne fashion	

Per serving: Calories 236 (From Fat 171); Fat 19g (Saturated 8g); Cholesterol 30mg; Sodium 632mg; Carbohydrate 6g (Dietary Fiber 1g); Protein 17g.

Chickpea Parsley Dip with Pita Chips and Celery and Carrot Sticks

Chickpeas are a good source of the extra protein you need to consume while you're pregnant. This snack is also very low in calories and has no saturated fat. The carrots are a good source of vitamin A and biotin.

Prep time: 45 min • **Yield:** 4 servings; serving is ½ cup

Ingredients	Directions
1 cup canned chickpeas, rinsed and drained (or more for thicker dip)	**1** Blend all ingredients in food processor until smooth.
½ cup low-fat plain yogurt	**2** Serve with pita chips, celery sticks, and carrot sticks.
½ cup chopped fresh parsley	
1 garlic clove, chopped	
1½ tablespoons fresh lemon juice	
1 tablespoon water	
¼ teaspoon salt	
Pita chips and celery and carrot sticks	

Tip: Feel free to add more garlic if you like a little more zip. You can also use the full can of chickpeas if you want your dip to be a bit thicker.

Per serving: Calories 80 (From Fat 12); Fat 1g (Saturated 0g); Cholesterol 2mg; Sodium 361mg; Carbohydrate 12g (Dietary Fiber 3g); Protein 5g.

Peanut Butter and Dried Fruit Bars

The whole-grain cereal in this recipe provides a good source of essential vitamins. The nuts have omega-3 fatty acids, which are good for your heart and good for your baby's development. The dried fruits contain antioxidants to keep you young. And, last but not least, the peanut butter gives you some extra protein.

Prep time: 30 min • **Baking time:** 10 min •
Yield: About 18 bars; 1 bar per serving

Ingredients	Directions
3 cups puffed whole-grain cereal **½ cup chopped nuts (such as pecans, walnuts, or almonds)** **¼ cup chopped pitted dates** **¼ cup chopped dried cranberries** **¼ cup raisins** **½ cup creamy peanut butter** **½ cup honey** **¼ cup light corn syrup**	*1* Preheat oven to 350 degrees F. Spray a 9-inch-square metal baking pan with non-stick spray. *2* Mix cereal, nuts, dates, cranberries, and raisins in a large bowl. *3* In a heavy, small saucepan, combine peanut butter, honey, and corn syrup. Bring to boil, whisking constantly until thickened, about 1 minute. *4* Pour peanut butter mixture over cereal mixture and stir. Transfer mixture to prepared pan. Press the mix into the pan. *5* Bake until golden, about 10 minutes. Cool; cut into squares.

Per serving: Calories 111 (From Fat 42); Fat 5g (Saturated 1g); Cholesterol 0mg; Sodium 28mg; Carbohydrate 17g (Dietary Fiber 1g); Protein 2g.

Fruit Smoothie

Try this recipe if you're looking for a drink snack instead of food. It's very satisfying because of its thickness. The calcium is great for fetal bone growth and development, and the fiber can help prevent constipation. It's also very low in fat and a great source of extra protein.

Prep time: 10 min • **Yield:** 1 serving; serving is about 2 cups

Ingredients	Directions
½ cup low-fat milk ½ cup low-fat vanilla yogurt	*1* Blend all ingredients in blender until smooth.
½ ripe banana	*2* Sit back and enjoy while reading your book!
1 teaspoon honey	
½ cup frozen fruit (such as strawberries, raspberries, or blueberries)	
1–2 ice cubes	
2 tablespoons powder (optional)	

Tip: You can also use soy milk instead of low-fat milk.

Per serving: Calories 271 (From Fat 27); Fat 3g (Saturated 2g); Cholesterol 11mg; Sodium 146mg; Carbohydrate 53g (Dietary Fiber 4g); Protein 11g.

Sunday Sundae

This is one of Keith's favorite snacks/drinks after a workout and is very satisfying. If you are dealing with gestational diabetes, you can modify the recipe to decrease the amount of carbohydrates and it still tastes just as good!

Prep time: 5 min • **Yield:** 1 large serving; serving is about 2 cups

Ingredients	*Directions*
1 ripe banana (if you have bananas that are overripe, freeze them for this recipe rather than throw them away — they work great here!) 1 cup low-fat milk or almond milk 1 scoop of vanilla protein powder (usually 70 mL scoop or about 2½ ounces for most brands) 1 heaping tablespoon of organic peanut butter (or peanut butter powder if you are watching your fat intake) 2 heaping tablespoons of wheat or oat bran 2 tablespoons of chocolate syrup 5–6 ice cubes	Place all ingredients in blender and blend until ice is crushed and drink is smooth. For those with gestational diabetes, zero-carb protein powders are available, along with the low-sugar chocolate syrup, to make this a more carb-friendly smoothie.

Per serving: Calories 479 (From Fat 115); Fat 13g (Saturated 4g); Cholesterol 75mg; Sodium 189mg; Carbohydrate 75g (Dietary Fiber 8g); Protein 22g.

Chapter 19

Ten Key Things You Can See on Ultrasound

In This Chapter

▶ Seeing what the sonographer sees

▶ Checking your baby's health from ultrasound

▶ Determining whether you're having a girl or a boy

*I*f you've ever had a parent-to-be show you an ultrasound picture of the baby, you know determining what you're looking at, let alone detecting a family resemblance, isn't always easy! But ultrasound pictures can be amazingly clear and useful — if you know what you're looking for. In this chapter, we show you what doctors and sonographers try to pick out on ultrasound to find out whether the baby is growing and developing well.

Measurement of Crown-Rump Length

The crown-rump length (CRL) is the distance from the top of the fetus's head *(crown)* to the buttocks *(rump)* during the first trimester (see Figure 19-1). It's the most precise sonographic measurement your practitioner can use to estimate gestational age. The other things that you can see in this image are a measurement of the nuchal translucency (NT) and the nasal bone (NB). (See Chapter 5.)

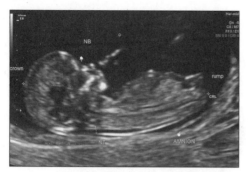

Image captured by Allison Borges, RDMS, and optimized by Kim Abruzese, RDMS

Figure 19-1: The crown-rump length is a first-trimester measurement used to determine how far along your pregnancy is.

The Face

Many people think the view of the fetus in Figure 19-2, taken during the second trimester, is sort of ghoulish. Some say that the baby looks like ET. But keep in mind that it's not a traditional photograph of the baby's face. The ultrasound beam passes through the fetus wherever it's directed and renders a picture of a "section" of the inside of the baby, not the surface.

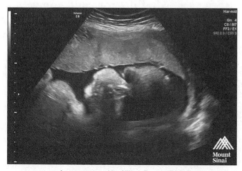

Image captured by Allison Borges, RDMS, and optimized by Kim Abruzese, RDMS

Figure 19-2: Smile for the camera!

The Spine

The spine is one area that even most novices at ultrasound can easily find. Take a look at it in Figure 19-3. In the second

trimester, imaging the entire spine is important in order to rule out neural tube defects (see Chapter 6).

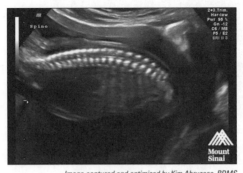

Image captured and optimized by Kim Abruzese, RDMS

Figure 19-3: You can easily see the fetal spine on ultrasound in the second trimester.

The Heart

The image in Figure 19-4 is the classic four-chamber view of the fetal heart that your practitioner looks for on ultrasound in the second trimester. You can clearly see two atria and two ventricles. A normal four-chamber view rules out the most major heart abnormalities. During an actual ultrasound, you can see the heart beating and the valves moving.

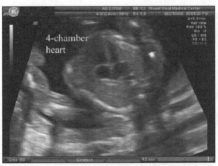

Image captured and optimized by Kim Abruzese, RDMS

Figure 19-4: In this picture, you can see the heart's four chambers. During the actual exam, you can also see the heart beating.

The Hands

In the second trimester, counting fetal fingers and toes is a challenge because the fetus moves constantly. But Figure 19-5 captures them all in the picture.

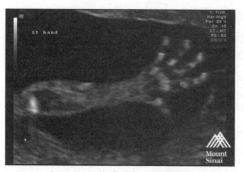

*Image captured by Cindy Candelario, RDMS, and optimized
by Kim Abruzese, RDMS*

Figure 19-5: All five fingers . . .

The Foot

Although you can't predict shoe size yet, you can see five toes on the foot in Figure 19-6, caught on ultrasound in the second trimester.

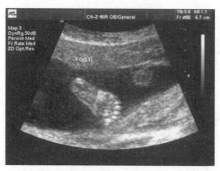

*Image captured by Cindy Candelario, RDMS, and optimized
by Kim Abruzese, RDMS*

Figure 19-6: . . . and all five toes.

The Fetal Profile

In Figure 19-7, you can see a fetus in the second trimester lying on her back. You can clearly see her forehead, nose, lips, and chin.

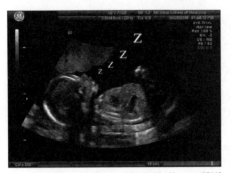

Image captured and optimized by Kim Abruzese, RDMS

Figure 19-7: In this ultrasound image, you can see the fetus resting in clear profile.

Three-Dimensional Image

In contrast to the other images in this chapter that are two-dimensional, this image is a different type of ultrasound that renders a picture of what the baby actually looks like. Figure 19-8 shows the baby's face with the arm in front of part of the mouth. 3-D ultrasound is one of the newest technologies available and provides amazing pictures, but hasn't replaced traditional two-dimensional scanning yet. 3-D images have limited use for routine evaluation of the baby at present.

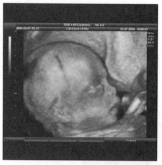

Image captured by Shyrwinka Williams, and optimized by Kim Abruzese, RDMS

Figure 19-8: You can actually see the baby's facial features clearly in this three-dimensional ultrasound.

It's a Boy!

As you can see in Figure 19-9, getting a very clear view of the developing penis is often possible.

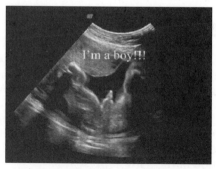

Image captured by Cindy Candelario, RDMS, and optimized by Kim Abruzese, RDMS

Figure 19-9: One look at this ultrasound image is enough to tell that the baby is a boy.

It's a Girl!

Figure 19-10 shows an easily recognizable image of the labia.

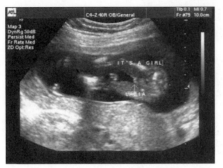

Image captured by Cindy Candelario, RDMS, and optimized
by Kim Abruzese, RDMS

Figure 19-10: The ultrasound image clearly shows this baby is a girl.

Index

• *G* •

• W •

• Y •

• Z •

About the Authors

Joanne Stone, MD, is a professor in the internationally renowned Department of Obstetrics and Gynecology at The Icahn School of Medicine at Mount Sinai in New York City. She is the director of the Division of Maternal-Fetal Medicine and also cares for patients with problem pregnancies. She has lectured throughout the country, is widely published in medical journals, and has been interviewed frequently for television and magazines on topics related to pregnancy, with a special emphasis on the management of multi-fetal pregnancies. She was a co-star in the critically acclaimed series *Pregnancy For Dummies* on the Discovery Health Channel. Away from the hospital she loves to spend time with her husband, George, and her two wonderful girls, Chloe and Sabrina.

Keith Eddleman, MD, works with Joanne at Mount Sinai. He is a professor in the medical school and the Director of Obstetrics at the hospital. He teaches medical students, residents, and fellows; lectures throughout the world; and appears often on television to discuss issues concerning the care of pregnant women. His areas of special expertise are ultrasound and reproductive genetics. He was also a co-star on the critically acclaimed series *Pregnancy For Dummies* on the Discovery Health Channel. His free time, when he has any, is split between spending time with his family at their apartment in Manhattan and at their country house in upstate New York.

Dedication

From Joanne: To my wonderful husband George, my beautiful children Chloe and Sabrina, and my amazing parents Regina and Philip, and in honor of my mother-in-law Celina and in memory of my father-in-law Nat. Thank you all for always being there for me.

From Keith: To Frank for many years of love and support, and to my mom Melba and in memory of my dad Alton for shaping me into the person I am.

Authors' Acknowledgments

Writing this book was truly a labor of love. We would like to thank everyone who played a part in the "birth" of this book, and specifically the following:

Tracy Boggier, Linda Brandon, Lynn Northrup, and the other folks at John Wiley & Sons, Inc., who conceived this idea and walked us through the whole process. Also, thank you to technical editor Aimee Chism Holland for her review, and to the National Association of Nurse Practitioners in Women's Health (NPWH) for recommending Aimee.

And to all our patients over the years whose inquisitive minds and need for accurate information inspired us to write this book.

Publisher's Acknowledgments

Acquisitions Editor: Tracy Boggier

Project Editor: Linda Brandon

(Previous Edition: Chad R. Sievers)

Copy Editor: Lynn Northrup

Technical Editor: Aimee Chism Holland

Art Coordinator: Alicia B. South

Project Coordinator: Lauren Buroker

Project Manager: Jennifer Ehrlich

Cover Photos: ©Mimi Haddon/ jupiterimages

Apple & Mac

iPad For Dummies, 6th Edition
978-1-118-72306-7

iPhone For Dummies, 7th Edition
978-1-118-69083-3

Macs All-in-One For Dummies,
4th Edition
978-1-118-82210-4

OS X Mavericks For Dummies
978-1-118-69188-5

Blogging & Social Media

Facebook For Dummies,
5th Edition
978-1-118-63312-0

Social Media Engagement
For Dummies
978-1-118-53019-1

WordPress For Dummies,
6th Edition
978-1-118-79161-5

Business

Stock Investing For Dummies,
4th Edition
978-1-118-37678-2

Investing For Dummies,
6th Edition
978-0-470-90545-6

Personal Finance For Dummies,
7th Edition
978-1-118-11785-9

QuickBooks 2014 For Dummies
978-1-118-72005-9

Small Business Marketing Kit
For Dummies, 3rd Edition
978-1-118-31183-7

Careers

Job Interviews For Dummies,
4th Edition
978-1-118-11290-8

Job Searching with Social Media
For Dummies, 2nd Edition
978-1-118-67856-5

Personal Branding For Dummies
978-1-118-11792-7

Resumes For Dummies,
6th Edition
978-0-470-87361-8

Starting an Etsy Business
For Dummies, 2nd Edition
978-1-118-59024-9

Diet & Nutrition

Belly Fat Diet For Dummies
978-1-118-34585-6

Mediterranean Diet For Dummies
978-1-118-71525-3

Nutrition For Dummies,
5th Edition
978-0-470-93231-5

Digital Photography

Digital SLR Photography
All-in-One For Dummies,
2nd Edition
978-1-118-59082-9

Digital SLR Video & Filmmaking
For Dummies
978-1-118-36598-4

Photoshop Elements 12
For Dummies
978-1-118-72714-0

Gardening

Herb Gardening For Dummies,
2nd Edition
978-0-470-61778-6

Gardening with Free-Range
Chickens For Dummies
978-1-118-54754-0

Health

Boosting Your Immunity
For Dummies
978-1-118-40200-9

Diabetes For Dummies,
4th Edition
978-1-118-29447-5

Living Paleo For Dummies
978-1-118-29405-5

Big Data

Big Data For Dummies
978-1-118-50422-2

Data Visualization For Dummies
978-1-118-50289-1

Hadoop For Dummies
978-1-118-60755-8

Language & Foreign Language

500 Spanish Verbs For Dummies
978-1-118-02382-2

English Grammar For Dummies,
2nd Edition
978-0-470-54664-2

French All-in-One For Dummies
978-1-118-22815-9

German Essentials For Dummies
978-1-118-18422-6

Italian For Dummies, 2nd Edition
978-1-118-00465-4

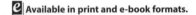 Available in print and e-book formats.

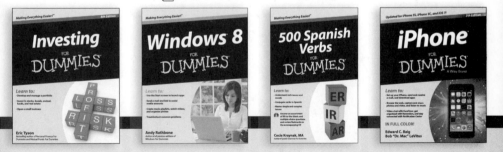

Available wherever books are sold.

For more information or to order direct visit www.dummies.com

Math & Science

Algebra I For Dummies, 2nd Edition
978-0-470-55964-2

Anatomy and Physiology For Dummies, 2nd Edition
978-0-470-92326-9

Astronomy For Dummies, 3rd Edition
978-1-118-37697-3

Biology For Dummies, 2nd Edition
978-0-470-59875-7

Chemistry For Dummies, 2nd Edition
978-1-118-00730-3

1001 Algebra II Practice Problems For Dummies
978-1-118-44662-1

Microsoft Office

Excel 2013 For Dummies
978-1-118-51012-4

Office 2013 All-in-One For Dummies
978-1-118-51636-2

PowerPoint 2013 For Dummies
978-1-118-50253-2

Word 2013 For Dummies
978-1-118-49123-2

Music

Blues Harmonica For Dummies
978-1-118-25269-7

Guitar For Dummies, 3rd Edition
978-1-118-11554-1

iPod & iTunes For Dummies, 10th Edition
978-1-118-50864-0

Programming

Beginning Programming with C For Dummies
978-1-118-73763-7

Excel VBA Programming For Dummies, 3rd Edition
978-1-118-49037-2

Java For Dummies, 6th Edition
978-1-118-40780-6

Religion & Inspiration

The Bible For Dummies
978-0-7645-5296-0

Buddhism For Dummies, 2nd Edition
978-1-118-02379-2

Catholicism For Dummies, 2nd Edition
978-1-118-07778-8

Self-Help & Relationships

Beating Sugar Addiction For Dummies
978-1-118-54645-1

Meditation For Dummies, 3rd Edition
978-1-118-29144-3

Seniors

Laptops For Seniors For Dummies, 3rd Edition
978-1-118-71105-7

Computers For Seniors For Dummies, 3rd Edition
978-1-118-11553-4

iPad For Seniors For Dummies, 6th Edition
978-1-118-72826-0

Social Security For Dummies
978-1-118-20573-0

Smartphones & Tablets

Android Phones For Dummies, 2nd Edition
978-1-118-72030-1

Nexus Tablets For Dummies
978-1-118-77243-0

Samsung Galaxy S 4 For Dummies
978-1-118-64222-1

Samsung Galaxy Tabs For Dummies
978-1-118-77294-2

Test Prep

ACT For Dummies, 5th Edition
978-1-118-01259-8

ASVAB For Dummies, 3rd Edition
978-0-470-63760-9

GRE For Dummies, 7th Edition
978-0-470-88921-3

Officer Candidate Tests For Dummies
978-0-470-59876-4

Physician's Assistant Exam For Dummies
978-1-118-11556-5

Series 7 Exam For Dummies
978-0-470-09932-2

Windows 8

Windows 8.1 All-in-One For Dummies
978-1-118-82087-2

Windows 8.1 For Dummies
978-1-118-82121-3

Windows 8.1 For Dummies, Book + DVD Bundle
978-1-118-82107-7

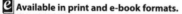 Available in print and e-book formats.

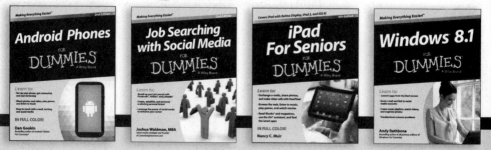

Take Dummies with you everywhere you go!

Whether you are excited about e-books, want more from the web, must have your mobile apps, or are swept up in social media, Dummies makes everything easier.

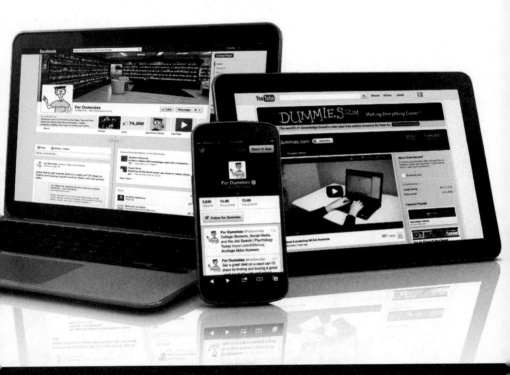

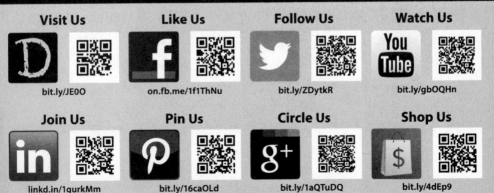

For Dummies is the global leader in the reference category and one of the most trusted and highly regarded brands in the world. No longer just focused on books, customers now have access to the For Dummies content they need in the format they want. Let us help you develop a solution that will fit your brand and help you connect with your customers.

Advertising & Sponsorships

Connect with an engaged audience on a powerful multimedia site, and position your message alongside expert how-to content.

Targeted ads • Video • Email marketing • Microsites • Sweepstakes sponsorship

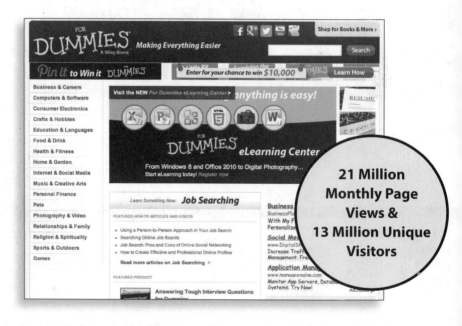

Dummies products make life easier!

- DIY
- Consumer Electronics
- Crafts
- Software

- Cookware
- Hobbies
- Videos

- Music
- Games
- and More!

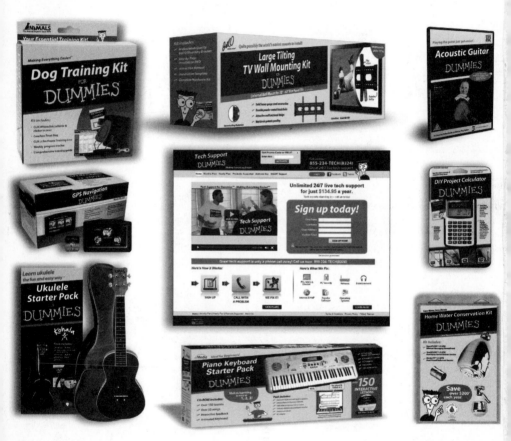

For more information, go to **Dummies.com** and search the store by category.

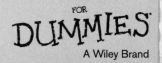

For Dummies is a registered trademark of John Wiley & Sons, Inc.

A Wiley Brand

# of For Dummies

Custom Publishing

Reach a global audience in any language by creating a solution, differentiate you from competitors, amplify your message, and encourage customers to make a buying decision.

Apps • Books • eBooks • Video • Audio • Webinars

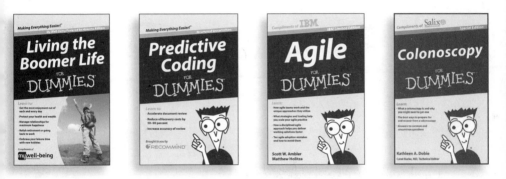

Brand Licensing & Content

Leverage the strength of the world's most popular reference brand to reach new audiences and channels of distribution.

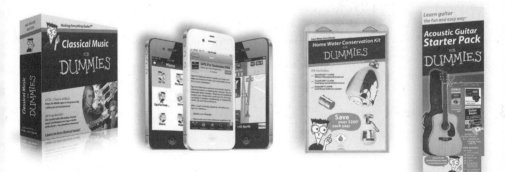

For more information, visit www.Dummies.com/biz

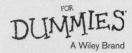

A Wiley Brand